MRCPCH PART 1
PAEDIATRIC QUESTIONS
WITH INDIVIDUAL
SUBJECT SUMMARIES

THIRD EDITION

Dr R M Beattie
Consultant Paediatric Gastroenterologist
Southampton General Hospital
Southampton

Dr Nick Brown
Consultant Paediatrician
Salisbury District Hospital
Salisbury

Dr Tracey Farnon
Specialist Registrar in Paediatrics
Wessex Deanery
Winchester

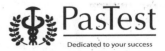

PasTest
Dedicated to your success

© 2006 PASTEST LTD

Egerton Court
Parkgate Estate
Knutsford
Cheshire
WA16 8DX

First edition 1997

Second edition 2000

Third edition 2006

ISBN 1904627692

A catalogue record for this book is available from the British Library.

The information contained within this book was obtained by the author from reliable sources. However, while every effort has been made to ensure its accuracy, no responsibility for loss, damage or injury occasioned to any person acting or refraining from action as a result of information contained herein can be accepted by the publishers or authors.

PasTest Revision Books and Intensive Courses

PasTest has been established in the field of postgraduate medical education since 1972, providing revision books and intensive study courses for doctors preparing for their professional examinations.

Books and courses are available for the following specialties:

MRCGP, MRCP Parts 1 and 2, MRCPCH Parts 1 and 2, MRCPsych, MRCS, MRCOG Parts 1 and 2, DRCOG, DCH, FRCA, PLAB Parts 1 and 2, Dental Students, Dentists and Dental Nurses.

For further details contact:

PasTest, Freepost, Knutsford, Cheshire WA16 7BR

Tel: 01565 752000   Fax: 01565 650264

www.pastest.co.uk   enquires@pastest.co.uk

Text prepared by Carnegie Book Production Ltd, Lancaster

Printed in the UK by the Alden Group

CONTENTS

CONTRIBUTORS

Dr R M Beattie, MRCP FRCPCH
Consultant Paediatric Gastroenterologist
Southampton General Hospital
Tremona Road
Southampton

Dr Nick Brown, MRCP, FRCPCH, MSc, DTM and H
Consultant Paediatrician
Salisbury District Hospital
Salisbury

Dr Tracey Farnon, MRCP FRCPCH
Specialist Registrar in Paediatrics
Wessex Deanery
Highcroft, Romsey Road
Winchester

Contributors to the First and Second Editions

Dr A B Acharya
Senior Registrar

Dr D L I Ellis
Senior House Officer

Dr L J Phillips
Senior House Officer

Dr A T Tidswell
Senior House Officer

Peterborough District Hospital
Thorpe Road
Peterborough

PREFACE TO THIRD EDITION

It is a pleasure to write the preface to the third edition of this book. The MRCPCH part one examination remains a major hurdle for aspiring paediatricians. The exam has changed considerably in the last 10 years with the disappearance of negatively marked MCQs and the introduction of new question types including Best of Fives and Extended Matching questions. The need for a thorough knowledge base of all aspects of paediatrics including applied basic science, however, remains. This book therefore uses all question types to aid revision with subject summaries providing structured and relevant teaching material after each question. This format which has been a major feature in the previous editions has, as the feedback I have received has shown, proved helpful for candidates in the preparation for the exam.

It is crucial for the candidate to be clear about what is expected in the exam and the Royal College of Paediatrics and Child Health website contains a considerable amount of information on the format of the exam, question types and subject material which needs to be covered.

I have been indebted to have considerable help in the production of previous editions from colleagues who have recently sat the exam and contributors who have helped with writing and checking questions. I am indebted to Nick Brown and Tracey Farnon for their enthusiastic help and support as co-authors of the third edition of the book.

I hope the book continues to prove helpful to candidates.

Best of Luck with the Exam!

R M Beattie
March 2006

ACKNOWLEDGEMENTS

My contribution to this book is dedicated to the memory of my wonderful mother, Ann. During stressful times, such as those faced when preparing for the MRCPCH, she would encourage me to tackle things '... *step by step, one day at a time*'. Just as her advice continues to guide me today, I hope it will also help you as you use this book to study for your forthcoming examinations.

Tracy Farnon
March 2006

INTRODUCTION

MRCPCH Part 1 Paediatric Questions with Individual Subject Summaries is designed to give you, the reader, the most effective exam practice. The questions in this book reflect the questions you will encounter in the exam – and include Best of Five and Extended Matching questions, recently incorporated by the Royal College.

Since January 2004, the MRCPCH examination has consisted of two papers:

Paper 1A
The first paper focuses on conditions that any practitioner who deals with children would encounter. This includes conditions that would be seen in a hospital, community or primary care setting. This is also known as the Basic Child Health paper.

Paper 1B
The written paper deals with more complicated problem solving skills, with an emphasis on the scientific knowledge underpinning child health care. This is also known as the Extended Paediatric paper. This paper is equivalent to the previous MRCPCH Part 1 paper.

Candidates must pass both papers in order to proceed to sit the MRCPCH Part 2 examination.

Both Papers 1A and 1B are set for 2½ hours and comprise:

35 Multiple True/False questions   each worth 5 marks

25 Best of Five questions   each worth 4 marks

8 Extended Matching questions   each worth 9 marks (3 marks per item)

The Multiple True/False question (MTF) (or MCQ) is the form of question with which most candidates are familiar – five separate questions under a stem with each of the five questions having a true or false answer.

The Best of Five question (BoF) has five options to match the heading statement or scenario. Of these options there is only one correct answer.

The Extended Matching question (EMQ) has ten associated options for which three scenarios or statements are given. For each of these there is only one correct answer.

There is no negative marking. Hence it is advised that all questions should be attempted.

The pass mark is calculated with regard to the predicted difficulty of each of the questions in the paper, and questions are graded into their appropriateness as being one of three categories; namely, essential, important or acceptable.

Access the RCPCH website to see examples of the examination and to keep up to date with any alteration in the examination that may occur: www.rcpch.ac.uk

questions

CARDIOLOGY

Multiple Choice Questions

1.   With regard to aortic stenosis

○   A   the commonest cardiac lesion in Down's syndrome
○   B   right ventricular hypertrophy is common
○   C   an ejection click suggests the stenosis is supravalvular
○   D   surgery is usually by valve replacement
○   E   there is an association with sudden death

2.   With regard to William's syndrome

○   A   the commonest cardiac lesion is an atrio-septal defect
○   B   is caused by a micro-deletion on chromosome 7
○   C   diagnosis can be confirmed by fluorescence in-situ hybridisation (FISH) studies
○   D   is associated with normal developmental milestones
○   E   hypercalcaemia is required to make the diagnosis

3.   Causes of a right-to-left shunt in the neonatal period include

○   A   Ebstein's malformation
○   B   perinatal asphyxia
○   C   critical aortic stenosis
○   D   tricuspid atresia
○   E   methaemoglobinaemia

4.   In the neonate presenting with central cyanosis

○   A   the hyperoxia test is used to confirm patency of the ductus arteriosus

○   B   acrocyanosis is indicative of central cyanosis

○   C   a physiological right-to-left shunt must be present

○   D   more than 5 g/dl of haemoglobin is in the reduced state

○   E   prostaglandin therapy may be appropriate

5.   In Down's syndrome

○   A   the commonest cardiac lesion is an atrial septal defect

○   B   echocardiography is indicated even if a murmur is not present

○   C   20% have associated heart defects

○   D   tetralogy of Fallot is a recognised association

○   E   the cardiac defects are the sole cause of pulmonary vascular disease

6.   Transposition of the great arteries

○   A   is associated with increased pulmonary blood flow

○   B   is the commonest cause of cyanotic congenital heart disease in the neonatal period

○   C   is associated with a metabolic alkalosis

○   D   can be corrected by the Jatene (arterial switch) procedure

○   E   has atrio-ventricular block as a recognised complication

7.   In tetralogy of Fallot

○   A   the murmur becomes louder during cyanotic spells

○   B   polycythaemia is a recognised finding

○   C   an atrial septal defect is a component of the tetralogy

○   D   clubbing develops within the first 3 months

○   E   right ventricular hypertrophy is present

8. **Which of the following conditions can present in the neonatal period with central cyanosis?**

○ A Eisenmenger's syndrome

○ B pulmonary atresia

• ○ C hypoplastic left heart

○ D transposition of the great arteries

○ E aortic stenosis

9. **Regarding the paediatric ECG**

○ A neonates have right axis deviation

○ B complete heart block is associated with maternal systemic lupus erythematosus

○ C right bundle branch block is seen in coarctation of the aorta

○ D Romano–Ward syndrome produces prolongation of the PR interval

○ E a resting heart rate in newborns of 180 is a tachycardia

10. **Which of the following chest X-ray findings would support the paired diagnosis?**

○ A atrio-septal defect and coeur en sabot (heart in a boot)

○ B patent ductus arteriosus (PDA) and rib notching

○ C truncus arteriosus and absent thymus

○ D total anomalous pulmonary venous drainage and cottage loaf appearance

○ E scimitar syndrome and dextrocardia

11. **Which of the following conditions are associated with an increased incidence of heart disease?**

○ A Kawasaki's disease

○ B congenital rubella

○ C Marfan's syndrome

○ D Turner's syndrome

○ E petit mal epilepsy

cardiology

12. Which of the following statements are true?

- ○ A the commonest congenital cardiac lesion is an ASVD
- ○ B tetralogy of Fallot is associated with plethoric lung fields
- ○ C the Blalock–Taussig shunt gives rise to a continuous murmur
- ○ D nitrous oxide can be used to treat persistent pulmonary hypertension
- ○ E Ebstein's anomaly is an anomaly of the tricuspid valve

13. Which of the following statements concerning atrial septal defects are correct?

- ○ A ostium secundum defects are commoner than ostium primum defects
- ○ B atrial fibrillation is a recognised associated complication
- ○ C in a secundum defect the ECG shows right bundle branch block and left axis deviation
- ○ D the pulmonary vascular resistance increases in early childhood
- ○ E a left-to-right shunt of more than 2:1 is an indication for surgical closure

14. Ventricular septal defects

- ○ A are usually located in the muscular part of the ventricular septum
- ○ B in the neonate will always cause a flow murmur across the defect which is present from birth
- ○ C infective endocarditis is a complication in 10%
- ○ D are associated with a higher oxygen content in the blood of the right ventricle than the right atrium
- ○ E are associated with right ventricular volume overload

15. Eisenmenger's syndrome can result from:

- ○ A pulmonary artery stenosis
- ○ B total anomalous pulmonary venous drainage
- ○ C tetralogy of Fallot
- ○ D aorto-pulmonary window
- ○ E ventricular septal defect

16.   Patent ductus arteriosus

- ○   A   is commoner in females
- ○   B   is commoner in pre-term infants
- ○   C   can be treated with prostaglandins
- ○   D   usually closes spontaneously in term infants
- ○   E   may present as recurrent apnoea

17.   Concerning the fetal circulation

- ○   A   the umbilical vein carries deoxygenated blood to the placenta from the fetus
- ○   B   fetal superior vena caval blood preferentially flows across the foramen ovale into the left atrium
- ○   C   40% of right ventricular outflow enters the lungs
- ○   D   the descending aorta is connected to the pulmonary artery via the ductus venosus
- ○   E   gas exchange occurs in the fetal lungs

18.   Which of the following statements are true?

- ○   A   patients with cyanotic congenital heart disease grow normally
- ○   B   immunisation is contraindicated in children with congenital heart disease
- ○   C   the oral contraceptive pill is contraindicated in patients with prosthetic heart valves
- ○   D   2% of patients with congenital heart disease have a chromosomal abnormality
- ○   E   30% of infants with chromosomal defects have heart defects

19.   Coarctation of the aorta

- ○   A   is associated with bicuspid aortic valves
- ○   B   is associated with rib notching in infancy
- ○   C   is a feature of Edward's syndrome
- ○   D   is more common in females
- ○   E   may be associated with blood pressure discrepancy in the upper limbs

cardiology

20. Which of the following cardiac defects and teratogens are correctly paired:

○ A alcohol and transposition of the great arteries
○ B sodium valproate and tetralogy of Fallot
○ C furosemide and PDA
○ D phenytoin and coarctation of the aorta
○ E lithium and Ebstein's anomaly

21. In childhood hypertension

○ A systolic pressure greater than the 75th centile for age and sex is the correct definition
○ B primary is more common than secondary hypertension
○ C irrespective of age the commonest cause is renal artery stenosis
○ D children with primary hypertension are usually symptomatic
○ E there is little point in obtaining blood or urine for analysis

22. Which of the following are causes of circulatory failure in the first week of life?

○ A arrhythmias
○ B hypoplastic left heart
○ C birth asphyxia
○ D severe anaemia
○ E fluid overload

23. Concerning infective endocarditis

○ A *Escherichia coli* is the commonest cause
○ B antibiotic prophylaxis is indicated to cover dental procedures in a child with an ostium secundum atrial septal defect
○ C splinter haemorrhages in the nail beds are an almost universal finding
○ D the diagnosis is excluded if echocardiography is normal
○ E it is usually the right side of the heart that is affected

24. Which of the following are correct?

○ A hypertrophic obstructive cardiomyopathy can be inherited as an autosomal dominant

○ B dilated cardiomyopathy is associated with doxorubicin toxicity in children

○ C restrictive cardiomyopathy is the commonest cardiomyopathy in childhood

○ D endocardial fibroelastosis is a form of hypertrophic cardiomyopathy

○ E there is an increased incidence of dilated cardiomyopathy in infants of diabetic mothers

25. With regard to rheumatic fever

○ A it occurs secondary to infection with β-haemolytic *Streptococcus* group A

○ B it causes a pancarditis

○ C it is associated with upper socio-economic class

○ D PR prolongation on the ECG is one of the major diagnostic criteria

○ E prophylactic antibiotics should be stopped after 3 months

26. The following support the diagnosis of an innocent murmur

○ A present only in diastole

○ B fixed splitting of S2

○ C heard only in high output states

○ D heard all over the praecordium

○ E variable with position and posture

27. Cardiac emergencies

○ A asynchronous DC shock is the appropriate treatment for a supraventricular tachycardia

○ B DC shock is the appropriate treatment of electromechanical dissociation

○ C atropine is the first-line drug for asystole

○ D ventricular fibrillation is a common cardiac arrhythmia in childhood

○ E lidocaine may be given via an intraosseous needle

cardiology

28. Features of Wolff–Parkinson–White syndrome include

○ A delta wave

○ B shortened PR interval

○ C association with sudden death

○ D prolonged QRS

○ E re-entry tachycardia

29. Which of the following are true

○ A the PR interval is prolonged in hyperkalaemia

○ B the normal PR interval in infancy is 0.2–0.3 s

○ C myxomas are the commonest cardiac tumours in childhood

○ D cerebral abscess is a rare complication of congenital heart disease under the age of two years

○ E a third heart sound can be normal in childhood

30. Causes of QT prolongation

○ A cisapride

○ B hyperkalaemia

○ C erythromycin without concurrent administration of cisapride

○ D head injury

○ E chlorphenamine

Best of Five Questions

31. **Which is the MOST appropriate diagnostic criterion for Kawasaki's disease?**

- ○ A Gall bladder infarct
- ○ B Intermittent low-grade fever
- ○ C Thrombocytopenia
- ○ D Petechial rash
- ○ E Conjunctivitis

32. **Which ONE is a sign of subacute bacterial endocarditis (SBE)?**

- ○ A Splinter haemorrhages
- ○ B Extensor surface nodules
- ○ C Eosinophilia
- ○ D Cervical nodes
- ○ E Renal artery bruit

33. **A 3-month-old baby boy is admitted to hospital breathless with poor feeding. On arrival main findings are: pale with pulse of 240/min, liver enlarged at 3 cm below costal margin and saturation in air of 88%. Which is the MOST appropriate first action?**

- ○ A iv adenosine
- ○ B iv β-blocker
- ○ C Application of ice pack over face
- ○ D Oxygen
- ○ E Intranasal adenosine

34. **A 4-day-old baby girl is admitted from home with increasing cyanosis. On examination, she is deeply cyanosed (saturation in air 78%), and had mild subcostal recession. She is alert and not distressed. What is the MOST likely diagnosis?**

○ A Large ventricular septal defect

○ B Tricuspid atresia

○ C Diaphragmatic hernia

○ D Persistent fetal circulation (PFC)

○ E Transposition of great arteries

35. **A 4-month-old is referred to the outpatient clinic with stridor since birth and faltering growth. The baby is thin with a soft ejection systolic and diastolic murmur. What is the MOST appropriate investigation?**

○ A Echocardiogram

○ B Barium swallow

○ C Direct laryngoscopy

○ D ECG

○ E Arteriography

36. **A 2-year-old fully immunised boy is referred with suspected measles. He has a week long history of fever and malaise and has developed a generalised morbilliform rash. On arrival he is miserable, febrile (temperature 40.1°C), cervical lymphadenopathy, conjunctivitis, desquamation over palms. Bloods apart from a high plasma viscosity are normal. What is the MOST appropriate first line management?**

○ A Full infection screen including lumbar puncture and urine and broad-spectrum antibiotic cover

○ B Vitamin A

○ C High-dose aspirin and parenteral immunoglobulin

○ D Parenteral steroids

○ E High-dose aspirin alone

Extended Matching Questions

37. Theme: Illness with cardiac manifestations

○ A Cardiomyopathy
○ B Endocarditis
○ C Rheumatic fever
○ D Pericarditis
○ E Malaria
○ F Nephritic syndrome
○ G Juvenile chronic arthritis
○ H Intrauterine infection
○ I None of the above

Choose the best options from the list above for the three situations described below. Each option may be used once, more than once or not at all.

1. A 14-year-old boy, treated for a rhabdomyosarcoma at age 3 years with complete recovery, presents with shortness of breath over some months. On examination he appears tired and tachypnoeic. There is triple rhythm and raised jugular venous pressure.

2. A 2-week-old presents with a gradual onset of tachypnoea, tachycardia and enlargement of the liver. Heart failure is suspected. Chest X-ray, ECG and echo show some ventricular dilation but a structurally normal heart. Other basic investigations including full blood count, biochemistry and culture of blood, urine and cerebrospinal fluid (CSF).

3. A 5-year-old Kenyan boy is referred from his village to the local clinic. He has had occasional jerky limb movements and a rash. He is afebrile, has a palpable spleen and a mid-diastolic murmur.

cardiology

38. Theme: Cardiac investigations

○ A 24-hour ECG
○ B Echo cardiography
○ C Cardiac catheter
○ D Thoracic computed tomography (CT) scan
○ E Thoracic magnetic resonance imaging (MRI) scan
○ F Chest X-ray
○ G Arterial compliance studies
○ H None of the above

Choose the best investigation from the list above for the three situations described below. Each option may be used once, more than once or not at all.

1. A 2-year-old boy sent to outpatients with a murmur. He is well and pink with normal pulses. There is a soft systolic murmur at the right supraclavicular area louder on sitting.

2. A 14-year-old girl with recurrent 'panic attacks' with a fast heart rate of 'at least 120 at rest'. On examination she is well with a normal cardiac examination.

3. A 5-year-old boy, who had an aortic stenosis repaired at age 18 month, presents with increasing shortness of breath. There is a systolic murmur on examination best heard over the 'aortic' area.

COMMUNITY PAEDIATRICS AND CHILD PSYCHIATRY

Multiple Choice Questions

39. Concerning anorexia nervosa

○ A   it is commoner in pupils of fee-paying schools
○ B   concordance is higher in monozygotic twins than in dizygotic twins
○ C   it is rarely associated with depression
○ D   continuing weight loss is an indication for hospital admission
○ E   less than 1% of cases are boys

40. Concerning childhood autism

○ A   there is an increased incidence of epilepsy in adolescence
○ B   it is caused by poor parenting
○ C   Asperger's syndrome represents a sub-group with more severe disease
○ D   it is commoner in girls
○ E   20% of cases are associated with a medical disorder

41. Features of attention deficit hyperactivity disorder include

○ A   impulsiveness
○ B   poor response to drug therapy
○ C   restlessness
○ D   auditory hallucinations
○ E   inattention

community paediatrics and child psychiatry

42. Concerning attention deficit hyperactivity disorder

○ A it is successfully controlled by dietary restriction

○ B it can lead to poor academic achievement

○ C it can be exacerbated by anticonvulsant treatment

○ D it is commoner in boys

○ E the use of drug therapy commonly causes sleep disturbance

43. School refusal

○ A is different from truancy

○ B is commonly associated with physical symptoms

○ C is associated with anxiety and depression

○ D can be treated with antidepressants

○ E generally has a poor outcome

44. Concerning childhood squints

○ A they occur in 4% of pre-school children

○ B they often cause amblyopia of the affected eye

○ C they are an absolute indication for tests of visual acuity

○ D paralytic squint is commoner than non-paralytic squint

○ E non-paralytic squints rarely require corrective surgery

45. In the assessment of hearing

○ A a history of cleft palate is relevant

○ B pure tone audiometry testing can be used in children of any age

○ C auditory brain stem evoked responses are affected by sedation

○ D deafness may be associated with a family history of sudden death

○ E a history of prematurity is significant

46. Munchausen's by proxy

- A should be suspected in cases of childhood hypoglycaemia
- B has about a 10% risk to the child of death or disability
- C is commoner in pre-verbal children
- D is associated with a family history of sudden infant death
- E symptoms do not occur when the parent or primary care-giver is away from the child

47. Psychiatric referral is indicated for

- A a 15-year-old girl who has taken an overdose of paracetamol
- B a 14-year-old boy off school with recurrent morning headaches
- C grief reaction in a 6-year-old boy lasting for a year
- D a 9-year-old who is afraid of the dark
- E encopresis in a 7-year-old boy where constipation has been excluded

48. In childhood depression

- A sleep is characteristically increased
- B a family history is common
- C girls are more likely to have depression than boys at all ages
- D auditory hallucinations are a recognised feature
- E parasuicidal behaviour is very rare

49. Concerning sudden infant death syndrome

- A prematurity is a risk factor
- B the risk is increased with increasing maternal age
- C it is commoner in females
- D it is associated with parental smoking
- E it is associated with sleeping on plastic mattresses

50. Concerning child sexual abuse

○ A   it occurs in up to 10% of children

○ B   child sexual abusers often have a history of being abused
       as a child

○ C   girls are 20 times more likely to be abused than boys

○ D   it is associated with an increased incidence of anal
       fissures

○ E   reflex anal dilatation is pathognomonic

51. Concerning physical abuse in children

○ A   fathers are more likely to be abusers than mothers

○ B   it is commoner in first born children

○ C   handicapped children are at increased risk

○ D   the head and neck are the commonest sites of injury

○ E   the majority of non-accidental fractures occur in children of
       school age

52. Concerning childhood schizophrenia

○ A   it is rare

○ B   long-term remission occurs in 90%

○ C   delusions are a feature

○ D   family history is often positive

○ E   it is associated with a lifetime increased risk of suicide

53. Speech delay is

○ A   commoner in females

○ B   common in autism

○ C   associated with tongue tie

○ D   commoner in first born children

○ E   associated with a family history of speech delay

54. **Causes of developmental regression include**

○ A Down's syndrome
○ B cerebral palsy
○ C Gaucher's disease
○ D subacute sclerosing panencephalitis
○ E human immunodeficiency virus (HIV) infection

55. **A child of 8 months would be expected to**

○ A transfer from hand to hand
○ B roll from back to front
○ C build a tower of three bricks
○ D say two words with meaning
○ E sit without support

56. **A child of 18 months would be expected to**

○ A throw a ball without falling
○ B spontaneously scribble
○ C wave bye-bye
○ D feed with a spoon
○ E speak in sentences

57. **A child of three years would be expected to**

○ A copy a square
○ B name two colours
○ C ride a tricycle
○ D go up stairs one foot per step
○ E build a tower of six cubes

community paediatrics and
child psychiatry

58. A child of 12 months would be expected to

○ A pick up a sugar cube between the finger and thumb
○ B be dry during the day
○ C feed with a biscuit
○ D use at least two different words with meaning
○ E wave bye-bye

59. Causes of toe walking include

○ A habit
○ B peroneal muscular atrophy
○ C spastic diplegia
○ D spina bifida
○ E tendo-Achilles shortening

community paediatrics and
child psychiatry

Best of Five Questions

60. **You receive a referral letter for your general paediatric clinic from a GP to see a 12-year-old girl who attends the local fee-paying grammar school. She complains of excessive tiredness for the last 4 months and her school attendance has fallen to less than 20% of expected. She experiences frequent waking overnight and daytime drowsiness. There is no history of weight loss or any systemic symptoms of note. Examination is unremarkable. The GP has already requested the following blood tests, all of which are normal: full blood count (FBC) and film, erythrocyte sedimentation rate (ESR), C-reactive protein (CRP), urea and electrolytes (U&E), liver and thyroid function tests (LFT and TFT), creatine kinase (CK), glucose and Ebstein–Barr virus serology. Urinalysis is also normal. The GP thinks the diagnosis is one of chronic fatigue syndrome. Which course of action would be MOST appropriate?**

- A Pass the referral to the Child and Adolescent Mental Health Services (CAMHS) so that they can institute family therapy and explore the possibility of an underlying depressive illness.

- B See in clinic prior to requesting ongoing follow-up by the physiotherapiststo commence a graded exercise programme to try to restore a more normal level of day to day activity for the child.

- C After thorough history and examination in clinic, reassure the family and patient that there is no evidence of serious underlying pathology. Explain variable timescale and prognosis. Develop a management plan with patient and family agreement that addresses issues of concern, and arrange regular reviews of progress.

- D Assess in clinic and arrange further investigations to rule out underlying pathology. At review, reassure patient and family that no organic cause has been found and problems will resolve with time.

- E After review in clinic, prescribe low-dose anti-depressants to try to normalise sleep pattern in an attempt to improve school attendance.

61. **Choose the MOST appropriate statement regarding separation anxiety from the list below.**

○ A   It is developmentally normal until the age of approximately 8 years.

○ B   It is commoner in girls than boys.

○ C   Presence of separation anxiety disorder in teenagers is most likely to present as school refusal and somatic symptoms.

○ D   Separation anxiety disorder has a poor prognosis even with early intervention and treatment.

○ E   To be diagnosed as a disorder (according to Diagnostic and Statistical Manual of Mental Disorders (DSM)-IV criteria), symptoms must have been present for a minimum of 3 months.

62. **Select the MOST appropriate statement from the following regarding somatoform disorders in childhood.**

○ A   They are often appropriately managed solely by the mental health services.

○ B   They rarely have any long-term consequences for the child or family.

○ C   They overlap with factitious disorders and malingering.

○ D   They occur more frequently in children whose parents suffer physical illness.

○ E   Medical investigations are rarely helpful.

63. **The following statements refer to sleep disorders in childhood. Select the MOST appropriate statement.**

○ A   Melatonin is a drug licensed for treating sleep disturbance in children.

○ B   Sleep laboratory studies are helpful in defining the nature of the majority of sleep disorders in childhood.

○ C   Sleepwalking is rare in prepubertal children.

○ D   Insomnia is the most frequent sleep disorder seen in post-pubertal children with depression.

○ E   Night terrors are short-lived episodes occurring during the first few hours of sleep, that terminate spontaneously and of which the child has poor recollection the following day.

64. **A school nurse discusses a 6-year-old boy with you who teachers have noticed appears to be more clumsy than his peers in the classroom and on the playground. He struggles in particular with his handwriting and he is not achieving at the same level as his classmates. What would be the MOST appropriate course of action to recommend.**

○ A Request educational psychology opinion to look for the presence of underlying learning difficulties.

○ B Make direct contact with teachers to establish level of concern prior to arranging a multi-disciplinary assessment of child's abilities with the consent of the parents.

○ C Referral to paediatric neurologist to rule out a possible underlying neurological disorder.

○ D Assess in clinic to obtain a full history and perform examination in order to make an application for a Statement of Special Educational Needs.

○ E Ask for an occupational therapy assessment and treatment programme to be drawn-up to follow in the classroom for improving the child's fine motor skills.

65. **In prospective cohort studies, the BIGGEST drawback is:**

○ A Bias
○ B Confounding
○ C Need for frequent measures
○ D Tolerability of intervention
○ E Loss to follow-up

66. **In randomised controlled trials, the MAIN aim of randomisation is to:**

○ A Reduce bias
○ B Reduce cost
○ C Increase compliance
○ D Reduce confounding
○ E Increase generalisability

community paediatrics and
child psychiatry

Extended Matching Questions

67. Theme: Trial design

○ A Ecological

○ B Case–control

○ C Prospective cohort

○ D Nested case–control

○ E Randomised controlled trial

○ F Cross-sectional

○ G Retrospective cohort

○ H Case report

Choose the best option from the list above for each of the three situations described below. Each option may be used once, more than once or not at all.

1. Generating hypothesis for the importance of regional differences in alcohol consumption and oral cancers.
2. Studying the relation between rare trace element deficiencies pre-conceptually and abdominal wall defects.
3. Ascertaining association between head circumference at birth and IQ at the age of 40 years.

68. Theme: Statistical methods

○ A *t* test

○ B Mann–Whitney rank sum test

○ C Pearson's correlation coefficient

○ D Survival analysis

○ E Odds ratio

○ F Relative risk

○ G Chi-squared

○ H Multiple regression

Choose the best method from the list above for each of the three situations described below. Each option may be used once, more than once or not at all.

1. Comparing growth parameters between two groups.
2. Comparing time to readmission after discharge with asthma on two different treatments.
3. Examining relation between body mass index (BMI) and peak flow rates.

69. Theme: Accidental injury

○ A Burns and scalds
○ B House fire
○ C Choking
○ D Poisoning
○ E Drowning
○ F Falls
○ G Baby walkers
○ H Road traffic accidents
○ I Cycling

Choose the best option from the list above for each of the three statements given below. Each option may be used once, more than once or not at all.

1. The cause of the largest number of accidental deaths of children in the home each year.

2. The cause behind the largest number of non-fatal accidental injuries in children under the age of 15 years.

3. The cause of the majority of childhood accidental deaths per annum.

community paediatrics and child psychiatry

25

70. Theme: Developmental problems

○ A Genetic studies for fragile X syndrome
○ B Chromosomal analysis for Down's syndrome
○ C Blood lead level
○ D Genetic studies for Rett's syndrome
○ E Genetic studies for William's syndrome
○ F Genetic studies for Wolf-Hirschhorn syndrome
○ G Plasma very long chain fatty acid levels
○ H Neuroimaging

Choose the most appropriate diagnostic test from the list above for each of the three case scenarios described below. Each option may be used once, more than once or not at all.

1. A 6-week-old baby girl is referred by the GP after attending for routine developmental assessment. The GP is concerned about the presence of dysmorphic features and poor growth. The baby has frontal bossing and a high frontal hairline in association with a broad, beaked nose and hypertelorism. The growth chart reveals that the weight is only just maintained on the 2nd centile and the head circumference has dipped beneath the 0.4th centile.

2. A 3-year-old boy is referred by the health visitor due to concerns regarding behaviour and development. The health visitor has been unable to review the child for over 6 months as the family have been in temporary accommodation out of area while waiting to be re-housed. The health visitor is concerned that his development appears to have regressed and in particular, he is still managing to use single words only when communicating. His mother complains that he seems to be much more short tempered than previously and he has developed problematic constipation.

3. You are referred a 2-year-old girl by her GP. Parents report an abrupt deterioration in her language skills over the previous 6 weeks so that she is now communicating by grunts and gestures whereas she had previously been able to put two words together with meaning. She has developed a tendency to bring her hands repeatedly to her mouth but is no longer able to feed herself or hold a beaker. They also describe episodes where she is hyperventilating and stares with no response to her parents' voice.

DERMATOLOGY

Multiple Choice Questions

71. Regarding scabies

○ A it is caused by infestation with the mite *Sarcoptes scabiei*

○ B failure to respond to treatment is usually due to incorrect diagnosis

○ C in children under the age of 2 years, the head and neck area should be omitted when applying scabicide treatment

○ D lindane is the treatment of choice

○ E itching may persist for up to 6 weeks after successful treatment

72. Concerning mastocytosis

○ A 75% of cases occur in childhood

○ B majority of patients have pruritic cutaneous lesions

○ C late-onset disease carries a better prognosis

○ D serum tryptase levels are typically elevated

○ E systemic symptoms of flushing, wheezing, diarrhoea and vomiting may occur

Best of Five Questions

73. **A pregnant lady with atopic eczema and asthma, who has a 4-year-old child with moderately severe eczema, requests advice regarding reducing the risk of eczema in her unborn child. Select the MOST appropriate advice from the following.**

○ A There is good clinical and epidemiological evidence to support the delayed introduction of potential food allergens in weaning foods (eg milk protein and eggs).

○ B In high-risk families, evidence exists to support prolonged exclusive breast-feeding (ie beyond 6 months) as a preventive measure.

○ C If breast-feeding is not possible, soya-based formulae should be used in preference to cow's milk preparations.

○ D Removing certain known food allergens from the mother's diet during pregnancy does not reduce the risk or prevent the onset of atopic eczema.

○ E Taking measures to minimise exposure to house dust mite have been shown to reduce the risk of the development of eczema after birth.

74. **A 6-week-old baby attending for developmental assessment is noted to have a well-circumscribed lesion on the bridge of his nose measuring 5 mm diameter and with a bluish hue. The GP refers the child to the ward. The mass feels firm to the touch. Her parents say it was not present at birth and have noticed that it temporarily increases in size when the baby cries. Appearances are consistent with a capillary haemangioma. What is the MOST appropriate advice to give to these parents?**

○ A Inform parents that no further follow-up is required as the majority spontaneously involute by school age.

○ B Referral to a plastic surgeon is required for consideration of removal of the lesion.

○ C Commence a course of oral steroids to limit the growth of the lesion.

○ D Reassure parents that it is likely to heal without scarring with time.

○ E Arrange follow up for the child in the out-patient clinic to monitor the growth of the lesion over the coming weeks.

Extended Matching Question

75. Theme: Infections

○   A   *Staphylococcus aureus*

○   B   *Mycoplasma pneumoniae*

○   C   Epstein–Barr virus

○   D   Coxsackie virus

○   E   *Candida albicans*

○   F   Group A streptococcus

○   G   Herpes simplex virus

○   H   Adenovirus

Choose the most likely causative infective agent from the list above for each of the three case scenarios described below. Each option may be used once, more than once or not at all.

1. A 4-month-old baby boy has a 72-hour history of low-grade fever and bilateral purulent conjunctivitis. Large flaccid bullae are present in the groins and axillae, with some areas of sloughing on the neck revealing a moist, erythematous base.

2. A 2-year-old girl is admitted with a high fever and refusal of any oral intake for 24 hours. Florid vesicles with an erythematous base are noted on the lips, gums and palate. Cervical lymphadenopathy is present. Inflammation and vesicle formation is also noted around the nail bed of one thumb.

3. A 6-year-old boy is seen with a blanching, urticarial-looking rash present for 48 hours. It commenced on the palms of both hands, spreading proximally and now involves the trunk and face. It is confluent in places. His mother describes lesions as starting off as discrete, raised areas which blister centrally before developing central pallor. There is no mucosal involvement. The child is otherwise well with normal systemic examination.

dermatology

ENDOCRINOLOGY AND SYNDROMES

Multiple Choice Questions

76. Concerning Addison's disease

○ A   it can present with hypoglycaemia if in crises

○ B   it is commoner in males

○ C   serum renin is characteristically low

○ D   the short synacthen test is normal

○ E   fatigue is a common presenting feature

77. Down's syndrome is associated with an increased incidence of

○ A   Alzheimer's

○ B   coeliac disease

○ C   acute leukaemia

○ D   Hirschsprung's disease

○ E   oesophageal atresia

78. Features of classic homocystinuria include

○ A   autosomal dominant inheritance

○ B   hyper-extendable joints

☑ C   normal at birth

☑ D   predisposition to vascular thrombosis

○ E   aortic root dilatation

79.   Congenital hypothyroidism

○   A   is usually due to dyshormonogenesis

○   B   is usually symptomatic in the neonatal period

○   C   incidence is 1 in 4000

○   D   high thyroid stimulating hormone (TSH), normal T_4 on treatment suggests poor compliance

○   E   screening is at the 6-week check

80.   Concerning Klinefelter's syndrome

○   A   karyotype is 47 XYY

○   B   there is increased risk of leukaemia

○   C   infertility is rare

○   D   gynaecomastia is a common finding in adolescents

○   E   testes are large

81.   In Turner's syndrome

○   A   fetal loss in the first trimester is common

○   B   hypogonadotrophic hypogonadism is a feature

○   C   infants are usually born small for dates

○   D   spontaneous puberty is never seen

○   E   horseshoe kidney is a recognised association

82.   Concerning phenylketonuria

○   A   the infant is normal at birth

○   B   the urine is odourless

○   C   it is caused by a deficiency of phenylalanine hydroxylase

○   D   seizures can occur

○   E   untreated individuals have a low IQ

83. Causes of a delayed bone age are

A   obesity

B   growth hormone deficiency

C   central precocious puberty

D   social deprivation

E   chronic asthma

84. Features of Noonan's syndrome include

A   webbing of the neck

B   pulmonary valve stenosis

C   mental retardation in 80%

D   delayed puberty

E   normal final adult height

85. Causes of gynaecomastia include

A   normal child

B   Klinefelter's syndrome

C   Noonan's syndrome

D   growth hormone deficiency

E   cimetidine

86. Features of Prader–Willi syndrome include

A   autosomal dominant inheritance

B   hypogonadism

C   hyperphagia

D   normal IQ

E   normal life expectancy

87. Concerning 21-hydroxylase deficiency

A   the gene defect is known

B   hypertension is common   *11-β hydroxylase deficiency*

C   a raised serum 17-OH progesterone is characteristic

D   plasma chloride is low in salt losers

E   can present as precocious puberty in males

88. Growth hormone will increase the final adult height in the following circumstances

A   growth hormone deficiency

B   familial short stature

C   hypothyroidism

D   Turner's syndrome

E   achondroplasia

89. The following are known to stimulate growth hormone secretion

A   glucagon

B   arginine

C   aldosterone

D   thyroxine

E   insulin

90. Concerning central (true) precocious puberty

A   it is commoner in boys than in girls

B   computed tomography (CT) head scanning is indicated in all boys

C   it is usually idiopathic in girls

D   testicular volume would be expected to be increased in boys

E   it is gonadotrophin independent

91. Fragile X syndrome

A   occurs as a consequence of allelic expansion

B   is a cause of macro-orchidism in boys

C   is asymptomatic in carrier females

D   causes increasingly severe mental retardation with successive generations

E   is associated with small ears

endocrinology and syndromes

92. Galactosaemia

A   has an incidence of 1 in 1000 live births
B   can cause congenital cataracts
C   can present with hypoglycaemia in the neonatal period
D   is associated with mental retardation even with early diagnosis
E   is treated with a lactose-free diet

93. Aldosterone

A   secretion is stimulated by a fall in serum sodium
B   is secreted in response to a rise in blood pressure
C   deficiency is a cause of hypokalaemia
D   acts on the ascending limb of the loop of Henlé
E   levels are normal in pseudohypoaldosteronism

94. During puberty

A   breast hypertrophy occurs in up to 40% of boys
B   onset of the growth spurt in boys occurs at stage 4–5 of testicular enlargement
C   peak height velocity in girls often occurs *precedes* after menarche
D   elongation of the eye can occur causing short sightedness
E   the first sign of puberty in girls is the appearance of pubic hair
    Breast ↑

95. Type 1 (insulin dependent) diabetes

A   has a peak incidence at 9–10 years of age
B   is commoner in children who possess the HLA-B3 antigen   *HLA B8 – DR3 – 4 RW15*
C   is associated with islet cell antibodies in 30% at diagnosis   *80–90%*
D   has a peak incidence during the summer months in the UK
E   is associated with an increased risk of diabetes in siblings of the affected case

96. Complications of type 1 diabetes include

○   A   tall stature
○   B   hypoglycaemia
○   C   lipoatrophy
○   D   proximal myopathy
○   E   cataract

97. Features of Graves' disease include

○   A   inappropriate weight gain
○   B   association with HLA DR3
○   C   diarrhoea
○   D   poor concentration
○   E   male predominance

98. The following conditions are associated with deletions of the listed chromosome

○   A   Down's syndrome − chromosome 21
○   B   Wolf−Hirschhorn syndrome −chromosome 4
○   C   DiGeorge (Catch 22) − chromosome 22
○   D   cri du chat − chromosome 4
○   E   William's syndrome − chromosome 13

99. In achondroplasia

○   A   bowing of the legs is common
○   B   length of the vertebral spine is decreased
○   C   diagnostic radiological features are present at birth
○   D   inheritance is autosomal recessive
○   E   macrocephaly occurs

endocrinology and
syndromes

Best of Five Questions

100. The following statements refer to type 2 diabetes in childhood. Choose the MOST appropriate statement.

○   A   It does not pose a significant problem to Western society.

○   B   It is usually associated with weight loss at presentation.

○   C   It is seen in association with acanthosis nigricans.

○   D   It is rarely associated with the microvascular complications seen in type 1 diabetes.

○   E   It is always treatable with dietary measures and oral hypoglycaemic agents.

101. Select the MOST appropriate statement regarding hypoglycaemia in neonates.

○   A   Im glucagon is the treatment of choice.

○   B   Increased glycogen stores in large-for-date babies, such as infants of diabetic mothers (IDM), are protective.

○   C   The best time to take blood and urine samples is after the correction of a hypoglycaemic episode.

○   D   Long-term consequences include lowered IQ and decreased head size.

○   E   A bolus of 2.5 ml/kg of 50% dextrose should be used to correct the abnormality.

102. Regarding McCune–Albright syndrome, which is the MOST appropriate statement?

○   A   Precocious puberty caused by this condition is more commonly seen in girls than boys.

○   B   Fibrous dysplasia commonly results in pathological fracture.

○   C   Café au lait pigmentation is typically present at birth.

○   D   Precocious puberty is primarily due to central gonadotrophin dependent causes.

○   E   A family history of café au lait pigmentation supports the diagnosis.

endocrinology and syndromes

37

103. An infant is born with ambiguous genitalia. Select the MOST appropriate statement from the following.

○ A Gender identity should be determined by the phenotypic appearance.

○ B Gonadal differentiation in utero occurs in the second trimester.

○ C Hypospadias co-existing with bilateral cryptorchidism should raise the suspicion of an intersex condition.

○ D Investigations to determine the underlying diagnosis should not be performed rapidly in order to ensure adequate time to counsel parents.

○ E If palpable gonads are present, the infant can be assigned the male sex.

104. Select the MOST appropriate statement listed below regarding obesity in childhood.

○ A The various strategies that are used to tackle obesity (ie dietary modification and increased physical activity) have a strong evidence base supporting their use.

○ B It is defined as a body mass index (weight in kg/height in metres²) greater than 30.

○ C Weight loss is the most frequently recommended course of action to prevent long-term health complications.

○ D It is a greater problem in girls than boys in the UK population.

○ E It may result in subclinical coronary artery sclerosis and atherosclerosis in childhood.

Extended Matching Questions

105. Theme: Growth and development

○   A   Russell–Silver syndrome
○   B   Turner's syndrome
○   C   Constitutional delay of growth and puberty
○   D   Kallmann's syndrome
○   E   Familial short stature
○   F   Growth hormone deficiency
○   G   William's syndrome
○   H   Noonan's syndrome
○   I   Hypopituitarism

Choose the best diagnoses from the list above for each of the case scenarios described below. Each option may be used once, more than once or not at all.

1.   A 13-year-old girl is seen in clinic for an opinion with regards to her short stature and pubertal development. Her growth chart reveals she was of low birth weight (2.2 kg). Her height had been maintained on the 2nd centile for age until the age of 11 years when it fell beneath the 0.4th centile. She is currently 130 cm tall. She has stage 2 pubic hair, but no breast bud development. Her mother is 173 cm tall and her father is 181 cm tall. The target centile range given the parents' heights is calculated as between the 25th and 98th centiles. The result of a bone age X-ray requested by the GP has already been reported and has the appearances equivalent to 12 years and 8 months of age. She has elevated levels of FSH and LH.

2.   A 10-week-old baby girl is referred by the health visitor with feeding problems and faltering growth. The baby was of low birth weight (2.4 kg at term) and is struggling to take the suggested volumes of high-energy formula to maintain adequate weight gain along the 0.4th centile, although the head circumference is increasing steadily along the 25th centile. The health visitor feels the baby appears slightly dysmorphic with a high forehead and micrognathia, giving a triangular appearance to the facies. The baby is noted to be slightly floppy on handling. Her parents report she has been smiling for the last 2 weeks. A murmur was heard on the post-natal check but an echocardiogram revealed no abnormality and the murmur has since resolved. Serum electrolytes including calcium levels and a 24-hour blood glucose profile are within normal limits.

3.   A 15-year-old boy is seen in clinic due to short stature. Growth
     charts, which are available from birth, show that his birth weight
     and length were on the 50th centile. Over the first year of life his
     height and weight fell to the 9th centile where his growth was
     maintained until the last 18 months when his height has fallen to
     just beneath the 2nd centile. Examination reveals testicular volume
     of less than 10 ml with the presence of sparse pubic and axillary hair.
     There are no dysmorphic features and systemic examination is
     otherwise unremarkable. Random growth hormone levels requested
     by the GP are just beneath the lower end of the normal range for his
     age. Thyroid function is normal, along with full blood count,
     biochemical profile and erythrocyte sedimentation rate (ESR). Bone
     age is delayed 3 years. His mother recalls that her menarche
     occurred at the age of 16 years.

106. Theme: Hypocalcaemia

○   A   Hypoparathyroidism

○   B   DiGeorge syndrome

○   C   Vitamin D deficiency

○   D   Pseudohypoparathyroidism

○   E   Chronic renal failure

○   F   Pseudopseudohypoparathyroidism

○   G   Fanconi's syndrome

Choose the best diagnosis from the list above for each of the three scenarios described below. Each option may be used once, more than once or not at all.

1. A 4-week-old baby is referred by the GP with a history of twitching movements. The baby has also only just regained his birth weight and is described by mum as difficult to feed. A murmur is heard and he is noted to have low-set ears on examination.

2. A 15-month-old girl is referred by the health visitor with concerns regarding delayed development. The child is on the 91st centile for weight and the 2nd centile for height. The fourth and fifth digits of both hands appear shorter than the other fingers and both radii are slightly bowed. Parents do not report any abnormal movements. Baseline biochemistry including full blood count, renal function, calcium, phosphate, alkaline phosphatase and thyroid function are all within normal limits. Chromosomal analysis is also normal.

3. A 3-year-old eastern European refugee girl attends Accident and Emergency (A&E) after a fall. An X-ray is taken of her tibia and fibula due to localised tenderness over this area. The bones appear osteopenic but no other bony abnormality is seen. She is referred for a paediatric opinion as she appears thin and malnourished. In view of the X-ray appearances, the A&E doctors have requested a bone profile which reveals a low corrected serum calcium and elevated serum phosphate. Parathyroid hormone levels returned subsequently are elevated.

endocrinology and syndromes

41

GASTROENTEROLOGY AND NUTRITION

Multiple Choice Questions

107. Familial adenomatous polyposis coli

- ○ A has autosomal recessive inheritance
- ○ B has yellow nails as one of the recognised features
- ○ C is pre-malignant
- ○ D is associated with peri-oral pigmentation
- ○ E is the commonest cause of polyposis in childhood

108. *Helicobacter pylori*

- ○ A is a Gram-positive bacterium
- ○ B causes chronic antral gastritis
- ○ C causes a nosocomial infection
- ○ D is best diagnosed on culture
- ○ E is a common cause of recurrent abdominal pain

109. Characteristic features of Crohn's disease include

- ○ A aphthous mouth ulcers
- ○ B ankylosing spondylitis
- ○ C sclerosing cholangitis
- ○ D raised inflammatory indices
- ○ E growth retardation

110. The following milks are protein hydrolysates:

O   A   Nutramigen

O   B   Prematil

O   C   Maxijul

O   D   Neocate

O   E   Paediasure

111. Meckel's diverticulum

O   A   is a remnant of the vitello-intestinal duct

O   B   can contain ectopic pancreatic tissue

O   C   is located within the jejunum

O   D   can present with massive blood loss per rectum

O   E   is a cause of intussusception

112. Absolute contraindications to breast feeding include

O   A   infants with galactosaemia

O   B   maternal tuberculosis

O   C   maternal human immunodeficiency virus (HIV)

O   D   atenolol

O   E   cytotoxic drugs

113. Recognised consequences of abetalipoproteinaemia include

O   A   failure to thrive

O   B   autosomal dominant inheritance

O   C   ataxia secondary to vitamin D deficiency

O   D   child is normal at birth

O   E   retinitis pigmentosa

gastroenterology and nutrition

114. Characteristic features of acrodermatitis enteropathica include

- ○ A malabsorption of copper
- ○ B autosomal dominant inheritance
- ○ C recurrent infections
- ○ D alopecia
- ○ E rapid response to treatment with zinc sulphate

115. Vitamin A

- ○ A deficiency is the commonest cause of visual loss worldwide
- ○ B is fat soluble
- ○ C has an important role to play in resistance to infection
- ○ D is present in milk
- ○ E is beneficial in the management of severe measles

116. Breast feeding reduces the incidence of

- ○ A atopy in infants born to mothers with a history of atopy
- ○ B gastrointestinal infection
- ○ C nappy rash
- ○ D respiratory infection
- ○ E infantile colic

117. Concerning vitamin K

- ○ A in the newborn period an oral dose is as effective as an intramuscular dose in all babies
- ○ B there is an association between intramuscular vitamin K and childhood cancer
- ○ C it is a fat soluble vitamin
- ○ D 1 mg of vitamin K im ensures adequate prophylaxis in term infants
- ○ E liver is a good dietary source

gastroenterology and nutrition

118. The xylose tolerance test

○ A   is a reliable test in children
○ B   is likely to be normal in cystic fibrosis
○ C   is dependent on the surface area of the small intestine
○ D   is abnormal in coeliac disease
○ E   requires a blood test

119. Serum folate levels are likely to be

○ A   reduced in gluten-sensitive enteropathy
○ B   reduced following resection of the terminal ileum
○ C   reduced on treatment with anticonvulsants
○ D   low in pernicious anaemia
○ E   reduced as part of the acute phase response

120. The content of human milk at term per 100 ml is as follows:

○ A   50 kcal
○ B   1.3 g protein
○ C   0.65 mmol sodium
○ D   4.2 g fat
○ E   7.0 g carbohydrate

121. Features of carbohydrate intolerance include

○ A   usually inherited
○ B   characterised by explosive stools
○ C   usually transient
○ D   reducing substances in the stool are negative
○ E   commonly follows *Salmonella* infection

122. Pre-term compared with term formula

○ A   contains more kcal per ml
○ B   has a lower sodium content
○ C   contains more calcium
○ D   contains more iron
○ E   has the same protein content

gastroenterology and nutrition

123. Human (breast) milk compared with unmodified cow's milk contains more

○ A protein
○ B sodium
○ C calories per 100 ml
○ D fat
○ E calcium

124. The following statements are true of nutritional supplements

○ A Maxijul is a glucose polymer
○ B Caloreen is a fat emulsion
○ C Duocal contains carbohydrate and protein
○ D Calogen contains 450 kcal per 100 g
○ E whey-based infant formulae contain more calories than casein-based infant formulae

125. Immunoglobulin A

○ A makes up 50% of serum immunoglobulins
○ B predominates on respiratory and gastrointestinal surfaces in its secretory form
○ C selective deficiency is rare with a prevalence of less than 1 in 10 000
○ D deficiency is associated with an increased risk of infection
○ E deficiency is associated with an increased risk of atopic disease

126. Causes of failure to thrive include

○ A low birth weight
○ B Duchenne's muscular dystrophy
○ C inadequate intake
○ D renal tubular acidosis
○ E pre-term gestation

gastroenterology and nutrition

127. The following statements are true

  ○ A starch is a glucose polymer

  ○ B lactose is a disaccharide made up of galactose and glucose

  ○ C carbohydrate digestion is dependent on pancreatic secretion

  ○ D sucrase hydrolyses sucrose into glucose and fructose

  ○ E glucose, galactose and fructose are all absorbed by an active transport mechanism

128. The following are characteristic features of Wilson's disease

  ○ A low serum copper

  ○ B low serum caeruloplasmin

  ○ C poor response to copper chelation

  ○ D Kayser–Fleischer rings

  ○ E autosomal recessive inheritance

129. The following cause predominantly unconjugated hyperbilirubinaemia in the neonate

  ○ A gallstones

  ○ B polycythaemia

  ○ C ABO incompatibility

  ○ D biliary atresia

  ○ E glucose 6-phosphate dehydrogenase deficiency

130. Causes of a flat duodenal biopsy include

  ○ A coeliac disease

  ○ B glucose–galactose malabsorption

  ○ C giardiasis

  ○ D cystic fibrosis

  ○ E cow's milk allergy

gastroenterology and nutrition

131. Coeliac disease

○ A incidence is 1 in 300 in the UK

○ B a negative IgA endomysial antibody test in a child taking a normal diet excludes the diagnosis

○ C duodenal biopsy is inadequate to make the diagnosis

○ D crypt hypertrophy is seen on small bowel biopsy

○ E there is an increased risk of malignancy

132. Hepatitis B

○ A is a DNA virus

○ B transmission is faeco-oral

○ C treatment of acute infection is by passive immunisation

○ D interferon gamma is a recognised treatment of the chronic carrier state

○ E anti-HBs antibodies suggest a chronic carrier state has developed following acute infection

133. Concerning hepatitis A

○ A chronic liver disease commonly follows acute infection

○ B it is transmitted by the faeco-oral route

○ C passive immunisation produces life-long immunity to infection

○ D it is an RNA virus

○ E diagnosis of acute infection is by stool culture

134. Hepatitis C virus can be transmitted by

○ A iv drug use

○ B blood transfusion

○ C faeco-oral route

○ D recombinant factor VIII therapy

○ E vertical route

gastroenterology and nutrition

135. The following are likely to cause bloody diarrhoea

- A rotavirus infection
- B *Campylobacter pylori* infection
- C ulcerative colitis
- D cystic fibrosis
- E *Giardia lamblia*

136. *Giardia lamblia*

- A is a bacterium
- B infestation is usually asymptomatic
- C can cause failure to thrive and chronic diarrhoea
- D symptomatic infection should be treated with erythromycin
- E can cause partial villous atrophy

137. Concerning intussusception

- A it is a known complication of Henoch–Schönlein purpura
- B it is commonest in babies under the age of 6 months
- C barium enema is contraindicated
- D if it presents over the age of 2 years an underlying cause is likely
- E pallor is often seen

138. Gilbert's syndrome

- A causes unconjugated hyperbilirubinaemia
- B causes bilirubinuria
- C can progress to cirrhosis
- D has a prevalence of 6%
- E episodes of jaundice are precipitated by acute infections

139. Features of ulcerative colitis include

○　A　arthropathy
○　B　transmural bowel inflammation
○　C　erythema nodosum
○　D　family history of inflammatory bowel disease
○　E　backwash ileitis

140. The following make a non-organic cause of recurrent abdominal pain more likely

○　A　3-year history
○　B　night pain
○　C　family history of migraine
○　D　mouth ulceration
○　E　weight loss

141. Pre-hepatic causes of portal hypertension include

○　A　Budd–Chiari syndrome
○　B　constrictive pericarditis
○　C　schistosomiasis
○　D　portal vein thrombosis
○　E　biliary atresia

142. The following are properties of vitamin A

○　A　immune enhancement
○　B　epithelial generation
○　C　metabolic driver
○　D　bone matrix co-factor
○　E　embryological differentiation

gastroenterology and nutrition

Best of Five Questions

143. Which of the following statements regarding rectal prolapse is the MOST correct?

  ○ A It is associated with cystic fibrosis in the majority of cases.

  ○ B It is usually painful.

  ○ C It requires reduction under general anaesthetic.

  ○ D It is commonest in the pre-school age group.

  ○ E It can always be resolved with a short course of laxatives and dietary advice.

144. Which is the MOST appropriate statement regarding constipation.

  ○ A It is usually associated with an underlying medical condition.

  ○ B It occurs occasionally in the pre-school age group.

  ○ C It can be precipitated by a child's refusal to use school toilets.

  ○ D It should be investigated with rectal biopsy to exclude Hirschsprung's disease.

  ○ E It can always be resolved with a short course of laxatives and dietary advice.

145. Which is the MOST appropriate statement regarding pancreatitis in childhood?

  ○ A It is commonly caused by gallstones.

  ○ B It may be caused by treatment with sodium valproate.

  ○ C It is a frequent cause of admission to hospital with abdominal pain in childhood.

  ○ D It is characterised by an elevated serum amylase level in association with abdominal pain.

  ○ E It is accompanied by ultrasound findings of an enlarged, oedematous pancreas.

gastroenterology and nutrition

146. A 5-month-old baby with pH study-proved gastro-oesophageal reflux has not improved on treatment with Gaviscon. The centile chart now shows that the weight gain is beginning to falter. The next MOST appropriate stage of treatment would be:

○   A   Addition of an acid suppressant (H_2 blocker or proton-pump inhibitor).

○   B   Referral for fundoplication.

○   C   Trial of a soya-based formula milk.

○   D   Use of a prokinetic agent such as cisapride.

○   E   Reassurance that with weaning, symptoms should improve.

147. A 30-month-old girl is referred to clinic with a 6-month history of passing up to five watery stools per day. Mother is particularly concerned as there are frequently recognisable food particles in the stools. The child's centile charts reveal that she is steadily gaining weight along the 50th centile for both height and weight. Dietary history reveals that she is a slightly fussy eater, tending to graze throughout the day rather than eating three full meals. She drinks up to 2.5 l of fruit squash per day via a bottle. Examination is unremarkable. The MOST appropriate course of action is:

○   A   Collection of a stool sample for detection of reducing substances and implementation of a lactose-free diet.

○   B   Arrange blood tests for full blood count, total IgA and anti-gliadin antibodies.

○   C   Microbiological analysis of stool sample (culture and virology assessment) to exclude infective diarrhoea.

○   D   Advice about dietary intake, especially with regard to the amount and type of fluids being offered with further follow-up to assess weight gain.

○   E   Assay for faecal elastase to rule out pancreatic insufficiency.

gastroenterology and nutrition

Extended Matching Questions

148. Theme: Prolonged jaundice

○   A   Biliary atresia

○   B   ABO incompatibility

○   C   Breast milk jaundice

○   D   Congenital hypothyroidism

○   E   Idiopathic neonatal hepatitis

○   F   Rhesus haemolytic disease

○   G   Congenital cytomegalovirus infection

○   H   Glucose 6-phosphate dehydrogenase deficiency

○   1   Neonatal haemochromatosis

○   J   *Escherichia coli* septicaemia

Choose the most likely diagnosis from the list above for each of the three scenarios described below. Each option may be used once, more than once or not at all.

1. A 5-day-old term baby boy of Mediterranean parents is referred with jaundice and poor feeding. Total serum bilirubin is 380 μmol/l, conjugated fraction <10%. His full blood count reveals haemoglobin of 10g/dl, white cell count 12 (10^9/l, platelets 400 and CRP <10. Maternal blood group is A rhesus positive and baby is O rhesus positive. On examination, the baby is found to have splenomegaly.

2. A 6-week-old breast and formula fed baby girl, born at term to Asian parents after a delivery complicated by prolonged rupture of membranes, is seen by her GP for routine developmental assessment. She is gaining weight along the 2nd centile, consistent with her birth weight. She is noted by the GP to be jaundiced and have hepatosplenomegaly on examination but otherwise handles normally and does not appear acutely unwell. Since the introduction of formula 2 weeks ago, the parents comment that her stools appear lighter in colour.

3. A baby girl is delivered at 35 weeks due to poor CTG in association with intra-uterine growth retardation. The baby is in poor condition at birth, requiring intubation. Hepatosplenomegaly and petechiae are noted on initial examination. Broad-spectrum antibiotics are commenced after blood cultures have been taken. The baby becomes jaundiced within 24 hours of delivery and elevated liver enzymes are noted on liver function testing. A CT scan of the brain is performed subsequently revealing bright areas in the periventricular region.

149. Theme: Rectal bleeding

○   A   Gardner's syndrome

○   B   Constipation

○   C   Ulcerative colitis

○   D   Intussusception

○   E   Hirschsprung's disease

○   F   Meckel's diverticulum

○   G   Crohn's disease

○   H   Henoch-Schönlein purpura

○   I   Meconium ileus

○   J   Coeliac disease

Choose the most likely diagnosis from the list above for each of the three scenarios described below. Each option may be used once, more than once or not at all.

1. A 5-year-old boy is brought to accident and emergency with abdominal pains of recent onset and parents report passage of fresh red blood per rectum. He has also complained of a sore left ankle over the same period of time. Systemic examination reveals a well-grown child on the 75th centile for height and weight. There is a palpable blanching rash on the shins. No masses are palpable per abdomen.

2. An 8-month-old baby boy with a known small muscular ventricular septal defect is seen in the general paediatric out-patient clinic with a history of recurrent episodes of abdominal distension in association with infrequent passage of stool which have been present since birth. His weight has fallen from the 25th centile at birth to the 2nd centile at present. His mother describes frequent episodes of vomiting which have not improved with anti-reflux therapy. The cardiologists do not feel his poor weight gain is related to his cardiac abnormality.

3. A 2-day-old term baby girl, born at home with birth weight 2.75 kg, is referred by the community midwife with a history of bilious vomiting and failure to open her bowels since birth. On palpation of her abdomen, which is moderately distended, there is a palpable mass in the right iliac fossa. Abdominal X-ray shows distended small intestinal loops, with a lower gastrointestinal contrast study revealing a microcolon with pellet-like meconium in the terminal ileum.

gastroenterology and nutrition

HAEMATOLOGY, ONCOLOGY AND POISONING

Multiple Choice Questions

150. Iron deficiency anaemia

- ○ A is characterised by a low serum iron and a low total iron binding capacity
- ○ B is associated with pica
- ○ C is prevented by the early introduction of cow's milk
- ○ D never requires treatment under the age of 6 months
- ○ E in childhood is associated with chronic blood loss in most cases

151. Concerning idiopathic thrombocytopenia in childhood

- ○ A bed rest is indicated
- ○ B bone marrow examination is essential
- ○ C incidence is 1 in 1000 children per year
- ○ D platelet transfusion is necessary if the platelet count falls below 20
- ○ E intravenous immunoglobulin may be beneficial

152. Glanzmann's thrombasthenia

- ○ A is inherited as an autosomal dominant
- ○ B gene locus is known
- ○ C platelet count is normal
- ○ D requires long-term steroid treatment
- ○ E splenectomy may be beneficial

153. Features of hereditary spherocytosis include

○ A splenomegaly
○ B conjugated hyperbilirubinaemia
○ C gallstones
○ D haemolytic crises following fava bean ingestion
○ E X-linked inheritance

154. Glucose 6-phosphate dehydrogenase deficiency

○ A only occurs in males
○ B can cause chronic haemolytic anaemia
○ C co-trimoxazole can trigger a crisis
○ D results in spherocytosis
○ E causes neonatal jaundice

155. Features of Wiskott–Aldrich syndrome include

○ A autosomal recessive inheritance
○ B normal platelet count
○ C T cell defect
○ D death from acute haemorrhage in 20%
○ E eczema

156. Concerning vitamin B_{12}

○ A deficiency can cause ataxia
○ B pernicious anaemia commonly occurs following terminal ileal resection
○ C in deficiency the mean corpuscular volume is usually normal
○ D deficiency usually occurs in untreated coeliac disease
○ E extrinsic factor promotes absorption

haematology, oncology and poisoning

157. Sickle cell disease

  ○ A   is associated with an increased risk of gallstones

  ○ B   is associated with an increased risk of nocturnal enuresis

  ○ C   can be diagnosed antenatally

  ○ D   is an indication for prophylactic penicillin

  ○ E   is associated with episodes of acute anaemia

158. Concerning rhesus haemolytic disease

  ○ A   it cannot occur in first born children

  ○ B   it occurs as a consequence of the transplacental passage of IgM

  ○ C   the most common antibody type is anti-D

  ○ D   it can present as hydrops fetalis

  ○ E   it is an indication for premature delivery

159. In the anaemia of chronic disease

  ○ A   the haemoglobin is usually less than 8 g/dl

  ○ B   the total iron binding capacity is raised

  ○ C   the anaemia is usually normocytic

  ○ D   the serum iron is usually reduced

  ○ E   iron supplements are contraindicated

160. Neonatal thrombocytopenia

  ○ A   is an indication for cerebral ultrasound

  ○ B   is an absolute indication for platelet transfusion after delivery

  ○ C   may be caused by toxoplasmosis infection during pregnancy

  ○ D   can occur in infants born to mothers with systemic lupus erythematosus

  ○ E   may be associated with absent radii

haematology, oncology and poisoning

161. Concerning blood transfusion

○ A   pyrexia is an absolute indication for stopping the transfusion

○ B   back pain is an indication of severe transfusion reaction

○ C   hyperkalaemia is a well recognised complication

○ D   white cell filters are indicated if the patient is having regular transfusions

○ E   hydrocortisone and antihistamines minimise mild transfusion reactions in patients having regular transfusions

162. Causes of neutropenia include

○ A   hyperglycinaemia

○ B   cytotoxic drug therapy

○ C   chronic granulomatous disease

○ D   Kostmann's syndrome

○ E   X-linked hypogammaglobulinaemia

163. Causes of bone pain and anaemia include

○ A   vitamin C deficiency

○ B   neuroblastoma

○ C   Langerhans' cell histiocytosis

○ D   acute lymphoblastic leukaemia

○ E   sickle cell disease

164. Features of acute lymphoblastic leukaemia in childhood include

○ A   an incidence of 1 in 3500 in the first ten years of life

○ B   fever at presentation

○ C   neutropenia

○ D   a better prognosis if the age is less than 2 years at presentation

○ E   long-term survival in 70%

haematology, oncology and poisoning

165. Thrombocytosis (platelet count > 400 x 10^9/l) is seen in

○ A   the first week of Kawasaki's disease
○ B   iron deficiency anaemia
○ C   post-splenectomy patients
○ D   Bernard–Soulier syndrome
○ E   juvenile chronic arthritis

166. Aplastic anaemia can occur secondary to

○ A   radiation
○ B   chloramphenicol
○ C   hepatitis A
○ D   Epstein-Barr virus
○ E   parvovirus infection

167. Diseases with an increased risk of malignancy include

○ A   ataxia telangiectasia
○ B   Bloom's syndrome
○ C   xeroderma pigmentosum
○ D   Down's syndrome
○ E   Fanconi's anaemia

168. Features of von Willebrand's disease include

○ A   prolonged bleeding time
○ B   autosomal recessive inheritance
○ C   menorrhagia
○ D   normal platelet count
○ E   normal platelet aggregation with ristocetin

169. Causes of a prolonged bleeding time include

○ A   Bernard–Soulier syndrome
○ B   Henoch–Schönlein syndrome
○ C   haemophilia
○ D   von Willebrand's disease
○ E   idiopathic thrombocytopenic purpura

haematology, oncology and poisoning

61

170. Concerning X-linked agammoglobulinaemia

○ A   the gene locus is known
○ B   the thymus is hypoplastic or absent
○ C   T cell function is normal
○ D   IgA, G and M are all reduced
○ E   intravenous immunoglobulin therapy is indicated

171. DiGeorge syndrome

○ A   inheritance is autosomal recessive
○ B   the thymus is hypoplastic or absent
○ C   cardiac defects are common
○ D   the lymphocyte count is always reduced
○ E   hypocalcaemia is common

172. Osteosarcoma

○ A   usually presents in the first decade
○ B   outcome <10% survival overall
○ C   usually occurs in the metaphyseal region of growing bones
○ D   lung metastasis at presentation occur in 80%
○ E   fever at presentation is common

173. In accidental iron ingestion

○ A   hypotension may occur within two hours of ingestion
○ B   toxicity is unlikely if vomiting stops within two hours of ingestion
○ C   abdominal X-ray is a useful investigation
○ D   pyloric stenosis may present 2 weeks after ingestion
○ E   lactic acidosis may occur 12 hours post-ingestion

174. Carbon monoxide

○   A   combines with haemoglobin to form carboxyhaemoglobin

○   B   shifts the oxygen dissociation curve to the left

○   C   toxicity occurs if the carboxyhaemoglobin level is 3–5%

○   D   toxicity causes headache

○   E   increases the oxygen carrying capacity of the blood

175. In overdosage with tricyclic antidepressants

○   A   tachycardia usually precedes coma

○   B   dialysis is effective at removing the drug

○   C   death is usually due to cardiac arrhythmias

○   D   the pupils are dilated

○   E   multiple doses of charcoal therapy should not be used

176. Recognised complications of aspirin overdose

○   A   hypoglycaemia

○   B   hyperkalaemia

○   C   hypoventilation

○   D   vomiting

○   E   deafness

177. Lead poisoning can present with

○   A   coma

○   B   convulsions

○   C   constipation

○   D   peripheral sensory neuropathy

○   E   anaemia

haematology oncology
and poisoning

178. The following are typical feature of sickle cell anaemia

○ A massive splenomegaly at the age of 10 years
○ B short stature
○ C presentation in the first month of life
○ D increased susceptibility to group B streptococcal infections
○ E increased susceptibility to malaria

179. There are established population screening programmes for the following haematological disorders

○ A hereditary spherocytosis
○ B glucose 6-phosphate dehydrogenase deficiency
○ C β-thalassaemia
○ D pyruvate kinase deficiency
○ E sickle cell disease

180. Good prognostic signs in acute lymphoblastic leukaemia include

○ A less than 2 years at presentation
○ B male sex
○ C high white cell count at diagnosis
○ D common cell type ALL
○ E mediastinal widening in chest X ray

Best of Five Questions

181. **An otherwise well 2-year-old presents with extreme pallor. Growth and development are normal. The child is pale but there is no lymphadenopathy or splenomegaly. Full blood count shows haemoglobin 4 g/dl (40 g/l), MCV 59. Other indices are normal. The MOST appropriate management is:**

○ A   Start gluten free diet.

○ B   Small bowel technetium scan.

○ C   Chelation therapy for lead.

○ D   Bone marrow aspirate.

○ E   Dietary review.

182. **In a child presenting with lymphadenopathy, which of the following is the BEST indicator of need for excision node biopsy?**

○ A   Multiple anterior cervical nodes.

○ B   Single supraclavicular node.

○ C   Associated chronic fatigue.

○ D   Post-auricular nodes.

○ E   Known to have congenital heart disease.

183. **In chronic lead poisoning what is MOST likely to occur?**

○ A   Macrocytic anaemia.

○ B   Osteomalacia.

○ C   Pulmonary fibrosis.

○ D   Cardiomyopathy.

○ E   Delayed developmental milestones.

haematology, oncology and poisoning

Extended Matching Questions

184. Theme: Presenting symptoms of paediatric malignancies

○   A   Wilms' tumour
○   B   Medulloblastoma
○   C   ALL
○   D   Osteosarcoma
○   E   Rhabdomyosarcoma
○   F   Hepatoblastoma
○   G   Hodgkin's lymphoma
○   H   Histiocytosis X

Choose the most likely diagnosis from the list above for each of the three scenarios described below. Each option may be used once, more than once or not at all.

1.   Acute limp
2.   Proptosis
3.   Pleomorphic rash

185. Theme: Signs of poisoning

○   A   Mydriasis
○   B   Bradycardia
○   C   Haematemesis
○   D   Hyperacusis
○   E   Pruritus
○   F   Hypoventilation
○   G   Chorea
○   H   Abnormal odour

Choose the most likely sign from the list above for each of the three drug poisonings described below. Each option may be used once, more than once or not at all.

1.   Iron
2.   Aspirin
3.   Tricyclic antidepressants

INFECTIOUS DISEASES AND IMMUNOLOGY

Multiple Choice Questions

186. Regarding the polymerase chain reaction (PCR)

- ○ A a large amount of template DNA is required
- ○ B peripheral blood lymphocytes are an appropriate template
- ○ C the PCR product can be analysed by Southern blotting
- ○ D it is not possible to analyse RNA by PCR
- ○ E is used to aid in the prognosis of some cancers

187. The following are true of tumour necrosis factor

- ○ A exists in three principal forms
- ○ B can encourage tumour growth
- ○ C is implicated in the pathogenesis of septic shock
- ○ D contributes to the disease process in rheumatoid arthritis
- ○ E is synthesised by macrophages

188. Regarding IgE

- ○ A it can cross the placenta
- ○ B serum concentration is equal to that of IgG
- ○ C it is increased in people with asthma
- ○ D it associated with type II hypersensitivity
- ○ E it is present in high concentration in normal individuals

189. Concerning chronic granulomatous disease

○ A inheritance is autosomal dominant

○ B results from failure of phagocytes to generate oxygen free radicals

○ C most affected patients are asymptomatic

○ D may cause delayed separation of the umbilical cord

○ E is diagnosed by the nitroblue tetrazolium (NBT) test

190. *Chlamydia trachomatis* causes

○ A lymphogranuloma venereum

○ B psittacosis

○ C non-specific urethritis

○ D conjunctivitis

○ E pelvic inflammatory disease

191. Toxoplasmosis

○ A usually presents with pyrexia and a rash

○ B can cause chorioretinitis

○ C has an 80% risk of infecting the fetus if the mother is infected during pregnancy

○ D is a cause of atypical lymphocytosis

○ E infection is best diagnosed by serology

192. Concerning *Streptococcus pneumoniae* (pneumococcus)

○ A it is a Gram-positive organism

○ B it is the commonest cause of meningitis in childhood

○ C vaccination with Pneumovax is recommended in children with sickle cell disease

○ D there are four different serotypes

○ E it is the cause of Lyme disease

193. In atypical mycobacterial infection

○   A   contact tracing is essential

○   B   pulmonary involvement is commoner in children than in adults

○   C   lymphoma is part of the differential diagnosis

○   D   incision and drainage is the recommended treatment of an infected node

○   E   anti-tuberculous chemotherapy is indicated in all cases

194. Familial Mediterranean fever

○   A   is inherited as an autosomal dominant

○   B   amyloidosis is a recognised complication

○   C   colchicine can be used to suppress an attack

○   D   is a bacterial infection

○   E   is characterised by episodes of abdominal pain and fever

195. Which of the following are DNA-containing viruses

○   A   mumps

○   B   hepatitis B

○   C   molluscum contagiosum

○   D   hepatitis C

○   E   respiratory syncytial virus

196. Which of the following statements regarding cerebrospinal fluid (CSF) are correct:

○   A   a normal CSF glucose excludes bacterial meningitis

○   B   red cells are a normal finding in the CSF of a child over the age of 6 years

○   C   CSF protein is higher in the neonate than in the older child

○   D   a spinal cord tumour can cause a lymphocytosis

○   E   the white cell count is always raised in bacterial meningitis

Infectious diseases and immunology

197. Impetigo

A   is contagious
B   is best treated with topical antibiotics
C   can cause a bullous rash
D   causes a fever in the majority of cases
E   is usually due to staphylococcal infection

198. Features of infectious mononucleosis include

A   spread by transmission of oral secretions
B   heterophile antibodies in the blood
C   positive Paul Bunnell in all cases
D   atypical lymphocytosis
E   splenomegaly

199. Schistosomiasis

A   it is usually asymptomatic
B   it is a cause of obstructive uropathy
C   ·chronic granulomatous injury occurs with chronic infection
D   terminal haematuria is typical of *Schistosoma haematobium*
E   mebendazole is the drug of choice   Praziquantel

200. The following are notifiable diseases

A   respiratory syncytial virus positive bronchiolitis
B   mumps
C   yellow fever
D   hepatitis A
E   meningococcal septicaemia

201. Concerning measles

A   it is a DNA virus
B   Koplik's spots are pathognomonic
C   it is most contagious during the prodromal period
D   a fatal carditis can occur
E   a single vaccination provides life-long immunity

Infectious diseases and immunology

70

202. Concerning Lyme disease

- A transmission to humans is by infected ticks
- B erythema toxicum is characteristic
- C it can present with a VII nerve palsy
- D antibiotics are unhelpful
- E diagnosis is usually made by blood culture

203. Concerning parvovirus B19 infection

- A it is a cause of non-immune hydrops
- B it can cause aplastic crises in sickle cell disease
- C thrombocytopenia is a recognised complication
- D intravenous immunoglobulin is indicated in all cases
- E an arthropathy can occur

204. Concerning the vertical transmission of hepatitis B

- A it is more likely if the mother is hepatitis B 'e' antigen positive
- B it is reduced by passive immunisation at birth
- C active immunisation is affected by maternal IgG
- D active and passive immunisation is more protective than passive immunisation alone
- E vertical transmission occurs around the time of birth

205. Factors that suggest transient synovitis of the hip joint rather than septic arthritis include

- A age under 5 years
- B normal erythrocyte sedimentation rate (ESR)
- C normal hip radiograph
- D neutrophilia
- E pyrexia

Infectious diseases and immunology

71

206. Risk factors for the vertical transmission of HIV include

O A   advanced clinical disease in the mother
O B   high CD4 count
O C   pre-term delivery
O D   caesarean section
O E   prolonged rupture of membranes

207. The following are causes of erythema nodosum

O A   tuberculosis
O B   systemic lupus erythematosus
O C   inflammatory bowel disease
O D   Hodgkin's disease
O E   streptococcal infection

208. Concerning systemic lupus erythematosus

O A   antibodies to double stranded DNA are virtually diagnostic
O B   50% are anti-nuclear antibody (ANA)-negative
O C   a low C3 suggests renal disease
O D   Anti-Ro antibodies are present in neonatal lupus
O E   procainamide can induce ANA positivity

209. Concerning Perthes' disease

O A   it predominantly occurs in males
O B   it is always unilateral
O C   patients are usually older than 10 years at presentation
O D   the incidence is 1 in 2000
O E   obesity is common

Infectious diseases and immunology

210. The following are true regarding immunisations

○   A   MMR vaccine should not be given to HIV-positive children

○   B   live polio vaccine should not be given to siblings of children receiving chemotherapy

○   C   pertussis vaccine is contraindicated if a first-degree relative has convulsions

○   D   MMR vaccine is ineffective if given within 3 months of immunoglobulin therapy

○   E   influenza vaccination is not indicated in children with cystic fibrosis

211. The following are recognised side-effects of the following vaccinations

○   A   collapse following the acellular pertussis vaccine

○   B   parotid swelling in the third week after MMR

○   C   convulsions following pertussis

○   D   poliomyelitis following the Salk poliovirus vaccine

○   E   regional adenitis following bacille Calmette Guérin (BCG)

212. Concerning influenza immunisation

○   A   anaphylactic hypersensitivity to egg protein is a contraindication

○   B   routine immunisation of healthcare workers is recommended

○   C   the vaccine is live

○   D   the vaccine is given by intradermal injection

○   E   cystic fibrosis is a contraindication

213. Meningococcal infection

○   A   infection with group C is the commonest in the UK

○   B   mortality from infection is 10%

○   C   peak age 3–7 years

○   D   vaccination is part of the routine childhood immunisation programme in the UK

○   E   can present with a macular rash

Infectious diseases and immunology

214. Diseases associated with HLA B27 include

○ A ankylosing spondylitis

○ B diabetes mellitus

○ C psoriatic arthropathy

○ D Marfan's syndrome

○ E dermatomyositis

215. Characteristic early features of Kawasaki's disease include

○ A exudative conjunctivitis

○ B thrombocytosis

○ C palmar erythema

○ D lymphadenopathy

○ E coronary artery thrombosis

216. Complications of rubella infection include

○ A orchitis

○ B thrombocytopenic purpura

○ C arthritis

○ D encephalitis

○ E congenital cataract

217. Features suggestive of a humoral immunodeficiency

○ A oesophageal candidiasis

○ B frequent urinary tract infection

○ C chronic diarrhoea with failure to thrive

○ D recurrent skin abscesses

○ E recurrent cold sores

218. The folowing are live vaccines

○ A hepatitis B

○ B tetanus

○ C hepatitis A

○ D pneumococcal

○ E oral polio

Infectious diseases and immunology

219. Absolute contraindications to pertussis vaccination are

○   A   personal history of fits

○   B   personal history of gross motor delay

○   C   family history of absence seizures

○   D   fever of 39.1 °C after previous vaccination

○   E   none

Best of Five Questions

220. A 5-year-old Caucasian boy returned 10 days before from East Africa. He had been given advised anti-malarials. He was admitted with high fever and 'confusion' and the examination shows no focal findings. The MOST important first line test is:

○   A   Blood culture.

○   B   Anti-streptolysin O test (ASOT).

○   C   Thin film for malaria parasite.

○   D   Thick film for malaria parasite.

○   E   Lumbar puncture.

221. A 3-year-old Indian boy is suspected of having pulmonary tuberculosis on the basis of a chronic cough and fever. Chest X-ray is reported normal. The MOST useful next test is:

○   A   Sputum culture.

○   B   Bronchoscopy.

○   C   Heaf test.

○   D   Diagnostic trial of therapy.

○   E   Mantoux test.

222. A sibling of an inpatient on a ward with several immunosuppressed children visits and plays with the other patients. The following day she develops the first crop of chickenpox lesions. The BEST management is:

○   A   Zoster immunoglobulin (ZIG) to the high-risk contacts.

○   B   Vaccinate the child himself.

○   C   Vaccinate the at-risk children.

○   D   Oral aciclovir to the high-risk children.

○   E   No immediate action needed; observe for signs in the high-risk children.

Extended Matching Questions

223. Theme: Investigations

O   A   Blood culture

O   B   Bone marrow aspirate

O   C   Urine microscopy

O   D   Sputum culture

O   E   Immunoglobulins

O   F   HIV antibody test

O   G   Hepatitis B antigen

O   H   None of the above

Choose the most likely investigation from the list above for each of the three scenarios described below. Each option may be used once, more than once or not at all.

1. A 3-year-old with three episodes of pneumonia over the previous year.

2. An unwell 5-year-old Sudanese child with weight loss, fever and massive splenomegaly.

3. A 3-year-old child attending nursery presenting with jaundice and hepatomegaly to 4 cm.

224. Theme: Diagnosis

○ A Malaria
○ B HIV
○ C Severe combined immunodeficiency
○ D Miliary tuberculosis
○ E Lyme disease
○ F Brucellosis
○ G Cytomegalovirus infection
○ H Measles
○ I None of the above

Choose the most likely diagnosis from the list above for each of the three scenarios described below. Each option may be used once, more than once or not at all.

1. A 13-year-old with fatigue and cervical lymphadenopathy.

2. A 1-year-old with febrile illness, cervical adenopathy, misery and conjunctivitis. On examination the infant has maculopapular rash plus the above.

3. A 5-year-old with circumscribed rash, fatigue and knee pains.

NEONATOLOGY

Multiple Choice Questions

225. α-Fetoprotein is increased in the following conditions
○   A   Down's syndrome
○   B   threatened abortion
○   C   congenital nephrotic syndrome
○   D   anencephaly
○   E   Turner's syndrome

226. Polyhydramnios is a feature of
○   A   renal agenesis
○   B   oesophageal atresia
○   C   duodenal atresia
○   D   anencephaly
○   E   coarctation of the aorta

227. Nitric oxide
○   A   is a pulmonary vasodilator
○   B   causes systemic hypotension
○   C   is synthesised from L-arginine and oxygen
○   D   is released from vascular walls during stress
○   E   causes contraction of gastrointestinal sphincters

neonatology

228. The following are useful in the assessment of gestational age in pre-term infants

   A   presence of palmar creases

   B   breast size

   C   sacral oedema

   D   the scarf sign

   E   muscle tone

229. The following statements about pulmonary hypertension are true

   A   it is a recognised complication of group B streptococcal sepsis

   B   hyperventilation is an effective treatment

   C   tolazoline is a potent pulmonary vasoconstrictor

   D   radial arterial $P_a(o_2)$ is lower then umbilical artery $P_a(o_2)$

   E   birth asphyxia is a risk factor

230. Concerning air leak syndromes in the newborn

   A   an underwater seal drain is generally not required for ventilated babies

   B   in a term baby with a small pneumothorax giving oxygen at high concentration can worsen it

   C   increasing the I:E ratio in a ventilated baby decreases the risk of pneumothorax

   D   pneumomediastinum is usually fatal

   E   they can be asymptomatic

231. Recognised problems of neonates born at term small for gestational age include

   A   hypothermia

   B   sepsis

   C   polycythaemia

   D   hypoglycaemia

   E   retinopathy of prematurity

neonatology

232. Complications of steroid therapy in the neonate include

○ A leucopenia
○ B hypoglycaemia
○ C impaired cognitive function at 5 years of age
○ D sepsis
○ E gastric perforation

233. Concerning necrotising enterocolitis

○ A exchange transfusion is a predisposing factor
○ B *Clostridium welchii* is implicated in the pathogenesis
○ C it is commonest in neonates born under 1500 g
○ D oral antibiotics are useful
○ E complications include short bowel syndrome

234. The following statements are true

○ A fracture of the cervical spine can occur with breech deliveries
○ B waiter's tip positioning of the arm is seen with Klumpke's paralysis
○ C phrenic nerve palsy with diaphragmatic weakness occurs with Erb's palsy
○ D caput succedaneum is limited by suture lines
○ E the clavicle is the commonest bone to fracture during labour and delivery

235. Causes of recurrent apnoeas in pre-terms include

○ A sepsis
○ B gastro-oesophageal reflux
○ C bowel movement
○ D hypoglycaemia
○ E anaemia

neonatology

236. Concerning respiratory distress syndrome

○ A   maternal diabetes is a risk factor

○ B   it is characterised by reduced lung compliance

○ C   can be treated by endotracheal administration of surfactant

○ D   prognosis is better in males

○ E   steroids given within 4 hours of delivery reduce the incidence of respiratory distress syndrome

237. Phototherapy

○ A   reduces serum unconjugated bilirubin levels

○ B   is a substitute for exchange transfusion in small pre-terms

○ C   is not very effective in dark-skinned infants

○ D   can cause watery stools in the treated infant

○ E   increases fluid requirements

238. Infants of diabetic mothers

○ A   usually develop hypoglycaemia on the second day of life

○ B   are always large for gestational age

○ C   sacral agenesis is one of the congenital anomalies seen

○ D   are at increased risk of developing diabetes mellitus

○ E   have an increased incidence of respiratory distress syndrome

239. Concerning neonatal polycythaemia

○ A   it refers to a haemoglobin level of above 180 g/l

○ B   trisomy 21 is a predisposing factor

○ C   necrotising enterocolitis is a recognised complication

○ D   capillary packed cell volume is usually less than venous packed cell volume

○ E   there are no long-term complications

neonatology

240. The following statements are true about perinatal asphyxia

○ A multiple gestation is a risk factor

○ B it is the commonest cause of cerebral palsy in the UK

○ C persistent fetal circulation is a recognised complication

○ D seizures occur in grade I hypoxic ischaemic encephalopathy

○ E hypocalcaemia can occur

241. Bile stained vomit on the first day of life

○ A makes duodenal atresia unlikely

○ B with a history of meconium-stained amniotic fluid rules out intestinal obstruction

○ C suggests pyloric stenosis

○ D requires a barium enema to rule out malrotation

○ E if due to meconium ileus responds to Gastrografin enemas in half the cases

242. The following statements are true

○ A cord haemoglobin in a term infant is usually between 12 and 14 g/dl

○ B increased red cell breakdown is the main cause of the physiological anaemia of infancy

○ C fetal haemoglobin does not have a β-chain

○ D β-thalassaemia can present with anaemia in the neonatal period

○ E the Apt test differentiates fetal from maternal haemoglobin

243. Problems associated with pre-term gestation include

○ A pulmonary haemorrhage

○ B hyperglycaemia

○ C jaundice

○ D metabolic acidosis

○ E periventricular leukomalacia

neonatology

244. Causes of neonatal fits include

○ A Wilson's disease

○ B hypoglycaemia

○ C DiGeorge syndrome

○ D lead poisoning

○ E kernicterus

245. Risk factors for congenital dislocation of the hip include

○ A breech delivery

○ B spina bifida

○ C male sex

○ D positive family history

○ E being first born

246. Predominantly conjugated hyperbilirubinaemia occurs with the following

○ A breast milk jaundice

○ B Crigler–Najjar syndrome

○ C biliary atresia

○ D α–1 antitrypsin deficiency

○ E choledochal cyst

247. Chickenpox in the neonate

○ A is a contraindication to breast feeding

○ B requires treatment with iv aciclovir

○ C is infectious

○ D has a mortality untreated of 90%

○ E is suggestive of an underlying immunodeficiency

neonatology

248. Cataracts are associated with

O   A   galactosaemia

O   B   congenital cytomegalovirus infection

O   C   retinopathy of prematurity

O   D   Hunter's syndrome

O   E   Gilbert's syndrome

249. The following are associated with an increased risk of sudden infant death syndrome

O   A   maternal smoking

O   B   paternal smoking

O   C   lower parental age

O   D   prone sleeping position

O   E   use of, on average, fewer blankets

250. In a well, thriving, breastfed 3-week-old baby with normal stools and jaundice, the following are first-line investigations

O   A α_1 anti-trypsin deficiency

O   B   urine amino acids

O   C   thyroid function tests

O   D   international normalised ratio

O   E   split bilirubin

251. Oxygen transfer from the placenta to fetus is possible because of

O   A   relative left shift of oxygen dissociation curve in haemoglobin F

O   B   relative right shift of oxygen dissociation curve in haemoglobin F

O   C   relative polycythaemia of fetal compared to adult blood

O   D   osmotic gradient

O   E   higher fetal stroke volume/kg

neonatology

Best of Five Questions

252. A 29-week gestation baby is delivered after prolonged rupture of membranes of 4 days. Meconium is present at delivery. At 2 hours of age the baby is grunting and poorly perfused. Which is the MOST important pathogen to consider?

○ A group A *Streptococcus*

○ B *Klebsiella*

○ C *Escherichia coli*

○ D *Pseudomonas*

○ E *Listeria*

253. You are asked to review a 2-day-old baby with poor feeding. On examination the baby is floppy with absent reflexes although appearing otherwise well and alert. The single MOST useful investigation is:

○ A MR head scan

○ B Creatinine kinase

○ C Muscle biopsy

○ D Electromyography

○ E Lumbar puncture

254. A systolic murmur is heard in an asymptomatic, pink, term baby with normal pulses on the day 1 check. The MOST appropriate action is:

○ A Four limb saturations

○ B Four limb blood pressure

○ C Echo same day

○ D Chest X-ray

○ E Review on the following day

neonatology

Extended Matching Questions

255. Theme: Congenital syndromes

O   A   Beckwith–Weidemann syndrome

O   B   Trisomy 13

O   C   Prader–Willi syndrome

O   D   Turner's syndrome

O   E   DiGeorge syndrome

O   F   Hypothyroidism

O   G   VATER syndrome

O   H   Crigler–Najjar syndrome

Choose the most likely diagnosis from the list above for each of the three scenarios described below. Each option may be used once, more than once or not at all.

1. Antenatal scan showing horseshoe kidney and pedal oedema.

2. A term baby of appropriate birth weight is floppy and feeding poorly.

3. An antenatal scan of a term baby shows duplex kidney. The first feed is very 'gurgly'.

256. Theme: Neonatal thrombocytopenia

O   A   Neonatal alloimmune thrombocytopenia/NAIT

O   B   Maternal drugs

O   C   TORCH infection

O   D   Sepsis

O   E α-Thalassaemia

O   F   Rhesus disease

O   G   Renal vein thrombosis

O   H   Maternal systemic lupus erythematosus

Choose the most likely condition from the list above for each of the three scenarios described below. Each option may be used once, more than once or not at all.

1. A 1-day-old well-looking baby with platelet count $30 \times 10^9/l$, petechial rash and a palpable spleen.

2. A baby with intrauterine growth retardation with platelets $20 \times 10^9/l$ and with lens opacities.

3. A well baby with petechial rash, platelets $20 \times 10^9/l$ and bradycardia of 60/min.

neonatology

87

NEPHROLOGY

Multiple Choice Questions

257. Angiotensin II

○　A　increases renin
○　B　stimulates catecholamine release
○　C　increases aldosterone
○　D　reduces after load on the heart
○　E　is synthesised in the kidney

258. Causes of inappropriate anti-diuretic hormone (ADH) secretion include

○　A　HIB meningitis
○　B　Pneumococcal pneumonia
○　C　Vincristine
○　D　Renal tubular acidosis
○　E　Phenytoin

259. Features of cranial diabetes insipidus

○　A　polyuria
○　B　failure to thrive
○　C　hyponatraemia
○　D　weight loss during a water deprivation test
○　E　autosomal dominant inheritance in 85%

260. The following are used in the emergency treatment of hyperkalaemia

○ A   normal saline infusion
○ B   intravenous salbutamol
○ C   nebulised salbutamol
○ D   intravenous adenosine
○ E   intravenous hydrocortisone

261. Nocturnal enuresis

○ A   Drug treatment accelerates resolution
○ B   in children under the age of 10 years is commoner in boys than in girls
○ C   the prevalence in 10-year-olds is around 5%
○ D   is primary in 95%
○ E   the incidence is 10 times greater when either parent has had nocturnal enuresis

262. Berger's disease (mesangial IgA nephritis) is characterised by

○ A   male predominance
○ B   deafness
○ C   exacerbations associated with upper respiratory infections
○ D   end stage renal failure in 2 years
○ E   proteinuria in 50%

263. In a 2-year-old pre-renal rather than renal failure is suggested by

○ A   fractional excretion of sodium of 4%
○ B   urinary sodium 10 mmol/l
○ C   urine osmolality 250 mmol/l
○ D   urine:plasma creatinine ratio of 5
○ E   history of diarrhoea

264. Renal osteodystrophy

○ A   is a complication of chronic renal failure
○ B   is characterised by an increased plasma phosphate
○ C   is characterised by a reduced serum alkaline phosphatase
○ D   is characterised by a normal parathyroid hormone level
○ E   is familial

265. Renal involvement in Henoch-Schönlein purpura

○ A   occurs in 25–50%
○ B   is always present within 4 weeks of the onset of the disease
○ C   usually manifests as an acute nephritis
○ D   is usually associated with a low C3 and C4
○ E   is usually progressive

266. The following patterns of inheritance are correct:

○ A   nephrogenic diabetes insipidus – autosomal recessive
○ B   Alport's syndrome – X-linked dominant
○ C   Hartnup's disease – X-linked recessive
○ D   vitamin D resistant rickets (hypophosphataemic rickets) – autosomal dominant
○ E   cystinosis – X-linked dominant

267. Minimal change nephrotic syndrome

○ A   has a peak incidence in children under 2 years
○ B   is commonly associated with macroscopic haematuria
○ C   has a male predominance
○ D   is usually associated with low C3
○ E   does not occur in adults

268. Metabolic acidosis occurs in

○ A   pyloric stenosis
○ B   cystinuria
○ C   Bartter's syndrome
○ D   cystinosis
○ E   pseudohypoaldosteronism

nephrology

269. In urinary tract infection (UTI) in children

- O   A   Number of scars is proportional to the number of UTIs
- O   B   Prophylaxis after a single UTI is advisable until the age of 10 years
- O   C   Pseudomonas UTIs are associated with renal stones
- O   D   MCUG is investigation of first choice in a 3-year-old with first UTI
- O   E   Bathing in bubble bath is a useful adjunct to antibiotic prophylaxis

270. In children with haemolytic uraemic syndrome

- O   A   the C3 is usually low
- O   B   mortality is less than 1%
- O   C   thrombocytopenia is common
- O   D   the blood film is usually diagnostic
- O   E   dialysis is required in 50%

271. The following features are characteristic of proximal renal tubular acidosis:

- O   A   metabolic acidosis
- O   B   inability to acidify the urine after an acid load
- O   C   the condition usually occurs in isolation
- O   D   high urinary pH
- O   E   failure of tubular reabsorption of bicarbonate

272. Orthostatic proteinuria

- O   A   is benign
- O   B   is only present when the patient is upright
- O   C   can be large
- O   D   is commonly familial
- O   E   can be precipitated by upper respiratory tract infection

273. In the assessment of haematuria

- ○ A hypercalciuria is a recognised cause
- ○ B a family history of deafness suggests IgA nephropathy
- ○ C co-existent proteinuria makes a renal parenchymal problem more likely
- ○ D renal tract ultrasound is essential
- ○ E measurement of C3 is not usually helpful

274. Causes of hypertension in infancy include

- ○ A a small blood pressure cuff
- ○ B coarctation of the aorta
- ○ C 17-OH progesterone deficiency
- ○ D prazosin
- ○ E hypovolaemia

275. Concerning post-streptococcal glomerulonephritis

- ○ A it is characterised by a low C3 in the acute phase
- ○ B it follows non-haemolytic streptococcal infection in 50% of cases
- ○ C hypertensive encephalopathy is a recognised complication
- ○ D treatment with penicillin reduces the time course of the illness
- ○ E it usually occurs in children under the age of 2 years

276. Concerning undescended testis

- ○ A commoner in premature infants
- ○ B by 12 months 5% remain outside the scrotum
- ○ C orchidopexy can be safely left until the second decade
- ○ D there is an increased risk of infertility
- ○ E there is an increased risk of malignant change

277. The following are associated with an increased risk of Wilms' tumour

○ A   cystinosis
○ B   aniridia
○ C   neurofibromatosis
○ D   tuberous sclerosis
○ E   Beckwith–Wiedemann syndrome

278. Chloride

○ A   is a cation
○ B   serum levels are high in pyloric stenosis
○ C   serum levels are high in renal tubular acidosis
○ D   serum levels may rise if normal saline is infused
○ E   is lost in the stool in chloridorrhoea

279. Recognised causes of hyponatraemia include

○ A   diabetes insipidus
○ B   high solute diet
○ C   inappropriate antidiuretic hormone secretion
○ D   diuretics
○ E   cystic fibrosis

280. Membranous glomerulonephritis

○ A   accounts for 20–40% of adult nephrotic syndrome
○ B   can be associated with hepatitis A infection
○ C   is commoner in males than in females
○ D   is not improved by steroids
○ E   can be secondary to systemic lupus erythematosus

281. Concerning polycystic kidney disease

○ A it is X-linked

○ B it can present in the neonatal period

○ C adult presentation is associated with progression to renal failure in many cases

○ D ultrasound is not a useful investigation

○ E liver involvement with cysts is common

282. Concerning vesico-ureteric reflux

○ A occurs in less than 5% of children who present with a confirmed urinary tract infection

○ B is a risk factor for urinary tract infection

○ C is an indication for prophylactic antibiotics in children under 4 years old

○ D spontaneous remission is common

○ E can be diagnosed using a DMSA scan

283. The following cause hypercalciuria

○ A furosemide

○ B William's syndrome

○ C hypoparathyroidism

○ D distal renal tubular acidosis

○ E vitamin D deficiency

284. Features of Finnish-type congenital nephrotic syndrome include

○ A raised α-fetoprotein antenatally

○ B usually presents between 6 and 12 months

○ C good prognosis

○ D steroids are useful

○ E autosomal recessive inheritance

Best of Five Questions

nephrology

285. A 2-year-old girl is admitted following a short diarrhoeal illness with irritability. Parents have noticed she looks 'puffy' and that she has not passed urine for 24 hours. On examination she is apyrexial but irritable. She has pedal oedema and appears pale. The MOST appropriate initial management is:

- A   Transfusion of packed cells.
- B   Start diuretics and iron supplements.
- C   Start anti-diarrhoeals and arrange out-patient review.
- D   Admit for investigation and fluid balance.
- E   Arrange to start peritoneal dialysis.

286. A 2-week-old baby boy whose mother had no ante-natal care is referred for assessment of failure to thrive. History give few clues but he has a rather poor urine stream. On examination he is scrawny with a pre-auricular tag and has palpable loin masses. The NEXT step should be:

- A   Start antibiotics and arrange review.
- B   Urgent renal ultrasound.
- C   Catheterisation.
- D   Renal biopsy.
- E   Intravenous pyelography.

287. A 5-year-old boy is referred with a 2- week history of general malaise and facial swelling. There is a history of recent travel to the Mediterranean. On examination, he has generalised oedema with shifting dullness on abdominal percussion. There is a grade 2/6 systolic murmur at the left sternal edge. He has 4+ proteinuria with BP of 140/100 mmHg. The BEST initial management is:

- A   Start high-dose prednisolone.
- B   Infusion of human albumin solution.
- C   Blood films for malaria and start parenteral antimalarial treatment.
- D   High-dose oral furosemide.
- E   Dietary review and start high protein diet.

290. **A 4-year-old girl is referred with peri-umbilical pain and urinary frequency for some months. MSUs have been negative. She has regressed behaviourally. Other members of her family have been well. She has a new baby sister who is 6 months old. Examination is normal. The MOST appropriate approach would be:**

○   A   Start antibiotic prophylaxis for possible missed urinary tract infections while arranging a renal isotope scan and cystogram.

○   B.   Arrange a screen of blood tests and abdominal ultrasound.

○   C.   Arrange to be seen jointly with social services on suspicion of abuse.

○   D   Surgical opinion.

○   E   Reassure that this is a normal reaction to new siblings and that no investigation is needed.

Extended Matching Questions

289. Theme: Blood pressure

- A Renal artery stenosis
- B Acute glomerulonephritis
- C Post streptococcal glomerular nephritis
- D Henoch Schönlein purpura
- E Nephrotic syndrome
- F Haemolytic uraemic syndrome
- G Wilm's tumour
- H Renal tubular acidosis
- I Vesico-ureteric reflux with scarring in infancy

Choose the most likely diagnosis from the list above for each of the three scenarios described below. Each option may be used once, more than once or not at all.

1. A 2-year-old boy is admitted with diarrhoea. On examination he is pale with pedal oedema. His blood pressure is 140/100 mmHg and platelet count is 70 x 10⁹/l.

2. A 13-year-old girl complains of headaches since several months. Her blood pressure is 150/110 mmHg. An ultrasound shows bilaterally small kidneys.

3. A 3-year-old with one 'thin arm' since birth presents with intermittent haematuria. On examination he is pale with abdominal mass and hemihypertrophy. His blood pressure is 90/60 mmHg.

290. Theme: Investigations

○ A Micturating cysto-urethrography
○ B MAG 3 scan
○ C DMSA isotope scan
○ D DTPA scan
○ E Renal tract ultrasound
○ F Abdominal computed tomography (CT)
○ G Abdominal magnetic resonance imaging (MRI)
○ H Renal angiography
○ I Renal biopsy
○ J None of the above

Choose the most useful investigation from the list above for each of the three requirements described below. Each option may be used once, more than once or not at all.

1. Assessment of degree of renal scarring.
2. At initial presentation of nephrotic syndrome.
3. Assessment of suspected peri-nephric abscess.

291. Theme: The kidney in systemic disease

○ A Systemic lupus
○ B Juvenile chronic arthritis
○ C Diabetes
○ D Congenital hypothyroidism
○ E Rheumatic fever
○ F Scleroderma
○ G Duchenne's muscular dystrophy
○ H Asthma
○ I Hyperparathyroidism
○ J Amyloidosis

Choose the most likely diagnosis from the list above for each of the three conditions described below. Each option may be used once, more than once or not at all.

1. Renal failure with parotid enlargement.
2. Renal involvement at outset of illness.
3. Microalbuminuria.

NEUROLOGY

Multiple Choice Questions

292. In Sturge–Weber syndrome

sporadic

- O A inheritance is autosomal recessive
- O B the facial naevus is in the distribution of the facial nerve *V th*
- O C incidence is 1 in 5000 *50000*
- O D rail track calcification on the skull X-ray is characteristic
- O E the facial angioma is rarely present at birth

293. Concerning narcolepsy

- ✓ A it typically starts in the teenage years
- ✓ B it is familial
- ✓ C psychiatric problems are common
- ⊗ D rapid eye movement (REM) sleep does not occur
- ⊗ E associated cataplexy is unusual

294. In raised intra-cranial pressure

- ✓O A central syndrome describes herniation of the cerebellar tonsils through the foramen magnum
- ✓O B hyperventilation may occur
- ✓O C Cushing's triad is a late sign
- ✗O D decerebrate precedes decorticate posturing
- ✗O E papilloedema is an early sign

295. Carpal tunnel syndrome

- A is commoner in females
- B is due to entrapment of the ulnar nerve
- C pain is rarely a symptom
- D sensation over the thenar eminence is not affected
- E therapeutic options include diuretics

296. Gilles de la Tourette syndrome

- A is associated with obsessive compulsive disorder
- B learning difficulties are rare
- C symptoms disappear during sleep
- D responds well to treatment with haloperidol
- E may be induced by administration of methylphenidate

297. Nystagmus

- A may be inherited as an X-linked dominant
- B in cerebellar nystagmus the direction of the fast phase is contralateral to the lesion
- C in vestibular nystagmus the direction of the rapid phase is ipsilateral to the lesion
- D may be caused by phenytoin toxicity
- E if vertical suggests cataract is a possible

298. Concerning head injuries

- A they are the leading cause of death in children
- B conscious level should be assessed using the full Glasgow Coma Score in all children
- C raised intra-cranial pressure is less common in infants
- D all children with a Glasgow coma score of less than 9 should be intubated and ventilated
- E analgesia should not be given in order to allow continuous assessment of the patient's neurological status

neurology

299. Concerning Guillain-Barré syndrome

- ○ A implicated infectious agents include Coxsackie virus
- ○ B distal sensory loss may occur
- ○ C reduced reflexes are present
- ○ D weakness is usually asymmetrical
- ○ E autonomic involvement does not occur

300. In spinal muscular atrophy type I (Werdnig–Hoffmann disease)

- ○ A inheritance is usually autosomal recessive
- ○ B the genetic abnormality is localised to chromosome 5
- ○ C the usual presentation is with delayed walking
- ○ D creatinine phosphokinase is always raised
- ○ E survival beyond 3 months is rare

301. Concerning epilepsy

- ○ A in a complex seizure consciousness is lost
- ○ B simple refers to short duration
- ○ C partial seizures begin focally
- ○ D epilepsy that is difficult to control is classified as symptomatic
- ○ E an aura is necessary to make a diagnosis

302. Features of tuberous sclerosis include

- ○ A 50% recurrence risk in offspring
- ○ B adenoma sebaceum
- ○ C hypsarrhythmic change on the electroencephalogram (EEG)
- ○ D good response of seizures to treatment with vigabatrin
- ○ E the frequent occurrence of malignant tumours

303. Concerning cerebral palsy

- ○ A 75% of cases are idiopathic
- ○ B birth weight of less than 1500 g is a risk factor
- ○ C mental retardation occurs in 20%
- ○ D perinatal asphyxia accounts for more than 50%
- ○ E prevalence is 1%

neurology

304. Features of petit mal epilepsy (typical absence epilepsy of childhood) include

○ A   age under 2 years
○ B   characteristic inter-ictal EEG
○ C   good response to carbamazepine
○ D   long-term remission
○ E   long-term risk of tonic-clonic seizures

305. The following are causes of cerebral palsy

○ A   hypothyroidism
○ B   pre-term delivery
○ C   Werdnig–Hoffmann disease
○ D   neonatal meningitis
○ E   congenital cytomegalovirus infection

306. Concerning infantile spasms

○ A   they occur in the first year of life
○ B   EEG findings are non-specific
○ C   the symptomatic group has a worse prognosis
○ D   vigabatrin is frequently used as the drug of first choice
○ E   30% of cases are idiopathic

307. Causes of hypotonia in the infant include

○ A   Becker's muscular dystrophy
○ B   failure to thrive
○ C   subacute sclerosing panencephalitis
○ D   coeliac disease
○ E   Down's syndrome

308. Features of a parietal lobe lesion include

○ A   contralateral homonymous hemianopia
○ B   disinhibition
○ C   grasp reflex
○ D   receptive dysphasia
○ E   apraxia

309. Benign rolandic epilepsy

- ○ A represents less than 1% of childhood epilepsy
- ○ B carries a poor prognosis
- ○ C abnormal inter-ictal EEG
- ○ D nocturnal generalised seizures can occur
- ○ E there is a good response of seizures to sodium valproate

310. Manifestations of a IIIrd nerve palsy include

- ○ A ptosis
- ○ B pupil dilatation
- ○ C blindness
- ○ D diplopia
- ○ E failure of lateral gaze

311. Concerning Friedreich's ataxia

- ○ A the gene locus is known
- ○ B plantars are down going
- ○ C a third of patients develop malignancy
- ○ D onset is usually by the age of 5 years
- ○ E pes cavus is a recognised finding

312. The following conditions are inherited as autosomal dominant

- ○ A tuberous sclerosis
- ○ B ataxia telangiectasia
- ○ C colour blindness
- ○ D haemophilia
- ○ E myotonic dystrophy

313. In Duchenne's muscular dystrophy

- ○ A inheritance is autosomal recessive
- ○ B creatinine phosphokinase is usually elevated
- ○ C muscle biopsy is unhelpful
- ○ D the defect is on chromosome 6
- ○ E cardiac involvement can occur

neurology

314. Risk factors for simple febrile convulsions include

- A age less than 6 months
- B family history of epilepsy
- C family history of febrile convulsions
- D past history of asthma
- E previous febrile convulsion

315. Concerning complex partial seizures (temporal lobe epilepsy)

- A consciousness is impaired
- B ethosuximide is the drug of first choice
- C the EEG shows three per second spikes
- D they can present as drop attacks
- E they are the commonest form of childhood epilepsy

316. Myoclonic jerks are commonly seen in

- A Lennox–Gastaut syndrome
- B Janz syndrome
- C Landau–Kleffner syndrome
- D West's syndrome
- E Gilbert's syndrome

317. The radial nerve

- A supplies the small muscles of the hand
- B nerve root is T1
- C is responsible for elbow extension
- D lesion is called Klumpke's paralysis
- E palsy causes wrist drop

neurology

318. The following statements are true concerning primitive reflexes

○   A   it is normal for the Moro reflex to be present at 8 months of age

○   B   the palmar grasp reflex usually disappears by 3 months of age

○   C   persistence of the asymmetric tonic neck reflex is an early sign of cerebral palsy

○   D   the parachute reflex is present at birth

○   E   the plantar reflex is normally flexor by 4 weeks

319. The following conditions are associated with hydrocephalus

○   A   anaemia

○   B   Klippel–Feil syndrome

○   C   choroid plexus papilloma

○   D   Dandy–Walker malformation

○   E   mucopolysaccharidoses

320. The following conditions are associated with microcephaly

○   A   malnutrition

○   B   holoprosencephaly

○   C   meningitis

○   D   trisomy 13

○   E   thyrotoxicosis

321. Regarding brain tumours

○   A   change in personality can be the presenting feature

○   B   craniopharyngiomas can present with a visual field defect

○   C   metastatic tumours are common in childhood

○   D   oligodendrogliomas are the commonest brain tumours in childhood

○   E   brain tumours are the commonest malignancy in childhood

neurology

322. Concerning neurofibromatosis

- ○   A   acoustic neuromas are present in type 1
- ○   B   maternal folate deficiency is a risk factor
- ○   C   optic nerve gliomas are seen
- ○   D   it is usually associated with intellectual impairment
- ○   E   type 2 is commoner then type 1

323. The following are causes of facial weakness

- ○   A   hypertension
- ○   B   Epstein–Barr virus
- ○   C   Erb's palsy
- ○   D   birth injury
- ○   E   myasthenia gravis

324. Recognised causes of microcephaly include

- ○   A   chickenpox in the third trimester
- ○   B   Dandy–Walker syndrome
- ○   C   myotonia congenita
- ○   D   neurofibromatosis type 1
- ○   E   maternal phenylketonuria

325. Important investigations on admission of a 3-year-old child with a first afebrile tonic-clonic seizure are

- ○   A   computed tomography (CT) head scan
- ○   B   serum calcium
- ○   C   blood culture
- ○   D   urea and electrolytes
- ○   E   EEG

Best of Five Questions

326. Select the MOST appropriate statement regarding craniosynostosis.

○ A   In posterior plagiocephaly due to positional moulding, the ear position is more anterior on the side of the flattening, whereas in that due to synostosis of the lambdoid suture, the ear position is more posterior.

○ B   Secondary craniosynostosis caused by primary failure of brain growth is approximately twice as common as primary craniosynostosis caused by premature suture fusion.

○ C   The major morbidity associated with primary craniosynostosis affecting one or two sutures is raised intracranial pressure.

○ D   Normal skull growth occurs parallel to each suture.

○ E   In order to prevent the need for multiple operative procedures in children with multiple suture craniosynostosis, surgical intervention is best delayed until after 6 months of age.

327. Select the MOST appropriate of the following statements with regard to performing a lumbar puncture.

○ A   A lumbar puncture is always required to confirm the diagnosis of meningococcal meningitis.

○ B   A lumbar puncture can be safely performed in the presence of a Glasgow Coma Scale score of 12 in an adolescent.

○ C   Normal findings on CT or MRI scan of the brain confirm that it is safe to perform a lumbar puncture.

○ D   Abnormal posturing is a contraindication to performing a lumbar puncture.

○ E   Delaying lumbar puncture until after the administration of antibiotics results in negative CSF cultures and should therefore be avoided.

328. The following statements refer to migraine in childhood. Select the MOST appropriate.

○   A   Girls are more commonly affected than boys throughout childhood.

○   B   Pre-school children are not affected.

○   C   They are preceded by auras – most commonly visual.

○   D   When complicated by hemiplegia, the headache precedes the onset of the neurological weakness.

○   E   Propranolol and sodium valproate can be used as prophylaxis.

329. The following statements refer to juvenile myoclonic epilepsy (JME). Select the MOST appropriate.

○   A   Myoclonic jerks, generalised tonic-clonic seizures and absence seizures may all feature.

○   B   Seizure control is usually possible with low-dose anti-convulsant therapy and successful drug withdrawal is possible after a suitable seizure-free interval has been achieved.

○   C   Myoclonic jerks are typically experienced at night.

○   D   Sodium valproate, lamotrigine and carbamazepine can all be used successfully as monotherapy to control seizure activity.

○   E   JME is frequently associated with learning difficulties.

330. A 3-year-old Afro-Caribbean boy develops an acute onset right-sided hemiplegia after a fall. Select the MOST appropriate of the following statements.

○   A   The most likely cause of the hemiplegia is an ischaemic stroke secondary to arterial dissection caused by the fall.

○   B   The boy should be screened for sickle cell disease as this is associated with a significantly increased risk of cerebrovascular events.

○   C   A haemorrhagic event is more likely to be the cause than an ischaemic event.

○   D   Aspirin at a dose of 5mg/kg/day should be commenced if the diagnosis of stroke is confirmed.

○   E   The majority of children suffering from a stroke survive without long-term neurological or cognitive sequelae.

Extended Matching Questions

331. Theme: Hypotonia

○ A Muscle biopsy for congenital myopathy
○ B Serum creatine kinase for Duchenne's muscular dystrophy
○ C Genetic studies for 22q11 deletion
○ D Thyroid function tests
○ E Urine toxicology screen
○ F Plasma very long chain fatty acids
○ G Urinary reducing substances
○ H Chromosomal analysis for Down's syndrome
○ I Genetic studies for cri-du-chat syndrome

Choose the most likely diagnostic investigation from the list above for each of the three cases described below. Each option may be used once, more than once or not at all.

1. A hypotonic baby boy with large anterior fontanelle, hepatomegaly and seizures.
2. A hypotonic female neonate of low birth weight with high pitched cry, microcephaly, round face and full cheeks, heart murmur, epicanthal folds and short fingers.
3. A hypotonic male infant with generalised hyporeflexia and reduced muscle bulk. Mother reports reduced fetal movements in utero.

332. Theme: Meningitis

○ A Group B Streptococcus
○ B *Listeria monocytogenes*
○ C Pneumococcus
○ D *Escherichia coli*
○ E *Haemophilus influenzae* type b
○ F Herpes simplex virus
○ G *Neisseria meningitidis*
○ H *Pseudomonas aeruginosa*
○ I *Staphylococcus epidermidis*
○ J *Mycobacterium tuberculosis*

Choose the most likely infecting organism from the list above for each of the three scenarios described below. Each option may be used once, more than once or not at all.

neurology

1. A 6-week-old baby with fever and irritability has the following lumbar puncture result:
    - appearance – cloudy
    - red cell count – $5/mm^3$
    - white cell count – $1,407/mm^3$ (polymorphs 70%)
    - protein – 1 g/l
    - CSF glucose – 2.1 mmol/l
    - blood glucose – 5.6 mmol/l
    - Gram stain – Gram-negative bacilli.

2. A 5-year-old girl with known sickle cell disease who has had a recent upper respiratory tract infection treated with amoxicillin presents with headache and vomiting. The lumbar puncture result is as follows:
    - appearance – turbid
    - red cell count – $2/mm^3$
    - white cell count – $3,589/mm^3$ (lymphocytes 62%)
    - protein – 0.7 g/l
    - CSF glucose – 2.8 mmol/l
    - blood glucose – 7.4 mmol/l
    - Gram stain – no organisms seen.

3. A 33-week pre-term neonate born 72 hours after rupture of membranes develops seizures on day 5. After stabilisation, a lumbar puncture is performed with the following results:
    - appearance – blood stained
    - red cell count – $137/mm^3$
    - white cell count – $11,247/mm^3$ (lymphocytes 80%)
    - protein – 2.4g/l
    - CSF glucose – 1.8 mmol/l
    - blood glucose – 3.6 mmol/l
    - Gram stain – Gram-positive bacilli.

RESPIRATORY

Multiple Choice Questions

333. The following cause the oxyhaemoglobin dissociation curve to shift to the right

○ A   alkalosis
○ B   high altitude
○ C   the Bohr effect
○ D   increased temperature
○ E   low concentration of 2,3 diphosphoglycerate (2,3 DPG)

334. Lymphocytic interstitial pneumonitis

○ A   has an insidious onset in most cases
○ B   usually presents in the first year of life
○ C   has a mortality greater than 50%
○ D   is due to *Pneumocystis carinii* infection
○ E   responds to oral steroids

335. Clearance of theophylline is increased by

○ A   cirrhosis
○ B   fever
○ C   phenytoin
○ D   cigarette smoking
○ E   erythromycin

336. *Pneumocystis carinii* **pneumonia**

O   A   is a viral infection

O   B   rarely presents under the age of 1 year

O   C   can be treated with high-dose penicillin

O   D   has a high mortality

O   E   can be present with a normal chest X-ray

337. Signs of acute severe asthma include

O   A   pulsus paradoxus > 20 mmHg

O   B   cyanosis

O   C   intercostal recession

O   D   hyperexpanded chest

O   E   pyrexia

338. Pulmonary hypoplasia in the newborn

O   A   can be idiopathic

O   B   is associated with oligohydramnios

O   C   is seen in 1 in 10 000 births

O   D   can be unilateral

O   E   occurs in Potter's syndrome

339. Concerning acute stridor in childhood

O   A   the commonest cause is acute laryngotracheobronchitis

O   B   acute epiglottitis is a rare cause

O   C   antibiotics should be given if the diagnosis is acute laryngotracheobronchitis

O   D   steroids are helpful if bacterial tracheitis is the diagnosis

O   E   nebulised adrenaline can be used even if the diagnosis is not known

respiratatory

340. Concerning bronchiolitis

○ A   most cases are in children under 6 months
○ B   25% of cases are due to respiratory syncytial virus
○ C   antibiotics are indicated in all children under 3 months at presentation
○ D   nebulised ipratropium bromide may be beneficial
○ E   steroids are unhelpful

341. The following are characteristic of type II respiratory failure

○ A   hyperventilation
○ B   hypoxia
○ C   ventilation perfusion mismatch
○ D   raised P_aCO_2
○ E   head injury as a possible cause

342. Concerning laryngomalacia

○ A   it is the most common cause of persistent stridor in infancy
○ B   prognosis is poor
○ C   it is rarely present at birth
○ D   failure to thrive is a common manifestation
○ E   laryngoscopy is indicated in all cases

343. Useful agents taken immediately before exercise to prevent exercise-induced asthma include

○ A   sodium cromoglycate
○ B   salbutamol
○ C   fluticasone propionate
○ D   terbutaline
○ E   salmeterol

respiratatory

344. Rigid bronchoscopy is generally required to

○ A remove a foreign body
○ B exclude a vocal cord palsy
○ C diagnose tuberculosis
○ D assess persistent atelectasis
○ E remove a blood clot

345. Causes of a false-positive sweat test include

○ A ventricular septal defect
○ B adrenal insufficiency
○ C pseudohypoaldosteronism
○ D asthma
○ E chronic renal failure

346. In children with cleft lip and palate the following are true

○ A it is an abnormality of mesodermal development
○ B there are associated abnormalities in more than 75%
○ C micrognathia is common
○ D recurrence risk in siblings is 1 in 25
○ E grommets are usually required

347. Which of the following suggest epiglottitis rather than viral croup

○ A short history
○ B pyrexia
○ C good response to nebulised adrenaline
○ D neck extension
○ E toxaemia

348. The following methods of administration of β-agonists are appropriate in a 4-year-old with chronic asthma

O A nebuliser
O B inhaler with a spacer device
O C turbo haler
O D disc haler
O E oral medication

349. Primary ciliary dyskinesia

O A is an autosomally recessively inherited group of disorders
O B males are usually infertile
O C is a cause of conductive hearing loss
O D is associated with situs inversus in 75%
O E normal life expectancy is possible

350. Concerning cystic fibrosis

O A clubbing is a feature
O B inheritance is autosomal recessive
O C the gene is on chromosome 6
O D males are almost universally infertile
O E meconium ileus is the presenting feature in 50%

351. Cystic fibrosis in children

O A the ΔF 508 mutation is strongly associated with pancreatic disease
O B may present with rectal prolapse
O C the commonest gene defect is due to deletion of phenylalanine at position 508
O D children with pancreatic involvement usually have diabetes mellitus
O E in lung infections *Burkholderia cepacia* is commoner than *Pseudomonas aeruginosa*

respiratory

352. Causes of bronchiectasis include

O   A   cirrhosis
O   B   asthma
O   C   foreign body
O   D   cystic fibrosis
O   E   pneumococcal infection

353. Obstructive sleep apnoea

O   A   is an indication for adenotonsillectomy
O   B   results in episodes of hypoxia
O   C   is a cause of daytime sleepiness
O   D   causes left ventricular hypertrophy
O   E   can present with hypercapnia

354. In *Mycoplasma pneumoniae* infection

O   A   the infection is spread by droplets
O   B   erythromycin is the drug of choice
O   C   cold agglutinins are present in 50%
O   D   culture is easily obtained
O   E   headache at presentation is unusual

355. The following statements are true concerning tonsillitis

O   A   bacterial is commoner than viral infection
O   B   pus on the tonsils is diagnostic of bacterial infection
O   C   agranulocytosis is a recognised differential diagnosis
O   D   post-operative bleeding should be managed with local pressure
O   E   quinsy is an indication for tonsillectomy

356. The following are appropriate in the immediate management of anaphylactic shock

○ A   oral chlorphenamine maleate

○ B   iv hydrocortisone

○ C   nebulised salbutamol

○ D   im adrenaline

○ E   calcium gluconate

357. Concerning pulmonary tuberculosis

○ A   *Mycobacterium tuberculosis* is commonly found in the soil

○ B   it is a notifiable disease

○ C   pleural effusions may occur

○ D   most children develop cavitating lung disease

○ E   a positive Mantoux's test is diagnostic of infection with *Mycobacterium tuberculosis*

358. Which of the following are present in the lung in their adult quota at birth

○ A   alveoli

○ B   goblet cells

○ C   terminal bronchioles

○ D   pulmonary vessels

○ E   acini

359. The peak expiratory flow rate

○ A   is increased in obstructive airways disease

○ B   is effort independent

○ C   is a suitable measurement to attempt on a 3-year-old

○ D   is diagnostic of asthma if the value increases by 20% after administration of bronchodilators

○ E   is influenced by airway diameter

respiratory

Best of Five Questions

360. A 1-year-old child is admitted unwell. The following arterial blood gas is taken on arrival in 10 l/min mask oxygen:

○   A   pH   7.13

○   B P_{CO_2} 4.2 kPa

○   C P_{O_2} 11 kPa

○   D HCO_3 10 mmol/l

○   E   Base excess   −10

361. Which of the following statements BEST describes the use of congenital lobar emphysema:

○   A   Affects the right upper lobe in almost 50% of cases.

○   B   Usually presents with tachypnoea and signs of respiratory distress in the neonatal period.

○   C   Is associated with a cardiac abnormality in less than 5% of cases.

○   D   Should be treated by lobectomy in order to prevent secondary bacterial infection or pneumothorax.

○   E   Is secondary to an intrinsic deficiency of bronchial cartilage.

362. Select the MOST appropriate statement from the following with respect to Monoclonal antibody to respiratory syncytial virus/palivizumab:

○   A   Reduces admission rates to hospital and intensive care units in infants with bronchopulmonary dysplasia (BPD) when compared with placebo.

○   B   Is effective in preventing respiratory syncytial virus infection if given to babies with congenital heart disease.

○   C   Is licensed for children aged less than 2 years who are born at less than 35 weeks gestation.

○   D   Can be administered annually to protect the at risk infant throughout the respiratory syncytial virus season.

○   E   Can be administered as an alternative to ribavirin to reduce the duration of mechanical ventilation for the treatment of babies with BPD and known respiratory syncytial virus infection.

363. Which of the following statements about whooping cough is MOST true?

O A It is caused by infection with the Gram-positive bacillus *Bordetella pertussis*.

O B Immunisation has controlled the spread of disease in the developed world and it is no longer a public health concern.

O C The initial catarrhal phase is indistinguishable from common upper respiratory tract infections.

O D During the paroxysmal stage, patients have evidence of lower respiratory tract disease on examination.

O E Macrolide antibiotics are helpful in altering the clinical course and should be given at whatever stage in the illness the patient is at when the diagnosis is made.

364. A nine-year-old boy presents to accident and emergency with a 3-day history of cough and fever. On examination his respiratory rate is 20/min and oxygen saturations 97% in air. There is no evidence of dehydration. He has coarse crackles at the right base. He has a lobar pneumonia on chest X-ray. The MOST appropriate treatment would be:

O A Admission for broad spectrum intravenous antibiotics for 48 hours or until the fever settles.

O B Supportive treatment only as the most likely causative agent is viral.

O C Treatment with a macrolide antibiotic orally with a follow-up chest X-ray in 6–8 weeks.

O D Treatment with oral amoxicillin with a follow-up clinic appointment in 6–8 weeks.

O E Chest physiotherapy used in conjunction with antimicrobial therapy.

respiratory

365. **A 5-year-old boy with asthma is having frequent exercise induced and nocturnal symptoms despite good compliance with his current prescribed regimen of inhaled steroids (fluticasone 125 μg bd) and long-acting β-agonist (salmeterol 50 μg bd) taken via large volume spacer. The MOST appropriate alteration to his therapy would be:**

○   A   Change inhaled steroids to budesonide 200 μg bd.

○   B   Add montelukast at a dose of 4 mg od.

○   C   Change to dry powder device as drug delivery will be improved.

○   D   Advise administration of short acting bronchodilator prior to exercise.

○   E   Increase dose of inhaled fluticasone to 250 μg bd.

respiratory

Extended Matching Questions

366. Theme: Respiratory diseases

- ○ A Bronchiolitis obliterans
- ○ B α_1 antitrypsin deficiency
- ○ C Tracheo-oesophageal fistula
- ○ D Cystic fibrosis
- ○ E Pulmonary haemosiderosis
- ○ F Bronchomalacia
- ○ G Lobar sequestration
- ○ H Cystic adenomatoid malformation
- ○ I Asthma

Choose the most likely diagnosis from the list above for each of the three scenarios described below. Each option may be used once, more than once or not at all.

1. A 10-month-old child with a history of progressive tachypnoea, cough and wheeze and faltering growth is found to have patchy perihilar changes on chest X-ray. He is jaundiced with hepatosplenomegaly. He has a microcytic anaemia and his stools are positive for faecal occult bloods.

2. A previously well 3-year-old girl is seen in the outpatient clinic with a history of dry cough and being generally run down for the last 4 months. Mum reports that she appears more breathless on exertion than previously. Symptoms appeared to develop after a flu-like illness. Inhaled steroids (fluticasone 125 µg twice daily) have had no effect on symptoms. She has an elevated respiratory rate at rest. Chest X-ray shows hyperinflation with some patchy lower lobe infiltrates bilaterally.

3. A 10-year-old boy is seen in clinic for follow up 2 months after a recent admission to hospital with a left-sided pneumonia. Parents report that he is now back to normal but they are concerned as in the last few years he has required a number of courses of antibiotics from the GP for recurrent episodes of chest infection. A follow up chest X-ray shows persisting shadowing in the left lower zone. The results of a sweat test performed the week prior to clinic are sweat chloride 43 mmol/l with a sweat weight of 147 mg.

respiratory

367. Theme: Management of acute respiratory illness

○   A   Intravenous cefotaxime

○   B   Nebulised adrenaline

○   C   Oral erythromycin

○   D   Intravenous hydrocortisone

○   E   Supportive treatment only

○   F   Oral dexamethasone

○   G   Intravenous benzyl penicillin

○   H   Regular nebulised salbutamol

Choose the most appropriate initial treatment from the list above for each of the three scenarios described below. Each option may be used once, more than once or not at all.

1. A 3-year-old girl whose family have recently arrived in the UK seeking asylum presents to accident and emergency with stridor. You are unable to take a history as the family cannot speak English. On examination, she is febrile (38 °C), quiet, drooling, pale and has poorly perfused peripheries with oxygen saturations of 92% in air. She is tachypnoeic (respiratory rate 50/min) and has a continuous soft stridor with evidence of tracheal tug and intercostal recession.

2. A 4-month-old baby (who was born at 32 weeks gestation) is admitted to the paediatric ward on Christmas Day with a 3-day history of being off feeds, snuffly and coughing. On examination he has a temperature of 37.5 °C and oxygen saturations in air of 89%, with marked subcostal recession and respiratory rate of 60/min. He has fine inspiratory crackles bilaterally with diffuse wheeze.

3. A 7-year-old boy who has been previously fit and well is seen on the paediatric assessment unit with a 5-day history of being generally unwell. He has had a wheezy cough and intermittent headache helped by paracetamol. Examination reveals that his oxygen saturations are 97% in air with no evidence of increased work of breathing. His right tympanic membrane is moderately inflamed. He has occasional wheeze and crackles mainly on the right and his chest X-ray shows patchy interstitial shadowing on this side.

respiratory

answers and subject summaries

CARDIOLOGY ANSWERS

1.   Aortic Stenosis

Answer: E

Aortic valve stenosis

This accounts for 5% of congenital heart defects. It is commoner in males.

Associations of aortic stenosis:

- Turner's syndrome
- William's syndrome
- coarctation of the aorta
- other cardiac abnormalities, eg hypoplastic left ventricle, mitral valve abnormalities.

The stenosis can be either supravalvular, valvular or subvalvular. There is often an associated bicuspid valve. Aortic stenosis is usually asymptomatic but in its most severe form can cause congestive cardiac failure, arrhythmias and sudden death in infancy (rare). The murmur is best heard in the aortic area and radiates to the neck. An ejection click suggests valvular stenosis. A palpable thrill is usually present in the suprasternal notch. Although left ventricular hypertrophy is common the electrocardiogram (ECG) can be normal.

Assessment of severity:

- symptoms – angina-like pain
  - syncope/dizziness on exertion
  - palpitations on exertion
- ECG evidence of left ventricular strain
- exercise test positive
- ST and T wave changes on the ECG during exercise.

Treatment:

Treatment is conservative in most cases avoiding valve replacement in the young patient. If the gradient across the valve is greater than 60 mmHg treatment is indicated. This is usually in the form of a balloon valvoplasty at cardiac catheter, or surgical valvuloplasty.

2.　William's syndrome

Answers: B C

William's syndrome is a neurodevelopmental disorder. It is caused by a micro-deletion on chromosome 7. Diagnosis can be confirmed by FISH studies.

Features:

- characteristic elfin facies
- characteristic affect – over-friendly with better verbal than visuospatial skills
- behavioural problems with poor concentration and distractibility
- normal birth weight with post-natal growth retardation secondary to poor feeding (failure to thrive)
- neurodevelopmental delay with delayed motor milestone and IQ in the 50–60s
- idiopathic hypercalcaemia – resolves at age 2 years. Management is with low calcium and vitamin D intake. Aetiology unknown.
- hypercalciuria
- squints
- hernia
- rectal prolapse
- cardiovascular abnormalities (75%)
  - supra-valvular aortic stenosis
  - peripheral pulmonary artery stenosis
  - others including valvular and septal defects have been reported
  - hypertension.

3.　Right-to-left shunt

Answers: A B D

Causes of a right-to-left shunt in the neonatal period include:

- normal heart
- persistent pulmonary hypertension
- transient myocardial ischaemia
- abnormal heart
- transposition of the great arteries
- tetralogy of Fallot
- pulmonary atresia with an intact ventricular septum
- pulmonary stenosis
- tricuspid atresia
- Ebstein's anomaly
- truncus arteriosus.

4.   Neonatal cyanosis

Answers: D E

The hyperoxia test is used to help differentiate between cardiac and non-cardiac causes of cyanosis. Cyanosis is indicative of more than 5 g/dl of haemoglobin being in the reduced state. The test is performed as follows: once cyanosis is confirmed by either an arterial blood gas or pulse oximetry the infant is given 100% oxygen to inspire. The baby with a respiratory cause for cyanosis will generally show a good increment ($P_a(O_2)$ > 20 kPa) whereas the infant with cyanotic congenital heart disease and a right-to-left shunt will not. There are some exceptions to this including total anomalous pulmonary venous drainage (due to pulmonary oedema) in which a moderate but not complete response to the hyperoxia test will be seen.

Acrocyanosis is peripheral cyanosis of the hands, feet and occasionally trunk. It is very common in the first 24 hours of life. If a duct-dependent cardiac lesion is suspected then a prostaglandin infusion should be started which prolongs patency of the ductus arteriosus pending transfer to a cardiac unit. Side-effects of prostaglandin include apnoea and therefore the child needs to be ventilated.

Differential diagnosis of cyanosis in the newborn:

- cardiac causes
- respiratory disease
- central nervous system depression
- methaemoglobinaemia.

Methaemoglobinaemia

The iron of both oxygenated and deoxygenated blood is normally in the ferrous state — this is essential for its oxygen-transporting function. Oxidation of the haemoglobin iron to the ferric state yields methaemoglobin. Methaemoglobin is non-functional and in sufficient quantities can cause cyanosis. It imparts a brown colour to the blood. Methaemoglobinaemia can be hereditary or acquired. Acquired methaemoglobinaemia occurs secondary to ingestion of substances that oxidise haemoglobin including dapsone, chloroquine and nitrites. Treatment is with ascorbic acid and methylene blue.

5.   Down's syndrome

Answers: B D

Cardiac lesions in Down's syndrome

Cardiac lesions are present in 30–50% of children with Down's syndrome. Of these defects, 30% are atrio-ventricular septal defects (AVSDs) and 30% are isolated ventricular septal defects (VSDs). Other cardiac lesions commonly seen include tetralogy of Fallot and PDA. Of all children with an AVSD, 25% have Down's syndrome. All children with Down's syndrome should have an echocardiogram.

Pulmonary vascular disease in children with Down's syndrome

There is an increased incidence of pulmonary vascular disease in children with Down's syndrome. The principal aetiology is cardiac (increased pulmonary flow). Other contributing factors include upper airway obstruction (laryngomalacia and adenotonsillar hypertrophy) and an increased incidence of intrinsic lung disease.

Atrio-ventricular septal defect

AVSD can be classified as partial or complete. In the partial form an ostium primum ASD is present with or without a cleft in the mitral valve. In the complete form there is a common atrio-ventricular valve with clefts in both the pulmonary and mitral valves.

6.   Transposition of the great arteries

Answers: A B D E

Transposition of the great arteries (TGA) represents about 6% of all congenital heart disease. It is the commonest cause of cyanotic congenital heart disease in the neonatal period. It is commoner in males than females.

In TGA the aorta arises from the right ventricle and carries deoxygenated blood to the body, and the pulmonary artery arises from the left ventricle and carries oxygenated blood to the lung. A lesion that mixes the two circulations is essential for survival (examples include PDA, ASVD, VSD). The child is usually cyanotic from or shortly after birth. The lesion is duct dependent and the infant's condition deteriorates when the duct closes. There is usually a metabolic acidosis at presentation. Arrhythmias of all types are common. ECG shows a right-sided axis and right ventricular hypertrophy. The chest X-ray shows cardiomegaly and increased pulmonary vascularity.

Surgical management of TGA

- palliative – atrial septostomy
- physiological repair (permanent palliation) – Mustard, Senning
- anatomical:
    - Jatene arterial switch (corrective)
    - Rastelli conduit (needs replacement).

7. Tetralogy of Fallot

Answers: B E

This accounts for 10% of congenital heart disease.

Components of tetralogy of Fallot:

- ventricular septal defect
- right ventricular outflow obstruction
- right ventricular hypertrophy
- over-riding aorta

The severity of the right ventricular outflow obstruction will determine the clinical picture.

- Mild obstruction – pink Fallot's – left-to-right shunt across the VDS – murmur ejection systolic (pulmonary stenosis) – cyanotic later as the shunt reverses.
- Moderate obstruction – presents with cyanosis – right-to-left shunt across VSD – murmur is ejection systolic due to pulmonary stenosis, VSD silent.
- Severe obstruction – duct dependent, presenting with cyanosis in the neonatal period.

ECG shows right ventricular hypertrophy and right axis deviation in cyanotic Fallot's. The ECG in acyanotic Fallot's shows right ventricular hypertrophy because the right ventricular pressure is high. Cyanotic spells usually begin around 4–6 months of age. They are due to functional infundibular spasm and potentially fatal. Features include worsening cyanosis and a reduction in the intensity of the murmur.

Treatment of cyanotic spells:

- bring baby's knees to chest (reduces venous return)
- β-blockers
- morphine
- sodium bicarbonate if acidotic
- vasoconstrictors

Surgical management of Fallot's is either palliative (systemic-to-pulmonary shunt) or complete. Total correction, if technically possible, is the preferred option. This is usually done at around 6 months.

Complications of Fallot's:

- polycythaemia
- subacute bacterial endocarditis
- cerebral abscess, cerebral thrombosis
- retardation of growth and development
- clubbing – usually appears after 1 year of age.

cardiology

8. Neonatal cyanosis

Answers: B C D E

Eisenmenger's syndrome is an acquired defect secondary to pulmonary hypertension. Cyanosis occurs in the hypoplastic left heart syndrome secondary to circulatory failure and worsens when the duct closes. Severe (critical) aortic stenosis can present in the neonatal period with cyanosis by the same mechanism.

Cardiac conditions presenting with neonatal cyanosis:

- decreased pulmonary flow
  - pulmonary atresia
  - Fallot's tetralogy
  - Ebstein's anomaly.
- increased pulmonary flow
  - hypoplastic left heart
  - tricuspid atresia
  - truncus arteriosus
  - total anomalous pulmonary venous drainage
  - double outlet ventricle
  - single ventricle
  - poor mixing
  - transposition of the great arteries.

9. Paediatric ECGs

Answers: A B C E

Mean QRS

- At birth – 125 degrees
- 1 month – 90 degrees
- 3 years – 50 degrees.

The right axis deviation seen in newborns is due to right ventricular dominance in the fetus. Right ventricular deviation in older children implies right ventricular hypertrophy. Left axis deviation (superior axis) in the neonatal period is seen in the following cardiac lesions:

- tricuspid atresia
- ASVD
- pulmonary stenosis.

Right bundle branch block

Right bundle branch block is the commonest conduction disturbance seen in children. The abnormality is usually due to right ventricular overload prolonging right ventricular depolarisation due to lengthening of the conduction pathway.

Criteria for right bundle branch block:

- prolonged QRS
- right axis deviation
- terminal slurring of the QRS over the right ventricular leads V3R, V4R and V1
- ST depression and T wave inversion is commonly seen in adults but rarely in children.

Causes of right bundle branch block:

- ASVD
- Ebstein's anomaly
- coarctation of the aorta (infants)
- endocardial cushion defects
- post right ventriculotomy
- partial anomalous pulmonary venous drainage
- normal variant.

Congenital heart block

Congenital complete heart block (ie complete atrioventricular dissociation) occurs in infants of mothers with systemic lupus erythematosus, particularly those with anti-Ro (SS-A) and anti La (SS-B) antibodies. The damage to the conduction pathway is irreversible. Antenatal diagnosis is possible because of persistent fetal bradycardia; 50% have an associated structural defect, usually congenitally corrected transposition. The condition is usually well tolerated and often does not require a pacemaker.

Heart rate

Heart rate varies with the age and status of the patient. A rate of 110–150 is normal in the newborn and the adult rate of 60–100 is achieved by the age of 6 years.

cardiology

10. Chest X-rays

Answers: C D E

Coeur en sabot (heart in a boot)

This is seen in tetralogy of Fallot and is due to hypoplasia of the main pulmonary artery and the consequent up turning of the apex away from the diaphragm. A right-sided aortic arch is seen in 25%.

Rib notching

This is a feature of coarctation of the aorta and occurs as a consequence of the increase in size of the intercostal vessels which function as collaterals. The upper two or three ribs are spared because their posterior intercostal arteries do not arise from the aorta. Rib notching is rarely seen in children under the age of 5 years.

Other chest X-ray changes of coarctation

- Dilation of the ascending aorta, descending aorta (post stenotic dilatation)
- Cardiomegaly
- Increased pulmonary vascular shadowing

Truncus arteriosus

The features on chest X-ray include a right-sided aortic arch, absent thymus (30% of cases have DiGeorge syndrome), cardiomegaly, and a prominent ascending aorta.

Total anomalous pulmonary venous drainage

There are two types:

- unobstructed – cardiomegaly, increased pulmonary vascular markings
- obstructed – normal heart size, increased pulmonary vascular markings (severe pulmonary oedema).

The lesion may be supra-cardiac, cardiac, infra-cardiac or mixed. Obstructed lesions are usually infra-cardiac. In the supra-cardiac unobstructed total anomalous pulmonary venous drainage, dilation of the left and right superior vena cava and the left innominate vein give rise to a 'cottage loaf' or 'snowman' appearance on chest X-ray.

Scimitar syndrome

This is a form of partial anomalous pulmonary venous drainage whereby the veins from the right lung drain directly into the inferior vena cava. The right lung is hypoplastic as a consequence and this allows movement of the heart to the right. The single vein draining the right lung produces a scimitar shape on the PA chest X-ray as it heads towards the right cardio-diaphragmatic angle.

11. Conditions associated with an increased risk of heart disease

Answers: A B C D

Kawasaki's disease

The cardiac lesions appear in the second week of the illness as proximal coronary artery aneurysms healing by fibrosis and thrombosis. Lesions are most common on the left side. Protection is offered by the early administration of intravenous immunoglobulin. Other cardiac lesions can occur including aortic and mitral regurgitation, myocarditis, pericarditis, pericardial effusion and myocardial infarction.

Congenital rubella

Infection with rubella during the first trimester causes the classic triad of deafness, cataracts and cardiac anomalies. Cardiac defects include peripheral pulmonary artery stenosis, PDA and septal defects. Other abnormalities seen in the congenital rubella syndrome include microcephaly, microphthalmia, intra-uterine growth retardation, hepatitis and neonatal thrombocytopenia.

Marfan's syndrome
- Mitral valve prolapse
- Dilation/dissection of the ascending aorta
- Aortic regurgitation
- Pulmonary artery aneurysm
- Mitral valve regurgitation

Turner's syndrome

The commonest cardiac lesion is coarctation of the aorta (15–30%). Other cardiac lesions seen include aortic stenosis, ASVD, and bicuspid aortic valves. Hypertension is not uncommon. Lesions commonly seen in Noonan's syndrome include pulmonary stenosis and obstructive cardiomyopathy. For examination purposes it is worth remembering that in Noonan's syndrome right-sided heart lesions are seen and in Turner's syndrome left-sided heart lesions are seen.

There is no increase in the incidence of congenital heart disease in petit mal epilepsy.

12.   Congenital heart disease

Answers: C E

The commonest congenital heart disease is a VSD. The lung fields are oligaemic in tetralogy of Fallot.

Blalock–Taussig shunt

This is an anastomosis between the subclavian artery and the pulmonary artery and is used for palliation of tetralogy of Fallot. The murmur is continuous. Continuous murmurs characteristically pass through the second heart sound into diastole.

Ebstein's anomaly

This is displacement of the septal and posterior leaflets of the tricuspid valve causing atrialisation of part of the right ventricle. In severe cases, children can present with cyanosis and cardiac failure. Arrhythmias are common including Wolff–Parkinson–White. Lithium during pregnancy is a risk factor.

Nitric and not nitrous oxide is used to treat persistent pulmonary hypertension.

Causes of plethoric lung fields

Acyanotic:

- ASVD
- VSD
- PDA
- endocardial cushion defect
- partial anomalous pulmonary venous drainage.

Cyanotic:

- single ventricle
- truncus arteriosus
- hypoplastic left heart
- transposition of the great arteries
- total anomalous pulmonary venous drainage.

Causes of continuous murmurs

- Blalock–Taussig shunt
- AV malformation
- aneurysm
- collateral vessels
- PDA
- venous hum
- peripheral pulmonary stenosis.

cardiology

13. Atrial septal defects

Answers: A B E

Isolated atrial septal defects (ASDs) account for 8% of congenital heart disease. The defect is commoner in females and there are three types:

- ostium secundum (commonest)
- ostium primum
- sinus venosus.

Ostium secundum defects are usually asymptomatic with pulmonary hypertension and right ventricular failure occurring in the third and fourth decades. Atrial arrhythmias occur in adulthood but are rare in childhood. Antibacterial prophylaxis is unnecessary for a secundum ASD. An ostium primum defect is likely to present earlier usually as a component of an endocardial cushion defect and requires antibiotic prophylaxis.

ECG appearance of atrial septal defects:

- ostium primum – right bundle branch block, left axis deviation
- ostium secundum – right bundle branch block, right axis deviation.

The presence of right bundle branch block is not diagnostic but its absence makes the diagnosis unlikely. A high proportion of ostium secundum ASDs close spontaneously by the age of 5 years. The risk of pulmonary hypertension and its sequelae increases with shunt size. Surgical repair is indicated if the pulmonary-to-systemic flow ratio is greater than 2:1. High pulmonary vascular resistance is a contraindication to surgery.

Fixed splitting of the second heart sound is characteristic of an ASD. This is due to the defect producing a constantly increased right ventricular volume and prolonging ejection time. The murmur of an ASD is not due to flow across the defect but due to increased flow across the pulmonary valve as a consequence the shunt.

cardiology

14. Ventricular septal defects

Answer: D

VSDs are the commonest congenital heart defect. The defect can occur in the membranous or muscular part of the septum. Defects in the membranous septum are more common and are usually single. Defects in the muscular part of the septum are usually multiple. The signs and symptoms depend on the haemodynamics of the defect, which is dependent on the size of the defect and the pulmonary vascular resistance. With a small defect, the murmur is rarely present at birth but appears as the pulmonary vascular resistance falls.

Untreated, a large shunt will result in high pulmonary flow and can progress to pulmonary hypertension and the Eisenmenger's syndrome. The second heart sound is loud if pulmonary hypertension is present. Infective endocarditis occurs in less than 2% of cases. It is the left and not the right ventricle that is volume overloaded. The shunt occurs mainly during systole when the right ventricle is contracting, and so the shunted blood enters the pulmonary circulation. The right atrium contains deoxygenated blood, the right ventricle contains deoxygenated blood from the right atrium and oxygenated blood from the left ventricle. At cardiac catheterisation, the oxygen content of blood in the right ventricle is greater than that in the right atrium. 30–60% close spontaneously in the first 6 months and many more subsequent to that. Surgery is required if the left-to-right shunt is such (usually quoted as > 2:1) that pulmonary hypertension has or is likely to develop.

15. Eisenmenger's syndrome

Answers: B D E

Eisenmenger's syndrome is pulmonary hypertension at a systemic level due to fixed elevation of pulmonary vascular resistance (ie pulmonary vascular disease) with a reversed or bi-directional shunt at the atrial, ventricular or aorto-pulmonary level. Cardiac defects associated with the development of Eisenmenger's syndrome include any cause of increased pulmonary artery flow with increased pulmonary artery pressure:

- VSD
- AVSD
- PDA
- aorto-pulmonary window
- total anomalous pulmonary venous drainage
- truncus arteriosus
- endocardial cushion defects
- double outlet right ventricle
- transposition of the great arteries with a VSD.

Symptoms of pulmonary vascular disease do not usually develop until the second or third decade. The following are risk factors for the earlier development of pulmonary hypertension:

- cardiac defect with large shunt
- perinatal asphyxia
- recurrent chest infections
- chronic upper airway obstruction
- Down's syndrome
- birth at or living at high altitude.

Symptoms and signs of Eisenmenger's syndrome:

- dyspnoea
- syncope
- haemoptysis
- arrhythmias
- clubbing
- raised jugular venous pressure
- right ventricular heave
- loud P2.

Heart-lung transplant is the only surgical option. Cardiac abnormalities presenting with cyanosis and reduced pulmonary flow are protected from the development of pulmonary vascular disease – pulmonary atresia, pulmonary stenosis, tetralogy of Fallot. Pulmonary valve stenosis is associated with:

- Noonan's syndrome
- trisomy 18
- fetal valproate syndrome
- maternal rubella
- neurofibromatosis
- LEOPARD syndrome
- William's syndrome

Critical/severe pulmonary stenosis presents in the neonatal period with cyanosis and right-sided heart failure which worsens with duct closure. Arrhythmias are common. Management is difficult and has high morbidity and mortality. The treatment of choice is stabilisation with prostaglandins followed by balloon dilatation or surgery.

16.   Patent ductus arteriosus

Answers: A B E

This accounts for 5–10% of congenital heart defects excluding extremely pre-term infants. It is present in 40–50% of pre-term infants whose birth weight is less than 1750 g, 30% of which have a significant ductus with congestive cardiac failure. The reason for the higher incidence in pre-term infants is that the responsiveness of ductal smooth muscle is gestation dependent. In term infants functional closure occurs within 10–15 hours of birth with complete anatomical closure by 2–3 weeks of age.

Presentation of PDA in the pre-term infant:

- cardiac failure
- apnoea
- increased ventilatory requirements.

Presentation of PDA in the term infant:

- small shunt:
  - asymptomatic
- large shunt:
  - poor weight gain
  - tachypnoea
  - tachycardia
  - cardiac murmur.

Findings on examination:

- continuous machinery murmur
- full pulses
- loud P2.

In the preterm infant the murmur may be limited to systole.

Management of PDA

In the pre-term infant this is dependent upon symptoms. Spontaneous closure is likely if the duct is asymptomatic. In symptomatic infants the management is fluid restriction, diuretics, maintenance of normal haemoglobin, indometacin and surgical ligation. In the term infant indometacin is not helpful and the principal therapeutic option is surgery with a catheter closure of the duct being performed between 6 months and 2 years of age. Spontaneous closure is not likely in term infants (persistence of the duct for 3 months:PDA).

17.   Fetal circulation

Answer: None correct

Oxygenated blood from the placenta returns to the fetus via the umbilical vein: 50% enters the hepatic circulation and 50% bypasses the liver via the ductus venosus. Most of the inferior caval blood as it enters the right atrium is directed through the foramen ovale into the left atrium. The right atrium contains blood from the superior vena cava, coronary sinus and some from the inferior vena cava. Right atrial blood enters the right ventricle, and 85% of right ventricular blood passes into the descending aorta via the ductus arteriosus and 15% enters the fetal lungs.

Changes in the fetal circulation occur at birth. The ductus venosus closes and loss of the low resistance placenta results in an increase in systemic vascular resistance. There is a functional closure of the foramen ovale. Lung expansion results in a fall in pulmonary vascular resistance, increased pulmonary blood flow and increased delivery of blood to the left atrium. Flow through the ductus arteriosus changes from the pulmonary to systemic to the systemic to pulmonary circulation. The high concentration of oxygen in the blood causes smooth muscle contraction of the duct and closure.

18.   Congenital heart disease

Answers: C E

Poor growth (height and weight) is common in children with cyanotic congenital heart disease. Catch-up growth after corrective surgery is common. The contraindications to immunisation are as for the normal population. The oral contraceptive pill is contraindicated in girls with cyanotic congenital heart disease due to the risk of thrombosis. The coil is also contraindicated as it is a potential focus of infection predisposing to endocarditis. A chromosomal abnormality is present in 6–10% of children with congenital heart disease and 30% of newborn infants with chromosomal abnormalities have heart defects.

19.   Coarctation of the aorta

Answers: A C E

This accounts for 10% of congenital heart disease. It is commoner in males (2:1). Associated cardiac anomalies include:

- bicuspid aortic valve (70%)
- mitral valve disease
- sub-aortic stenosis
- VSD.

cardiology

The coarctation is usually just after the origin of the left subclavian artery (98%) at the level of the ductus arteriosus. It can occur proximal to the origin of the left subclavian artery in which case the blood pressure in the right arm will be higher than in the left arm; the classic discrepancy being between the upper and lower limb blood pressure. The murmur of coarctation is systolic. Continuous murmurs are occasionally heard from collaterals. Up to 10% of children with coarctation have berry aneurysms in the cerebral circulation. Rib notching does not appear until late childhood. Treatment is surgical by either balloon dilatation, graft or a subclavian flap. This is usually carried out soon after diagnosis.

Associations of coarctation of the aorta:

- trisomy 13
- trisomy 18
- Turner's syndrome
- valproate toxicity.

20. Teratogens

Answers: A B D E

The following are teratogens for the defects shown:

Alcohol	ASD, VSD, PDA, TGA
Amphetamines	ASD, VSD, PDA, TGA
Lithium	Ebstein's anomaly
Oestrogens/progesterones	VSD, TGA, Fallot's
Phenytoin	Pulmonary stenosis, aortic stenosis, PDA, coarctation, ASD, VSD
Thalidomide	Fallot's, truncus arteriosus
Sodium valproate	TOF, VSD
Warfarin	Fallot's, VSD

Maternal diseases linked to an increased risk of congenital heart disease include:

- diabetes – transposition, septal defects, coarctation, transient cardiomyopathy
- phenylketonuria – tetralogy of Fallot
- SLE – congenital heart block.

21. Hypertension

Answer: None correct

Childhood hypertension is defined as systolic or diastolic blood pressure greater then the 95th centile for age, recorded on three separate occasions. There are two types: primary (aetiology unknown) and secondary (aetiology known). Secondary hypertension is commoner in infants and younger children. Primary hypertension is commoner than secondary hypertension in adolescents and young adults when there is often a family history. Children with primary hypertension are rarely symptomatic. Obesity is associated with primary hypertension, and in 70–80% of children with secondary hypertension there is a renal cause. Initial investigations are aimed at detecting renal parenchymal disease.

22. Circulatory failure in the first week of life

Answers: A B C D E

Cardiac causes:

- critical aortic stenosis
- hypoplastic left heart
- coarctation
- myocardial ischaemia (hypoxic ischaemic encephalopathy, hypoglycaemia)
- severe anaemia
- cardiomyopathy
- arrhythmia
- arteriovenous fistula
- obstructed pulmonary venous drainage
- TGA with VSD

By the end of the first week when pulmonary vascular resistance falls left-to-right shunts become an important cause of heart failure including VSD, PDA, AVSD and truncus arteriosus. Non-cardiac causes of heart failure such as sepsis and fluid overload need to be considered.

23. Infective endocarditis

Answer: None correct

The commonest organism is *Streptococcus viridans*. Other causative micro-organisms include *Staphylococcus aureus* and *Enterococcus*. The infected lesions are usually left sided (apart from those in intravenous drug abusers). Most patients who develop infective endocarditis have either congenital or acquired heart defects. With the exception of an ostium secundum AVSD, all congenital heart defects increase the risk of endocarditis. The commonest source of the bacteria is the teeth. Good dental hygiene and antibiotic prophylaxis for dental procedures is essential.

The clinical manifestations are often difficult and non-specific. More than 80% have a fever; 50% have skin manifestations which include petechiae, Osler's nodes and splinter haemorrhages; and 50% have embolic phenomena. Haematuria is common. Finger clubbing may occur in chronic cases. A murmur is universal — either a new murmur or the change in character of an existing murmur. Diagnosis is on clinical suspicion, positive blood culture (which may need to be done repeatedly — three blood cultures have a 95% pick-up rate) and by the demonstration of valvular vegetations on echocardiography. Treatment is with long-term antibiotics. Surgery is occasionally required.

24. Cardiomyopathy

Answers: A B

Hypertrophic

Sixty per cent of cases of hypertrophic cardiomyopathy are inherited as an autosomal dominant. Of these, 50% are due to mutations of the β-cardiac myosin heavy chain genes. These cases can be detected using polymerase chain reaction prior to the onset of symptoms. Infants of diabetic mothers and infants on steroids for chronic lung disease experience a transient form. Sudden death occurs in 4–6% of affected children per year.

Dilated

Idiopathic/multifactorial is the commonest form. There is an X-linked type that presents in adolescence. The commonest cause is idiopathic (probably post viral). Other causes include doxorubicin toxicity, phaeochromocytoma, mitochondrial disease and carnitine deficiency.

Restrictive

This is rare in childhood. Associations include sarcoidosis, amyloidosis, haemochromatosis, Fabry's disease and Loeffler's syndrome.

Endocardial fibroelastosis

This is a form of dilated cardiomyopathy. Usually only the left side of the heart is affected. There are both hereditary and non-hereditary forms. This is rare in childhood.

Infants of diabetic mothers have a three times greater risk of congenital heart disease than the rest of the population. Defects seen include VSD, transposition, coarctation, persistent pulmonary hypertension and reversible hypertrophic cardiomyopathy.

25. Rheumatic fever

Answers: A B

Rheumatic fever develops secondary to infection with group A β-haemolytic *Streptococcus*. It is commoner in lower socio-economic classes and the peak incidence is between the ages of 5 and 15. Rheumatic fever is diagnosed by the Duckett-Jones criteria.

Major criteria:

- carditis – 50%
- chorea – 15%
- polyarthritis – 70%
- erythema marginatum – 10%
- subcutaneous nodules – 1%

Minor criteria

- arthralgia
- fever
- prolonged PR interval
- raised erythrocyte sedimentation rate (ESR), C-reactive protein (CRP)

Diagnosis is dependent on two major or one major and two minor criteria being present and there being evidence of recent streptococcal infection (raised ASO titres, anti-deoxyribonuclease B). The exceptions are:

- chorea – if no other cause is identifiable then chorea by itself is diagnostic
- insidious/late onset carditis with no other explanation
- rheumatic recurrence – the presence of one major or one minor criterion with evidence of prior streptococcal infection suggests recurrence.

Pancarditis occurs in 50%. Consequences of this include heart block, tachycardia, cardiomegaly, congestive cardiac failure and valve disease. It is only the carditis that produces sequelae which include mitral regurgitation, mitral stenosis, aortic regurgitation and tricuspid regurgitation. Aspirin is indicated in the acute phase, initially at 120 mg/kg for 14 days and then 70 mg/kg until the fever settles. Prednisolone is indicated in severe carditis. Antibiotic prophylaxis should be continued long term.

cardiology

26. Innocent murmurs

Answers: C E

Features of an innocent murmur:

- localised
- poorly conducting
- musical/vibratory
- soft grade 1–3/6*
- systolic*
- varies with posture
- present in high output states, eg febrile illness
- cardiac examination otherwise normal
- chest X-ray, ECG normal.

*Except venous hum.

Still's murmur

This is an early systolic murmur most commonly heard in children aged 2–6 years resolving towards adolescence. Grade 1–3 present in early systole, heart sounds normal. Maximum intensity is at lower left sternal edge. The murmur is vibratory and best heard with the patient flat reducing in intensity when they sit up.

Venous hum

This is a continuous murmur most commonly heard in children aged 2–6 years. The diastolic component is usually loudest. It is best heard over the supraclavicular fossa on the right with the head turned to the other side. It may radiate and is often heard on both sides. It disappears on lying flat or if the neck veins are compressed.

Pulmonary flow murmur

This is a very common murmur. Characteristically it is brief and in mid-systole. It is loudest with the patient supine and during expiration. Occurs in children and adolescents of all ages and is louder during hyperdynamic states such as fever and post exercise.

Innocent murmurs are commonly heard in the neonatal period.

cardiology

27. Cardiac emergencies

Answer: E

Supra-ventricular tachycardia

The commonest cardiac arrhythmia in the paediatric age group is a supra-ventricular tachycardia. Classically the onset is abrupt. It can last for a few minutes or several days. It is tolerated well by most children although the majority will develop cardiac failure if the arrhythmia persists for long enough. Management depends on whether the child is in shock as a consequence of the arrhythmia. Options include:

- vagal stimulation – facial immersion/carotid massage
- adenosine (can cause apnoea) – bolus doses given into a proximal vein – 50 µg/kg, 100 µg/kg, 250 µg/kg.
- digoxin, flecainide
- synchronous DC shock.

Management of asystole/electromechanical dissociation:

1 clear airway
2 ventilation with high concentration oxygen and cardiac massage
3 adrenaline – iv endotracheal, intra-osseous
4 fluid expansion
5 further adrenaline
6 exclude tamponade, pneumothorax, drug overdose.

Asystole is the commonest arrest rhythm in childhood.

Ventricular fibrillation

This is rare in childhood. Potential causes include tricyclic antidepressant toxicity, hypothermia, hyperkalaemia, myocarditis and myocardial infarction. Treatment is by asynchronous DC shock (after a praecordial thump) at 2 J/kg. This is repeated at the same dose if no output is produced and the dose then doubled. Adrenaline is given if there is still no response. A resuscitation circuit is then established including cardiopulmonary resuscitation (CPR), DC shock and adrenaline which is continued either until a response is obtained or resuscitation discontinued. All resuscitation drugs can be given intra-osseously except bretylium tosylate which is an anti-arrhythmic occasionally used in older children.

28. Wolff–Parkinson–White syndrome

Answers: A B C D E

Patients with this syndrome are prone to supra-ventricular tachycardia from pre-excitation due to an anomalous atrioventricular conduction pathway bypassing the junctional tissue. The accessory pathway allows a circuit to be formed which facilitates a re-entry tachycardia. The ECG characteristics include:

- shortened PR interval due to rapid anterograde conduction
- prolonged QRS caused by premature action of the ventricle through the accessory pathway followed by normal depolarisation through the AV node and the bundle of His
- delta wave – slurring of the upstroke to the QRS complex.

Usually associated with a structurally normal heart (70–80%). There is a recognised association with Ebstein's anomaly, corrected transposition and cardiomyopathy. There is a risk of sudden death. Digoxin is contraindicated. Appropriate anti-arrhythmics include verapamil and flecainide.

29. ECG

Answers: A D E

The PR interval varies with age:

- upper limit of normal in infants – 0.14 s
- upper limit of normal in older children – 0.16 s.

Causes of a prolonged PR interval:

- AVSD
- Atrio-ventricular canal defect
- Ebstein's anomaly
- myocarditis
- ischaemia
- hypothermia
- hyperkalaemia
- Duchenne's muscular dystrophy
- digoxin
- quinidine.

Myxomas are the commonest adult cardiac tumour. They are rare in childhood. They are most commonly found in the left atrium. Rhabdomyomas are the commonest cardiac tumours in childhood. These are usually located on the ventricular septum and may be multiple. They are associated with tuberous sclerosis. They can cause obstruction to ventricular flow and arrhythmias. Spontaneous regression does occur. Cerebral abscess is rare under the age of 2 years. Cerebral thrombi are more common (albeit still very rare). The third heart sound occurs as a consequence of rapid ventricular filling during diastole. It occurs in up to 20% of normal children. It is loud in conditions with decreased ventricular compliance secondary to ventricular dilatation, for example cardiac failure secondary to a VSD.

30. Causes of QT prolongation

Answers: A D

- QT prolongation precipitates ventricular tachycardia and fibrillation.
- torsades de pointes:the ventricular tachyarrhythmia
- 25–30% sporadic:
  - autosomal dominant – Romano Ward
  - autosomal recessive – Jervell Lange Neilson (associated with congenital deafness)
- QT (in seconds) is measured from the start of the Q wave until the end of the T wave
  - Corrected QT:measured QT/square root of RR
  - > 0.44 is abnormal
  - Longer QT intervals have been reported in normal infants.

Management:

- β-blockers
- left cardiac sympathetic denervation
- occasionally pacemaker.

Situations that prolong the QT:

- hypocalcaemia
- hypomagnesaemia
- myocarditis
- central nervous system trauma
- drugs – cisapride, quinidine, terfenadine, astemizole, amiodarone, amitriptyline, phenothiazines, anti-malarials.

Association with sudden infant death

- Prolonged QT is more common in infants who have suffered sudden infant death – large prospective study.

- Association with cisapride

- Macrolide antibiotics and anti-fungals act by the cytochrome P450 system and inhibit cisapride breakdown. Macrolide antibiotics include erythromycin, clarithromycin; antifungals include fluconazole, itraconazole, ketoconazole and miconazole.

31.   E: Conjunctivitis

Conjunctivitis is the only criterion above. Kawasaki's disease is a clinical diagnosis. The generally accepted definition (American Heart Association 1990) is: fever of 5 days duration with no obvious underlying cause plus at least four of the following five:

- bilateral conjunctivitis
- oral changes (strawberry tongue, fissuring of the lips)
- peripheral extremity changes (desquamation of palms and soles)
- cervical adenopathy
- pleomorphic rash.

The platelet count often rises some 2 weeks into the illness and misery is a prominent (but not a diagnostic) feature. Some cases are complicated by gallbladder hydrops. Misery is the only symptom which fits. The fever is high, platelet count rises after 1–2 weeks, the rash is pleomorphic.

32.   A: Splinter haemorrhages

SBE is a serious systemic infection with a cardiac focus. Underlying cardiac abnormalities (of valves or septa) predispose but are not a *sine qua non*. Organisms include *Streptococcus viridans* and *Staphylococcus aureus*. Clinical signs include splinters, retinal haemorrhages and changing cardiac murmurs. Diagnosis rests on a positive blood culture (in practice several taken) and showing vegetations on echo. Treatment consists of prolonged antibiotic treatment (6 weeks standard), valve replacement in cases of irreversible damage and (arguably) lifelong antibiotic prophylaxis.

33.   D: Oxygen

This baby has supra-ventricular tachycardia and is compromised cardiovascularly. This is more likely to be due to a re-entry phenomenon than a structural defect. As in any cardio-respiratory emergency, an ABC approach is the priority followed by management to terminate the dysrhythmia. Vagal manoeuvres such as ice packs, carotid sinus massage (hard in a baby) and ocular pressure may help to terminate the dysrhythmia. Parenteral adenosine given rapidly in escalating doses is the drug treatment of choice if vagal methods fail, followed by synchronous DC shock. Recurrent SVT may require longer term anti-arrhythmic treatment (digoxin, or alternative). In more severe cases, pathway ablation is a final usually successful option.

34.   E: Transposition of the great arteries

This baby clinically has cyanotic congenital heart disease. The key features are deep cyanosis without major respiratory distress indicative of a physiological right-to-left shunt. The most likely diagnosis is transposition of the great arteries. Until the patent ductus closes there may be no symptoms or signs, but as the pulmonary–systemic connection reaches critical point, cyanosis becomes overt. Fallot's tetralogy, pulmonary atresia, tricuspid atresia anomalous pulmonary venous drainage and truncus arteriosus all give rise to a similar picture but are much less common. A VSD is unlikely to cause symptoms at this age and would manifest as heart failure without cyanosis. PFC and diaphragmatic hernias present with a much 'sicker' baby with respiratory signs and within the first few hours if not sooner.

35.   B: Barium swallow

Though 'simple' laryngomalacia is by far the commonest cause of early stridor (and almost always self resolving) the picture in this case is different. This child is failing to thrive (always significant) and has a murmur suggesting a vascular/aortic ring which is best elucidated by a barium swallow as it will compress the oesophagus.

Causes of stridor:

- Intrinisic, eg:
  - Laryngomalacia
  - Cord nodules/polyps
  - Haemangiomata of the cords
  - Cord palsies
  - Laryngeal nerve palsy
  - Subglottic stenosis after prolonged intubation
  - Laryngeal web

- Extrinisic, eg:
  - Vascular ring
  - Right atrial enlargement
  - Cystic hygroma (obvious)
  - Thyroid enlargement

cardiology

36.   C: High-dose aspirin and parenteral immunoglobulin

This child fulfils the criteria for Kawasaki's disease (see Q 31). The rash is often confused with measles (which was rare in the UK but is becoming more common again with the reduction in MMR vaccine uptake). However, the extreme misery, desquamation and cervical nodes point in another direction. Once suspected treatment should be started without delay due to the risk of coronary artery aneurysm developing or enlarging. Meta-analyses suggest that high-dose aspirin (50 mg/kg per day in divided doses) until defervescence and a single dose of immunoglobulin (2 g over 12 hours iv) is the best management pending echocardiography and this regimen is now accepted practice. Vitamin A at presentation is routine management of measles in developing country settings and reduces mortality by up to 50%.

37.   ILLNESS WITH CARDIAC MANIFESTATIONS

1.   A – Cardiomyopathy

This boy has anthracycline cardiomyopathy. In the past these drugs were widely used but are still needed in certain malignancies. Lifelong cardiac follow-up is need with annual echo because a proportion develop dilated cardiomyopathy which is dose dependent. There is often a gap of many years before the signs become overt. Treatment is supportive until transplantation is possible.

2.   I – None of the above

This child has high output failure though the underlying problem does not appear to be cardiac. Options are anaemia, sepsis or a vascular anomaly. The picture suggests a vein of Galen aneurysm or an arterio-venous malformation. The signs will include heart failure with a cerebral bruit. The aneurysm can be delineated by magnetic resonance imaging (MRI) or angiography.

3.   C – Rheumatic fever

This boy has classic rheumatic fever with a rash, chorea and a mitral murmur. It is post-streptococcal and ASO titre is likely to be raised. See Answer 25 for the Duckett-Jones criteria. For diagnosis either (a) two major or (b) one major and two minor plus evidence of a preceding streptococcal infection are needed. The splenomegaly is coincidental and unrelated to the rheumatic fever. It is likely to be due to recurrent episodes of malaria; in endemic areas the prevalence of splenomegaly is high. Management is symptomatic. Opinions vary with regard to the need for streptococcal treatment but most would give a short course of high-dose penicillin to eradicate the infection. After rheumatic fever, long term (at least into adulthood) low-dose prophylaxis is recommended.

38. CARDIAC INVESTIGATIONS

1. H –None of the above

This has all the features of an innocent murmur; soft, systolic, positional. Up to 30% of children have such a murmur detected at some stage often while they are being auscultated for other reasons. In this case the 'louder sitting' characteristic suggests a venous hum as opposed to a Still's murmur or pulmonary flow (both of which are best heard lying down). No investigation is needed and only parental reassurance is necessary.

2. A –24-hour ECG

Though these may be simple panic attacks the girl's complaint requires that supra-ventricular tachycardia is ruled out. A 24 hour tape may show runs of supra-ventricular tachycardia and it is helpful to carry this out with an event monitoring facility. A standard ECG may show signs of Wolf–Parkinson–White (short PR interval with a delta wave).

3. C – Cardiac catheter

This child's aortic valve is re-stenosing until proved otherwise. Doppler echo studies will be suggestive but the gold standard remains cardiac catheterisation. This child is likely to require percutaneous transluminal redilatation open repair should this fail.

COMMUNITY PAEDIATRICS AND CHILD PSYCHIATRY ANSWERS

39.   Anorexia nervosa

Answers: A B D

The characteristic features of anorexia nervosa are severe weight loss, excessive exercising, depression (in about 50%), self-induced vomiting and laxative abuse associated with a distorted self-image and a morbid fear of being fat. It is commoner in pubertal girls, in whom amenorrhea is usually present, than in pre-pubertal girls. The incidence is higher in pupils of fee-paying schools and children of higher socio-economic status. It is also higher in certain populations such as ballet dancers and fashion students. Concordance is greater in monozygotic than dizygotic twins. The prevalence of anorexia is 0.5–1.0%; 1 in 10 cases are boys; 50% make a complete recovery, 25% make a partial recovery with some residual minor eating problems and the remaining 25% persist with a chronic course of illness. Mortality is 5–10%.

Bulimia nervosa is characterised by binge eating followed by self-induced vomiting and laxative abuse. These individuals are not usually underweight but share the same fear as sufferers of anorexia nervosa of becoming fat. Dental caries are common. The prevalence is estimated at 1%. The severity is variable. It is commoner in late adolescence and early adult life than in childhood. The prevalence in childhood is much lower.

Medical problems:

- reduced metabolic rate with bradycardia, postural hypotension, peripheral cyanosis, cold intolerance and lethargy
- impaired resistance to infection with bone marrow suppression which can be marked
- amenorrhea, hypocortisolaemia, impaired thyroid function, lanugo hair, osteopenia
- hypoalbuminaemia, oedema, constipation
- electrolyte abnormalities including secondary to laxative abuse, raised urea secondary to reduced fluid intake, impaired liver function
- elevated amylase with parotid swelling or pancreatitis
- effects of vitamin deficiency including hair loss.

40. Autism

Answers: A E

Autism usually presents before 3 years of age and is characterised by speech delay, absence of pretend play, stereotyped repetitive behaviour, lack of social interest and poor social interactions with parents and other children. The disorder is a spectrum and often called autistic spectrum disorder. The incidence is 2–13 per 10 000. Boys are more commonly affected than girls by 3:1. There is a genetic association with 3% of siblings being affected. One in five cases are associated with a medical condition, fragile X syndrome and tuberous sclerosis being the commonest. Mental retardation is common, 70% have an IQ <70. The more severe the mental retardation the more likely the child will have epilepsy in adolescence (20–30%). There is no association with social class or poor parenting.

Of children with autism, 50% gain useful language by 5 years of age but there is odd use of language with delayed echolalia and stereotyped phraseology. Useful acquisition of language by the age of 5 years is a good prognostic indicator for function in adult life. Two-thirds of autistic children grow up to be adults with severe learning difficulties who are unable to look after themselves.

Asperger's syndrome

This is probably part of the autistic spectrum but a milder form with relatively normal IQ and language development. The prevalence is around 10–25 per 10 000. It is commoner in boys. Recognised personality traits include abnormalities of gaze, poverty of expression and gesture, unusual and narrow focus of intellectual interests and a lack of feeling for others. Most people with Asperger's are also clumsy.

41. Attention deficit hyperactivity disorder

Answers: A C E

42. Attention deficit hyperactivity disorder

Answers: B C D E

Hyperactivity in childhood is common but is considered a disorder when it interferes with social function, learning and development. Attention deficit hyperactivity disorder is characterised by inattention, overactivity and impulsiveness. It affects 1–4% of school-age children. It is commoner in boys than girls (ratio: 3:1). Inattention leads to brief interest in activities and problems with learning and development. Over-activity is the excess of movements with restlessness and fidgeting. Impulsiveness causes action without thinking, often acting dangerously leading to frequent accidents.

Behavioural therapy can lead to improvement but it is intensive. Drug therapy is with stimulant drugs such as dexamfetamine and methylphenidate. Their use is controversial. Side-effects of drug therapy are common and include insomnia, suppression of appetite and depression. Rare side-effects include psychosis, growth retardation, increased frequency of tics and worsening of epilepsy. Modification of diet has been reported to improve symptoms in a number of children but behavioural modification or drug therapy or both are much more widely used.

Assessment of symptoms and effect of treatment can be aided by use of the Connor Teacher's Rating Scale questionnaire to assess activity and attention at school. The condition is said to persist into adult life in 10–20%. Some other causes of hyperactivity in children are:

- normal variant
- understimulation/boredom
- sleep disturbance
- learning difficulties
- anxiety disorder
- autistic spectrum disorder
- temporal lobe epilepsy
- drugs, eg anti-epileptic medication, sedatives.

43. School refusal

Answers: A B C D

School refusal is due to an excessive degree of anxiety making it difficult for the child to attend school. It occurs in about 1–2% of children of school age. There is equal sex incidence. It is commonest at age 5–6 years and 11 years when a new school is started. Depression is present in about 50–70%. Physical symptoms are common. The outcome is very good with a programme of psychotherapy and flooding therapy (taking the child to school, often under supervision of the therapist). Drug therapy is not indicated in most cases, but tricyclic antidepressants, eg imipramine, have been shown to be of use when there is co-existent depression. Truancy is differentiated from school refusal as it is the willful avoidance of school and not due to anxiety about school attendance.

44. Squint

Answers: A B C

Childhood squint (strabismus) is the misalignment of the eyes during visual fixation. It is common in childhood affecting 4% of children < 6 years of age. If left untreated it can cause secondary visual loss (amblyopia) in the affected eye.

community paediatrics and
child psychiatry

Squint is divided into two categories:

- non-paralytic squint: where there is no abnormality of the extraocular muscles or nerves supplying them
- paralytic squint: where there is a weakness of one or more of the extra-ocular muscles leading to squint. This is less common and when it presents a cause must be sought.

Diagnosis:

- corneal light reflex test: the degree of squint can be assessed using prisms in front of the eye while doing the test (Krimsky method)
- cover testing
- visual acuity testing: this is mandatory to assess vision in both eyes
- eye movements.

Treatment of non-paralytic squint:

- correction of any refractive error
- patching the normal eye allowing the development of vision in the affected eye
- corrective surgery: this is largely cosmetic and involves strengthening or weakening the appropriate extra-ocular muscles to balance out the squint. Often a second operation is required to align the eyes fully.

45. Deafness

Answers: A D E

Deafness is either conductive, sensorineural or mixed. There are many causes of deafness and these should be learned.

A number of causes are listed below:

- congenital
  - autosomal dominant – 33%
  - autosomal recessive – 65%
  - X-linked – 2%
  - syndromes: Alport's syndrome (with renal failure); Treacher Collins syndrome; Klippel–Feil anomalies of the spine; Down's syndrome; Waardenburg's syndrome; Jervell–Lange–Nielson syndrome associated with prolonged QT interval and sudden death; Pendred's syndrome.

community paediatrics and child psychiatry

- Acquired
  - Pre-natal: congenital infection – rubella, cytomegalovirus; drugs such as thalidomide
  - Perinatal – it is common in pre-term infants with a prevalence in very low birth weight infants (< 1500 g) of 1%. Pre-term infants are particularly susceptible to hypoxia, hyperbilirubinaemia, intra-ventricular haemorrhage and the use of drugs such as gentamicin.
- Older children
  - Otitis media
  - Glue ear
  - Meningitis.

Assessment of deafness:

- Oto-acoustic emissions: these are emitted by normal ears in response to sound emitted by an aural probe. They are not emitted by ears with a hearing loss of > 30 dB, and it is an all or nothing response. They have a 100% sensitivity and 80% specificity for sensorineural hearing loss.
- Brain-stem evoked auditory responses: electrodes are placed over the skull and electrical activity is picked up in response to auditory stimulation. This is a useful test in babies under 6 months of age especially in those at high risk of deafness (jaundice, prematurity, low birth weight). The test is not affected by sedation.
- Distraction testing is used from 6 months to 1 year of age.
- Play audiometry can be used after 18 months to 2 years of age.
- Pure tone audiometry is used after 3.5 years of age as this is the age in which co-operation can be achieved.

Glue ear

This is the commonest form of deafness in children. Causes include acute otitis media, allergy and malformation of the eustachian tube (associated with cleft palate). These all lead to accumulation of fluid in the middle ear which may become infected. The fluid prevents equalisation of pressures between the middle ear and the atmosphere from occurring and damps the response of the ear drum to sound. A large proportion of cases resolve spontaneously or with a trial of decongestant therapy. If not, treatment is with grommet insertion. The main indications are speech delay and severe hearing loss.

community paediatrics and child psychiatry

46. Factitious or induced illness

Answers: A B C D E

Munchausen's by proxy, or factitious or induced illness (FII), is a disorder which can end with disability or even death. It involves fabrication of the child's symptoms by the parent or care-giver and simulation of physical signs. Clinical presentations include:

- poisoning
- drug ingestion or injection
- apnoea by suffocation
- physical injuries.

Often the parent has a background in health care, presents as a good parent, gets on well with medical staff and seems to be unconcerned about their child's symptoms. The parent may also interfere with ward investigations (blood in stool or urine samples, diluting urine, altering the temperature measurements). The diagnosis is often difficult to make but clues include:

- a persistent or recurrent illness which cannot be explained
- investigation results that do not correlate with the health of the child
- symptoms which do not occur while the parent is away
- the parent may not leave the child's bedside in hospital, even for short periods of time
- treatment is ineffective or poorly tolerated, even if appropriate for the suspected clinical problem
- inconsistent medical history.

Investigation depends on symptomatology. Samples should be collected by medical staff to prevent contamination. Covert video surveillance has been used successfully in a number of cases of apnoea caused by parental suffocation. Treatment involves protecting the child and siblings from potential harm. Involvement of social services at an early stage is essential.

47.   Indications for referral to a child psychiatrist

Answers: A C E

- Emotional or behavioural problems unresponsive to first-line counselling
- Deliberate drug overdose or attempted suicide
- Difficult child protection cases
- Difficult diagnostic problems where there is no obvious organic cause.

Included in behavioural problems are those which are common in childhood:

- separation anxiety
- soiling
- persistent grief reactions
- grief reactions causing severe disruption to the child or family environment.

A persistent grief reaction is one which has persisted beyond the normal age range. A general rule of thumb is that it is persistent if it lasts longer in months than the child's age in years. The prevalence of psychiatric disorder in childhood depends on the age range, the population studied and the diagnostic criteria used, however, prevalence is higher in urban than rural areas; conduct and hyperactivity disorders are commoner in boys at all ages; emotional disorders show an equal sex distribution in 4–11-year-olds, but are three times more common in girls between the ages of 12 and 16 years.

Risk factors and associations of psychiatric disorder:

- child
  - severe learning disability, up to 40%
  - low self-esteem and academic failure
  - physical illness: strong association with epilepsy and slight increase in most other illnesses
  - specific developmental delay, eg speech delay
  - bullying and peer group pressure
  - abuse.

- family
  - family breakdown (up to 80% incidence in children 1 year after divorce)
  - maternal ill health
  - paternal criminality, alcoholism
  - abuse
  - poverty
  - death and loss, including loss of friendships
  - inconsistent discipline
  - family history of psychiatric disorder.

community paediatrics and child psychiatry

48. Childhood depression

Answers: B D

Major depressive illness in children is uncommon (2 per 1000), but many children have depressive symptoms and the incidence of both increase during adolescence. Depression can be primary (isolated depression) or secondary (secondary to other psychiatric disorder or physical disease).

- Primary depression is often associated with a family history of depression.
- Pre-pubertal boys are twice as likely to have depression as pre-pubertal girls. This sex incidence is reversed after puberty.
- Suicidal behaviour (parasuicide) is common in children who suffer from depression.
- Successful suicide in childhood is extremely rare.

Symptoms characteristically include depressed mood and tearfulness, lethargy and loss of interest in usual activities, feelings of guilt and self-blame, diminished appetite and poor weight gain (but appetite can be increased), impaired sleep (but can be increased), social withdrawal, outbursts of aggression and delusional symptoms in the form of auditory hallucinations accusing the child of worthlessness.

49. Sudden infant death syndrome

Answers: A D

Sudden infant death syndrome (SIDS) is the unexpected and unexplained death of an infant (on post-mortem findings and on examination of the scene of death). The peak incidence is between 2 and 4 months of age with 95% of deaths occurring before 6 months of age. The incidence has been declining since 1989, when there were 1337 deaths, to 442 deaths in 1993. The incidence started declining before the government Back to Sleep campaign in 1991 which promoted sleep in the supine position, probably due to prior publicity of the need to put babies to sleep supine. The major risk factors for sudden infant death are:

- parental smoking – antenatal and post natal
- prone sleeping position
- male sex
- maternal age (younger)
- low birth weight
- prematurity
- febrile illness
- thermal stress (high temperature, over wrapping).

The use of apnoea monitors has not reduced the risk of SIDS. There is no proved association of SIDS with the type of mattress used.

community paediatrics and child psychiatry

50. Child sexual abuse

Answers: A B D

Child sexual abuse occurs when another person who is sexually mature involves the child in any activity which the other person expects to lead to their own sexual arousal. This includes exposure, pornography, sexual acts with a child and masturbation. The prevalence suggested by a MORI poll in adults asking whether they had been abused as children (UK 1985) is approximately 10% – this is probably an underestimate; 12% of females and 8% of males reported abuse. About 60% of child sexual abuse is by an immediate family member. There is often a history of generational abuse.

Current conviction rate of abusers taken to court is 5%. The court cases are extremely distressing to the child, they may be accused of lying or feel that they have not been believed if conviction does not occur. The worry about not being believed is probably one reason for lack of disclosure in school-age children who have been sexually abused. Child sexual abusers often have a history of child sexual abuse (approximately 27% sexually abused as a child and 17% witnessed child sexual abuse) but this does not mean that all children who are abused go on to abuse.

Facts about abusers:

- 31% – fathers
- 4% – mothers
- 10% – older brothers
- 7% – baby sitters
- 17% – unrelated men (who may be part of an organised paedophile ring)

Anal fissures are common in children who are sexually abused. In children who are sexually abused there is an increased incidence of anorexia, headaches, recurrent abdominal pain, encopresis, enuresis and behavioural problems. There is a higher prevalence of child sexual abuse in children with special educational needs. Reflex anal dilatation is not a normal reflex. It may occur in inflammatory bowel disease, in chronic constipation, with the use of enemas and after anal stretch surgery, but it also occurs after anal penetration. The conclusion of the Cleveland Inquiry (1988) was that 'the sign of anal dilatation is abnormal and suspicious and requires further investigation. It is not in itself evidence of anal abuse'. Strong indicators of child sexual abuse are pregnancy, sexually transmitted disease, lacerations or scars in the hymen, anal fissures and positive forensic tests (semen). Child sexual abuse is associated with physical abuse in 15% of cases.

community paediatrics and child psychiatry

51. Physical abuse in children

Answers: B C D

The reported incidence of physical abuse in children is 0.8/1000 (England and Wales 1983). It is characterised by a history inconsistent with the pattern of the injury. It is responsible for 200–300 non-accidental deaths per year in the UK. Mothers are more likely to be abusers than fathers, and handicapped children are at increased risk. It occurs in all social classes. Risk factors include large family size, first-born children (50%), low income, low parental intelligence, previous history of abuse in the parents and poor health of the parents (including alcohol and drug abuse). The commonest site of injury is the head and neck. There may be abnormal coagulation in up to 16% of children in whom abuse is suspected. Fractures are commoner in pre-school age children. Falls at home from about 1 m result in skull fractures of non-abused children in 1%. Almost 1 in 4 of all skull fractures seen in childhood are thought to be due to abuse, increasing to 1 in 3 of complex skull fractures. Intracranial injury is the commonest cause of death in abused children, and 95% of serious head injuries in the first year of life are due to abuse. This is usually due to shaking injury which can lead to intracranial bleeding and is associated with retinal haemorrhages. The shaken child may also be hit against a hard object resulting in skull fracture and severe acceleration/deceleration injury. Rib fractures are rarely seen in non-abused children. Periosteal new bone formation is seen on X-ray 7–10 days after the initial injury.

52. Schizophrenia

Answers: A C D E

Schizophrenia is characterised by particular abnormalities of thinking, perception and emotion. It is usually diagnosed between the ages of 15 and 35 years, but the onset may be in childhood: early onset < 17 years, very early onset < 13 years. The difficulty in diagnosing schizophrenia in childhood is that some symptoms are modified by the cognitive immaturity of the child and may not fit into the adult syndrome.

Symptoms include delusions, hallucinations, formal thought disorder (a disorder in the logic of thinking) and changes in affect. Immaturity of development particularly affects the severity of illogical thinking. Children with, or who go on to develop, schizophrenia may just seem odd. The stages of schizophrenia are usually divided into an active phase where they are psychotic (lasts 1–6 months, shortened by anti-psychotic drug therapy), a recovery phase where there is a degree of impairment often with depression and a residual phase where recovery is incomplete (80%) leaving a degree of social and psychological impairment. It may progress to the chronic stage when a person may not recover from the acute stage.

Schizophrenia is uncommon in children, becoming commoner after 15 years of age. Some of the difficulties in diagnosis in children may account for this. Whole life prevalence is 1%. Family history is often positive. Lifetime incidence is 8% with an affected sibling, 12% if a parent is affected, 40% if both parents affected and 55% if an identical twin has schizophrenia. The prognosis for recovery is 25–40% for adults, only a small minority recovering without further episodes. The prognosis is worse for early-onset schizophrenia. The prognosis is better in females. There is a lifetime suicide risk of 15%.

53. Speech delay

Answers: B E

Recognised causes of speech delay include:

- hearing defects
- mental retardation due to any cause for example congenital hypothyroidism, tuberous sclerosis, Down's syndrome, fragile X syndrome, intrauterine infections, and fetal alcohol syndrome
- cerebral palsy
- developmental expressive aphasia
- emotional deprivation
- autism.

The family history is usually of relevance. There is often a history of speech delay in the parents, girls tend to speak earlier than boys, first born children tend to speak earlier than subsequent children and twins speak later than singletons. Tongue-tie, cleft palate and malocclusion may affect speech quality but do not cause speech delay.

Milestones in the development of speech:

- 3–6 months: loud tuneful vocalisations.
- 6–12 months: babbles in long repetitive syllables. Syllables 'da', 'ma' may be used from 8 months initially inappropriately but use in correct context to parents by 12–14 months.
- 1–1.5 years: starts using words in appropriate context. Understands many more words.
- 1.5–2.5 years: many intelligible words mixed with jargon. Starts asking 'why', 'where' questions by two years. Joins two or more words in phrases by 2 years.
- 2.5–4 years: period of rapid speech development with the acquisition of many new words. Constantly asking questions. Stops talking to him or herself during play in favour of directing speech towards others.
- 4+ years: can narrate stories, correct grammatical usage by 4.5 years.

Delay in any of these areas is a warning that there is a problem with either hearing or in speech acquisition.

54. Developmental regression

Answers: C D E

This question distinguishes causes of developmental regression (the loss of previously acquired developmental milestones) from the causes of developmental delay (delay in acquisition of normal milestones). It is useful to distinguish the age of onset of regression. Regression before age of 2 years occurs in:

- HIV encephalopathy
- aminoacidurias
- hypothyroidism
- lysosomal enzyme disorders, eg mucopolysaccharidoses, sphingolipidoses (e.g. Gaucher's disease), glycoprotein degradation disorders, mucolipidoses
- mitochondrial disorders, eg Leigh's encephalopathy, Menkes' kinky hair syndrome
- neurocutaneous disorders, eg neurofibromatosis, tuberous sclerosis
- genetic disorders of white and grey matter
- progressive hydrocephalus.

Regression after 2 years of age occurs in subacute sclerosing panencephalitis. Late onset is seen in:

- lysosomal enzyme disorders
- mitochondrial disorders
- genetic disorders of white and grey matter.

55. Normal development

Answers: A B E

56. Normal development

Answers: A B C D

57. Normal development

Answers: B C D E

58. Normal development

Answers: A C D E

Normal developmental milestones

The reader is referred to a standard text book of development. Some useful milestones are:

- 4–6 weeks: smiles.
- 6 weeks: prone-pelvis flat. Ventral suspension-head up to plane of body momentarily. Fixes and follows in the horizontal plane.
- 12–16 weeks: prone supports on forearms. Fixes and follows in the horizontal and vertical plane.
- 20 weeks: full head control. No head lag when pulled to sit. Reaches for objects and grabs them.
- 6 months: prone weight bears on hands. Rolls prone to supine. Transfers hand to hand, chews, feeds with a biscuit.
- 7 months: rolls supine to prone. Sits hands held forwards for support.
- 9 months: finger thumb opposition. Sitting can lean forward and recover position. Waves bye-bye. Starting to stand with support from furniture.
- 1 year: walking with one hand held. Uses two words with meaning. Mouthing stops.
- 13 months: stands alone for a moment.
- 18 months: goes up and down stairs holding rail. Can throw a ball without falling. Domestic mimicry. Feeds with spoon. Spontaneous scribble. Takes off socks and shoes. Can follow simple orders. Uses many words, jargon still present. Tower of 3–4 cubes. Dry in day.
- 2 years: goes up and down stairs two feet per step. Kicks ball without falling. Washes and dries hands. Tower of six to seven cubes. Puts on socks, pants and shoes. Imitates vertical stroke. Turns pages one at a time. Joins two words in sentences.
- 2.5 years: jumps with both feet. Walks on tiptoes. Pencil held in hand not in fist. Knows sex and full name. Names one colour.
- 3 years: upstairs one foot per step, downstairs two feet per step. Rides tricycle. Attends to toilet needs without help. Dresses and undresses if helped with buttons and shoes. Names two colours. Constantly asks questions. Copies a circle.
- 4 years: up and downstairs one foot per step. Buttons clothes fully. Catches a ball. Copies a cross. Names three colours. Speech is grammatically correct and can give age. Eats with spoon and fork. Brushes teeth. Understands taking turns and sharing. Distinguishes past, present and future and right and left. Can hop for a few seconds on each foot.
- 5 years: can skip and hop. Drawing skills are improved – draws square (4.5 years) and triangle (5.5 years), can write a few letters. Names four colours. Can give home address. Distinguishes morning from afternoon. Dresses and undresses alone. Chooses own friends. Understands needs for rules in games and play.

59.   Toe walking

Answers: A B C E

Toe walking is common between the ages of 1 and 2 years. In most cases it is a habit and these children can stand on their heels without difficulty and ankle movements are normal. Other causes include:

- prematurity
- spastic cerebral palsy
- congenital shortening of the Achilles' tendon
- Duchenne's muscular dystrophy
- peroneal muscular atrophy
- infantile autism
- spinal tumour
- unilateral hip dislocation.

60.   C: Chronic fatigue syndrome

Prevalence is highest in adolescents, with females outnumbering males approx 3:1. Children are more likely to make a full recovery than adults although a small percentage may remain incapacitated for years. The onset may be gradual or sudden, with or without a preceding acute illness. Debilitating fatigue exacerbated by activity is the most commonly reported symptom Other symptoms are malaise, headaches, sore throat, sleep disturbance, myalgia, abdominal and joint pains. Depression, anxiety and other psychological conditions may co-exist.

Diagnosis is based on the impact of condition on a patient rather than the duration of symptoms per se. A thorough history is required to include family history and emotional dimensions of illness. Physical examination should include height, weight, head circumference, neurological assessment, lymph nodes and sinuses, lying and standing blood pressure and heart rate. Routine investigations to be performed in all cases are as stated in the question, with others dependent on any relevant findings on history and examination. Diagnosis should be made as soon as possible and communicated to the patient and family. Other appropriate professionals should be included in management and may include CAMHS, physiotherapy, dieticians, education and social services. In-patient admission and medication may need to be considered in a small minority. Prolonged bed rest should be avoided. Regular review is essential to monitor progress and revise management plan as needed.

The Royal College of Paediatrics and Child Health have published extensive evidence-based guidelines in 2004 for the management of children with chronic fatigue syndrome. These are available on the College website (www.rcpch.ac.uk).

community paediatrics and child psychiatry

61. C: Separation anxiety disorder

DSM-IV criteria state that separation anxiety consists of excessive anxiety beyond that expected for the child's developmental level related to separation or impending separation from the primary caregiver in children less than 18 years of age and lasting for at least 4 weeks. It is normal until the age of approximately 3–4 years. It is commoner in children who have suffered bereavement or who have over-protective parents. Incidence is approximately equal among boys and girls. The mean age of onset of separation anxiety disorder (SAD) is 7.5 years. Approximately three out of four children with SAD will go on to develop school refusal, which has a mean age of onset of 10 years. SAD manifests differently at different ages. In those aged under 8 years, it tends to present with unrealistic worry with regard to harm to parents and school refusal. In those aged 9–12 years, the commonest complaint is of excessive distress at times of separation such as overnight school trips. Those 12–16-year-old present with school refusal and somatic problems.

SAD symptoms are frequently reinforced by family members. It is more commonly found in children where there is a family history of anxiety disorder or if there is any history of early or traumatic separation from the attachment figure (such as divorce). Cognitive behaviour therapy and family therapy are helpful in returning the child to normal patterns of behaviour. Complications include depression and substance abuse, but in general the prognosis is good if detected and treated early.

62. D: Somatisation

Somatoform disorders are a group of psychological disorders where a patient experiences a physical symptom in the absence of an underlying medical condition. It is common for children to express emotional distress as physical pain and transient episodes do not affect overall functioning. However, the persistent experiences associated with a disorder will often interfere with school, home life and friendships. In contrast to factitious disorders or malingering where symptoms are intentionally produced or feigned, in somatoform disorders, intentional deception does not occur.

Headaches, stomach aches, dizziness, chest pain and nausea are the most commonly reported symptoms. Risk factors include presence of depression or anxiety disorder, female sex, family dysfunction and increasing age. It also occurs more frequently in children whose parents have non-life-threatening disease or medically unexplained symptoms. It is more likely to occur in children with a history of being abused. Exclusion of medical and neurological conditions is the major diagnostic concern, eg brain tumours and temporal lobe epilepsy. Families may be resistant to considering a psychological cause of the child's symptoms, so careful explanation and reassurance are essential at all stages. Treatment involves

community paediatrics and child psychiatry

ruling out concurrent physical problems and maintaining or improving the overall functioning of the patient. Mental health services are helpful in managing patients with more severe symptoms, often jointly with medical involvement.

63.   E: Sleep disorders

Up to one in four children have some type of sleep problem, the commonest being nightmares, sleepwalking and insomnia. Learning difficulties, attention deficit hyperactivity disorder, family dysfunction, depression and anxiety are commonly seen in association. Nightmares affect up to half of 3–6-year-olds, being common after stressful or frightening events. They usually occur during second half of the night and are well remembered the next day. Night terrors typically occur during first 3 hours of sleep and are associated with autonomic arousal (tachypnoea, tachycardia). They end spontaneously and the child quickly returns to sleep with poor recall the next day. Sleepwalking is seen most commonly in the 3–10 year age group, and can affect up to 30% of children. There is usually no recollection the next day.

Chronic insomnia is associated with the presence of another mental disorder in 35–50% of cases. Pre-pubertal children with depression are most likely to experience insomnia whereas their post-pubertal counterparts are more likely to complain of hypersomnia. Substance-induced sleep disorder (drugs or alcohol) should also be considered. Obstructive sleep apnoea is the commonest reason for referral for sleep studies. Other reasons include suspected narcolepsy, sleep-related seizure-like activity and snoring associated with daytime somnolence. The majority of childhood sleep problems can be managed with behavioural techniques including emphasising the need for good sleep hygiene (eg simple, consistent bedtime routine, dark, quiet room and removal of distractions such as a television) and techniques such as controlled crying. Medications are rarely needed. Melatonin is occasionally used but is not licensed in the UK for use in children with sleep disorders.

64.   B: Developmental co-ordination disorder

This is also known as dyspraxia and exists in varying degrees of severity with various associated comorbidities such as learning difficulties, attention deficit and other disabilities. Problem arises due to a failure to sequence information required to perform 'complex' tasks in a co-ordinated fashion. The problem area may be limited to certain fine or gross motor skills or include problems with speech and language or thought processing. The exact incidence unknown but likely that 5% of children worldwide have the disorder with up to 10% experiencing more minor forms of co-ordination difficulties. More males thought to be affected than females. Developmental progress in early childhood may suggest presence of the disorder but it typically comes to light during school years and the child's teacher is often the first person to raise concern. Crucial to the diagnosis is that no underlying neurological condition exists (eg cerebral palsy or muscular dystrophy) but this can usually be excluded without need for specialist input.

There are numerous strategies for evaluation of a child with suspected developmental co-ordination disorder. Much information can be gathered by observing a child performing routine daily tasks such as writing, using knife and fork and scissors, catching and throwing a ball and dressing and this is often done in an environment familiar to the child such as the classroom rather than in a clinic setting. In standardised tests, a child scoring below the 5th centile for age is thought to be indicative of a motor problem. Those involved in the assessment process, which should be multi-disciplinary, may include occupational therapists and physiotherapists, speech and language therapists, educational psychologists, teachers and parents. After identification of problem areas, individual intervention programmes can be devised to either allow acquisition of skills that are absent or to provide optimal coping mechanisms for deficiencies.

65.   E: Cohort studies

By far the biggest scientific problem in cohorts is the loss of subjects over time to migration, death from other causes or loss of interest. Provided selection is appropriate and subject similar in factors other than exposure, bias and confounding are less of a problem than in case–control studies. There are no interventions in cohort studies as they are observational.

community paediatrics and
child psychiatry

66. D: Randomisation

An RCT is essentially an experimental situation where the investigators manipulate the subjects' exposure. Randomisation if done properly ensures an equal mix of potential confounders between groups thereby eliminating their effect

67. TRIAL DESIGN

1. A – Ecological

Ecological studies look at regional differences in possible exposure with outcomes. This is on a population not individual basis and therefore can only be used to generate ideas.

2. D – Nested case–control

A nested case–control study is built in to a cohort and is used to selectively measure exposure retrospectively between cases and controls where the measurement is expensive. The usual design is to take samples on all participants (in this case for trace elements), store them and to measure only in cases (mothers with susbsequent babies with abdominal wall defects) and selected controls thereby reducing wastage and cost

3. G – Retrospective cohort

Provided that data are available, such a study with a long latency is best done by a retrospective cohort. Most studies using birth or exposure records many years before the measured outcome

68. STATISTICAL TESTS

1. A – *t* test

t tests are used to compare two groups of approximately equal size with variables of normal distribution.

2. D – Survival analysis

Any time to event study is best analysed by survival analysis, eg proportional hazards or a hazard ratio.

3. C – Pearson's correlation coefficient

The relation between one variable and another is best looked at by correlation. As both are near normal, in this case Pearson's.

69. ACCIDENTAL INJURY

1. B – House fire

2. F – Falls

3. H – Road traffic accidents

Accidents are the single biggest cause of death in children over the age of 1 year in the UK and a major cause of long-term disability and ill health. More than 2 million children are taken to hospital annually after an accident, half of which occur in the home. The numbers of accidents and accidental deaths in childhood are falling but children from lower social classes remain at greatest risk. Boys are twice as likely as girls to have accidents. The majority of accidents within the home occur to pre-school children.

Falls are the commonest cause of non-fatal injury, more than 2/3 occurring in the under-fives and approximately 60% being male. Scalds are most often as a result of spillage of hot drinks and are more frequent than burns. House fires are the commonest cause of death within the home. They may be caused by cigarettes, candles, chip pans, faulty wiring or children playing with matches or lighters. Accidental poisoning usually occurs in preschool children and is most commonly due to the ingestion of medications within the home, though the majority require little or no treatment. The risk of choking declines with age. Although the number of choking episodes is declining, the number of cases involving toys is increasing. Baby walkers are associated with more injuries than any other nursery equipment. At least a third of babies using baby walkers will be injured, whether as a result of a fall, burn, scald or poisoning. Road traffic accidents account for the largest number of serious injuries and fatalities – affecting both pedestrians and passengers. They constitute increasing proportions of accidental deaths as children get older. Reducing traffic speed, use of cycle helmets and correctly fitted child restraints have all been proved to reduce the risk of death and serious injury.

community paediatrics and child psychiatry

70. DEVELOPMENTAL PROBLEMS

1. F – Genetic studies for Wolf–Hirschhorn syndrome

The features described are typical of Wolf–Hirschhorn syndrome, which is caused by a deletion on chromosome 4p. Clinical features include developmental delay, seizures (50%), distinct facial appearance ('Greek warrior helmet' facies) and midline closure defects. It is usually diagnosed in neonatal period due to the dysmorphic features. It is associated with intra-uterine growth retardation, reduced fetal movements and microcephaly. Affected individuals typically develop ataxic gait and absence of speech and may have associated cardiac anomalies (ASD, VSD), diaphragmatic hernia and agenesis of corpus callosum. Approximately one in three die before the age of 2 years. If a child survives this period, slow but constant developmental progress is made.

2. C – Blood lead level

Long-term effect of lead exposure is greatest during first 2 or 3 years of life when the brain is developing and because lead is absorbed from the gastrointestinal tract more effectively in children than adults. The greatest public health risk is exposure to leaded paint. Symptoms of low level lead poisoning are non-specific and include temperamental lability, behavioural change, loss of developmental milestones and language delay. Increased exposure may cause abdominal pain and anorexia, constipation, headache, ataxia, lethargy and coma. The classic findings of lead lines on X-rays of long bones are rarely now seen so blood level estimation is the best approximation of lead exposure. Treatment involves removal of source of lead exposure with chelation therapy being required in only the more severe cases. See also Answer 179.

3. D – Genetic studies for Rett's syndrome

This history is a typical presentation of Rett's syndrome, which is thought to affect females only, being lethal in utero to affected males. Apparently normal initial development is followed by a period of stagnation and regression. The latter may occur acutely over days or insidiously over months and is characterised by loss of hand skills and oral language. Abnormal breathing patterns, seizures and gut motility problems are also features. Usually evident by age 2–4 years. After period of regression, children stabilise experiencing no further cognitive decline, progressing through puberty and often surviving into adulthood. Diagnosis is made if defined diagnostic clinical criteria are met. In 1999 a genetic mutation (*MECP2*) was identified on the X chromosome which has been found to be present in up to 80% of cases of Rett's syndrome. Treatment is supportive.

DERMATOLOGY ANSWERS

71. Scabies

Answers: A E

This is caused by the mite *Sarcoptes scabiei* with person-to-person spread. It is highly contagious. Papules, vesicles, pustules and nodules are usual presenting lesions. Intensely itchy although very young infants often do not scratch and just appear miserable with widespread eczematous erythema on the trunk. Pathognomonic burrows – most commonly found in finger web spaces and on thenar and hypothenar eminences. Children much more likely to have involvement of the head and neck than adults and therefore application of the first choice scabicide, permethrin, should include the scalp, neck, face and ears in those aged under 2 years. All household members should be treated with repeat application after 1 week. Malathion can also be used but lindane is no longer used in UK due to reports of aplastic anaemia.

Treatment failure is most commonly due to inadequate application of treatment in an individual or within a household (allowing re-infestation), or washing of hands during treatment period without re-application. Resistance to permethrin is also recognised. Treatment failure should not be presumed until 6 weeks have elapsed, as it can take this length of time for the eczematous reaction and subsequent pruritus to resolve completely.

72. Mastocytosis

Answers: A B D E

This is characterised by mast cell proliferation and accumulation within various organs, most commonly the skin. Urticaria pigmentosa is the commonest form, consisting of oval or round reddish-brown macules, papules or plaques which can vary in number from a few to thousands. Characteristic change seen on stroking a urticaria pigmentosa lesion is (called Darier's sign) the lesion becoming pruritic, oedematous and erythematous due to mast cell degranulation. The skeletal, haematopoietic, gastrointestinal, cardiopulmonary and central nervous systems may all be involved either directly or indirectly, with symptoms including headache, flushing, dizziness, tachycardia, hypotension, syncope, nausea, vomiting, abdominal pain and diarrhoea. Most cases of urticaria pigmentosa in children resolve spontaneously by puberty. Adolescent and adult onset urticaria pigmentosa is more likely to be persistent and involves greater risk of systemic involvement. Increasing age at onset also carries a greater risk of malignant transformation. Males and females are equally affected.

Skin biopsy is usually required to make the diagnosis. Serum tryptase levels are elevated as are urinary N-methylhistamine levels. Treatment is symptomatic and consists of H_1 and H_2 anti-histamines along with avoidance of agents known to precipitate mediator release such as non-steroidal anti-inflammatory drugs (NSAIDs) and opioids as well as physical stimuli such as emotional stress and extremes of temperature. Bone marrow biopsy may be required in the presence of an abnormal full blood count. Those with extensive systemic disease may require injectable adrenaline as a first aid measure to prevent anaphylaxis.

73. D: Atopic eczema

It affects 10–15% of children, and up to 50% of those who also have hay fever or asthma. Males and females are equally affected, and it often starts in infancy. Most will improve by teenage years but up to one in four will experience symptoms into adulthood. Typical distribution in infancy affects scalp and face, with extensor surfaces also involved in some. Older children and adults have predominantly flexural involvement. Features include pruritus and xerosis (dry skin). Genetic and environmental factors are involved and include contact irritants (soaps, detergents, wool), aeroallergens (house dust mite, pollen, dander), microbial agents (*Staphylococcus aureus*), food allergens (cow's milk, soya, egg) and psychological stress. Treatment consists of adequate skin hydration, avoidance of allergenic precipitants, topical corticosteroids, systemic antihistamines, antibiotic treatment of secondary infection and immunosuppression (prednisolone, ciclosporin) in extreme cases.

Evidence for the effectiveness of preventive measures is generally applicable in high-risk families only (ie family history of atopy in parents *and* siblings). Removal of certain foods from the pregnant mother's diet can be harmful and has not been shown to reduce the risk of eczema in the unborn child. Breast-feeding is protective against the development of allergies when compared with formula feeding, but there is no evidence to support its exclusive use beyond the age of 6 months. If breast-feeding is not possible in families at high risk of atopic disease, evidence exists to support the use of hydrolysed cow's milk formulae rather than cow's or soya milk-based products. Conclusive evidence to support delaying the introduction of common food allergens when weaning is lacking, although it is frequently recommended. No benefit has been shown of the preventive effect of avoiding house dust mite during pregnancy and after birth, although if combined with food allergen avoidance, some protection against atopic eczema in infancy may be gained.

74. E: Capillary haemangioma

Also known as a strawberry naevus, this is the commonest tumour in infancy and is seen in approximately 10% of white infants. The incidence is much lower in black and Asian babies. It is commoner in pre-term babies and when mothers have undergone chorionic villous sampling in pregnancy. Females ae three times more commonly affected than males. It presents at birth in 30%, and is a focal and solitary lesion in 80% — most commonly found on head and neck (60%), followed by trunk (25%) and extremities (15%). May appear initially as area of blanching of skin, followed by development of fine telangiectasia and then a red macule or papule. Colour depends on depth of lesion — red or crimson if superficial, purple/blue or flesh coloured if deep.

Proliferation of lesions occurs during first year of life, most rapidly during first few weeks and up to age of 6 months. Involution then occurs, typically from the centre. By age 5 years, 50% have completely resolved, and 70% by 7 years and 90% by 9 years. Approximately 50% leave some form of permanent skin change (eg telangiectasia, superficial dilated veins or epidermal atrophy). Treatment is required for certain lesions, ie those that impinge on vital structures (eg causing airway obstruction or impairment of visual fields), for ulcerated, bleeding or secondarily infected lesions and for those causing psychological distress often due to cosmetic disfigurement. Other indications for intervention include complications such as congestive cardiac failure (seen when multiple or visceral lesions present such as in diffuse neonatal haemangiomatosis) and in Kasabach–Merritt syndrome (consumptive coagulopathy and thrombocytopenia). Treatment options include medical therapy with systemic or intralesional steroids, subcutaneous interferon-alfa, laser or excision surgery. Close follow-up would be required in this particular case to ensure that any further growth of the naevus does not impinge on the infant's visual fields given its location over the nasal bridge.

dermatology

75. INFECTIONS

1. A – *Staphylococcus aureus*

The lesions described are those of Staphylococcal scalded skin syndrome, and are caused by exotoxin A and B producing *Staphylococcus aureus* phage type 2. The toxin causes red rash and separation of dermis beneath granular cell layer with resulting bullae formation and sheet-like desquamation. The infecting *Staph. aureus* organism may originate from skin, throat nose, mouth or umbilicus. There is associated general malaise, fever (not always present), irritability and skin tenderness. Erythematous rash accentuated in flexor creases. Peri-oral crusting often present. White cell count may be normal and blood cultures usually negative. Gram stain/culture from original infection site may confirm *Staph. aureus* infection. Frozen section of peeled skin confirms superficial site of cleavage, thus differentiating from toxic epidermal necrolysis where cleavage occurs deeper below epidermis. Treatment involves parenteral anti-staphylococcal antibiotics, wound care, analgesia and rehydration as appropriate.

2. G – Herpes simplex virus (HSV)

Most childhood HSV infections (outside the neonatal period) are due to HSV type 1, primarily transmitted via contact with infected saliva. Herpetic gingivostomatitis is the most frequent clinical presentation of primary infection in children, usually affecting those aged 6 months to 5 years. Herpetic whitlow is seen particularly in children who suck the thumb. The incubation period for HSV ranges from 2 to 12 days, while viral shedding from an infected individual may persist for up to 3 weeks. Usually an abrupt onset of illness with high fever and listlessness. Child typically refuses to eat or drink due to markedly swollen and sometimes bleeding gums with associated drooling of saliva. Vesicular lesions may develop on tongue, buccal mucosa, palate, lips and face. Tender submandibular and cervical lymphadenopathy also present. Children may require admission for intravenous fluids and analgesia. In severe cases or those caught early on in the illness, anti-viral therapy with aciclovir may be indicated. Children with eczema and those who are immunocompromised are at particular risk. Secondary bacterial infection may occur.

3. G – Herpes simplex virus

The child has a rash known as erythema multiforme, which is characterised by the target lesion but can present with a wide spectrum of severity. Erythema multiforme can be caused by an extensive array of infectious agents, drugs and other causes. HSV is thought to be the trigger for almost 100% of cases of erythema multiforme minor (see below) and is also thought to account for almost half of cases of erythema multiforme major. The precipitating HSV infection itself may be subclinical. Other causative agents include:

- infective – mycoplasma, staphylococcal species, *Pneumococcus*, Epstein–Barr virus, adenovirus, Coxsackie virus, parvovirus
- drugs – penicillin, cephalosporins, trimethoprim, anti-tuberculous therapy, carbamazepine, sodium valproate
- environmental – cold, sunlight, radiotherapy.

Erythema multiforme minor consists of localised skin eruption with little or no mucosal involvement whereas in Erythema multiforme major, the mucosal involvement is more extensive, with Stevens–Johnson syndrome representing the most severe form. Up to 70% of cases have mucosal involvement, primarily oral, but can also affect eyes and genitalia. Prodromal symptoms may be mild or absent in erythema multiforme minor, with 50% of patients with erythema multiforme major having non-specific symptoms that precede the eruption by 1 to 14 days. Skin lesions typically start as a dull red macule or urticarial plaque which develops a central papule or vesicle which then clears. The outer ring becomes raised and oedematous. The distribution is usually distal at first, spreading centrally and primarily affecting extensor surfaces. The palms, neck and face are frequently involved.

A punch biopsy will confirm the diagnosis but is not routinely indicated in milder cases. Treatment involves that of the underlying infective condition or withdrawal of suspected drug. Symptomatic treatment includes oral anti-histamines, analgesia and mouth/eye care for mucosal involvement. Immunosuppressive agents such as systemic corticosteroids and ciclosporin may be needed in severe cases. Erythema multiforme minor usually resolves within 2–3 weeks but episodes are frequently recurrent. Erythema multiforme major is often more protracted, lasting 3–6 weeks.

dermatology

ENDOCRINOLOGY AND SYNDROMES ANSWERS

76. Addison's disease

Answers: A E

- Incidence 1 in 10 000.
- Commonest cause is auto-immune.
- Familial incidence.
- Female preponderance.
- Auto antibodies usually present.
- Associated with other autoimmune conditions including hypothyroidism, hypoparathyroidism, diabetes mellitus, cirrhosis and alopecia.

Presenting features:

- hypoglycaemia
- lethargy
- muscle weakness
- fatigue
- gastrointestinal symptoms
- hyperpigmentation.

Investigations:

- hyponatraemia
- hyperkalaemia
- renin is elevated
- short synacthen test – no rise in cortisol at 60 or 120 minutes.

NB: Baseline cortisol may be normal.

Addisonian crisis:

- may be the presenting feature
- precipitated by intercurrent illness or stress
- dehydration, hypotension and collapse
- electrolyte disturbance as above.

endocrinology and syndromes

Management:

- Long-term treatment with oral hydrocortisone and fludrocortisone. Hydrocortisone needs to be increased at times of stress.
- Monitoring of growth and bone age.
- Addisonian crisis
  - normal saline with added dextrose
  - intravenous hydrocortisone.

Other causes of adrenal insufficiency:

- adrenoleukodystrophy.
- adrenal destruction, eg birth injury, Waterhouse–Friderichsen syndrome (associated with meningococcal septicaemia), tuberculosis, tumour metastases.
- congenital adrenal hyperplasia.
- congenital adrenal hypoplasia.
- steroid usage.
- steroid withdrawal.

77.   Down's syndrome

Answers: A B C D E

A thorough knowledge of the genetics, clinical features, management and complications of Down's syndrome and of the other common chromosomal disorders is necessary for the exam and can be found in any of the larger paediatric texts (see Bibliography). Down's syndrome is associated with an increased incidence of

- congenital heart disease (AVSD, VSD, PDA)
- oesophageal atresia
- duodenal atresia
- Hirschsprung's
- coeliac disease
- hypothyroidism
- obstructive sleep apnoea
- pulmonary hypertension
- immunodeficiency
- cataract
- cervical instability
- leukaemia
- Alzheimer's disease.

endocrinology and
syndromes

78. Homocystinuria and Marfan's syndrome

Answers: C D

Homocystinuria

The incidence of homocystinuria is 1 in 300 000. Inheritance is autosomal recessive, and prenatal diagnosis is possible. It is a disorder of the conversion of methionine into cystine with a consequent accumulation of homocystine. Clinical features of homocystinuria include:

- normal at birth
- marfanoid features, tall and thin with long fingers, the lower segment of the body longer than the upper segment and an arm span greater than height
- subluxed lens – downward and inward
- stiff joints
- connective tissue weakness – hernia, scoliosis
- propensity to vascular thrombosis
- progressive mental retardation (70%).

Diagnosis is based on plasma and urinary amino acids. Treatment aims to reduce the homocystine levels. Options include pyridoxine, folic acid, a low protein diet and aspirin as an anti-thrombolytic.

Marfan's syndrome

The incidence of Marfan's syndrome is between 1:16 000 and 1:60 000. Inheritance is autosomal dominant, with the gene locus on chromosome 15. Clinical features of Marfan's syndrome include:

- usually abnormal at birth
- long fingers, lower segment of the body longer than the upper segment, arm span greater than height
- subluxed lens – upwards and outwards, myopia, retinal detachment, glaucoma and cataract
- hyper-extendable joints
- connective tissue weakness – hernia and scoliosis
- mitral and aortic valve disease including aortic root dilatation
- pneumothorax.

Diagnosis is clinical. Slit-lamp examination and echocardiography are useful. Plasma amino acids exclude homocystinuria. Cardiac problems are a significant cause of morbidity.

Ectopia lentis

This is an isolated finding of a dislocated lens usually inherited as an autosomal dominant condition.

endocrinology and syndromes

79. Congenital hypothyroidism

Answers: C D

This has an incidence of 1 in 4000. It is usually asymptomatic until 6–12 weeks of age. The male to female ratio is 1:2. Symptoms and signs include poor feeding, constipation, lethargy, jaundice, large tongue, umbilical hernia and hoarse cry. Without treatment myxoedema (soft tissue accumulation) and failure to thrive will occur and cretinoid facies will develop. Neonatal screening is done with the Guthrie card test for phenylketonuria at 7–10 days. In most areas both T_4 and TSH are assayed. Usually T_4 will be low and TSH raised although in 10% the T_4 will be normal. Neonatal screening will not usually detect hypothyroidism due to TSH deficiency.

Congenital hypothyroidism is usually due to thyroid dysgenesis sometimes with ectopic thyroid tissue being present. Less commonly it occurs secondary to an inborn error of hormone synthesis (dyshormonogenesis). Treatment is lifelong with thyroxine. The dose is 100 μg/m^2/day. The best method of monitoring is by assessment of growth and development. A normal T_4 should be aimed for, but the TSH does not necessarily have to be normal. A high TSH and a normal T_4 may indicate poor compliance. Outcome is near normal (but not normal) development provided treatment is started early. Large cohort studies show a 5–10 point difference in IQ compared with a control population. The TSH at presentation is of prognostic importance with the higher levels being of greater concern.

80. Klinefelter's syndrome

Answers: B D

This has an incidence of 1 in 1000 males. The karyotype is 47 XXY. The aetiology is meiotic non-disjunction with the extra X chromosome coming from the father in 50% and the mother in the other 50%. Increased maternal age is a risk factor. There are a number of variants with more than two X chromosomes and mosaicism is common. Children are usually asymptomatic until the age of 5 years. After that they can present with behavioural problems or psychiatric disturbances. Intelligence is below average. The children are usually tall and thin. Puberty is delayed and infertility is common, and is due to azoospermia. The testes and phallus are small. Gynaecomastia is common (80%). There is an increased risk of pulmonary disease, varicose veins, breast cancer, leukaemia and mediastinal germ cell tumours. The prepubertal hormone profile is normal. By mid-puberty the follicle-stimulating hormone (FSH) and luteinising hormone (LH) levels are raised and the testosterone is low, and testosterone replacement is required. Elevated levels of oestradiol with a high oestradiol: testosterone ratio account for the development of gynaecomastia during puberty.

81.   Turner's syndrome

Answers: A C E

The incidence is 1 in 1500–2500 live born females. The karyotype is 45XO, 45XO/46XX. Mosaicism is present within most cell lines, and the paternal sex chromosome is lost. Loss of the maternal sex chromosome is a lethal deletion. There is no effect of increasing maternal age on incidence. Spontaneous fetal loss is common, usually in the first trimester.

Clinical features of Turner's syndrome:

- infants are usually small for dates
- lymphoedema and feeding difficulties in the neonatal period
- neck webbing
- cubitus valgus
- cardiac abnormalities – coarctation of the aorta, bicuspid aortic valve, aortic stenosis
- renal abnormalities – pelvic kidney, single kidney, pelvic-ureteric junction obstruction
- growth failure
- failure of puberty (hypergonadotrophic hypogonadism)
- pigmented naevi.

There are two options for management of growth failure:

- steroid treatment – oxandrolone, an anabolic steroid with minimal androgenic side-effects, if used in low dose will increase final adult height
- growth hormone – recombinant growth hormone is given as injections and increases final height (6–8 cm). Higher doses are needed than in growth hormone deficiency.

Management of pubertal failure

In 20% of cases of Turner's syndrome there is some ovarian function and development of some signs of puberty. Most require oestrogen replacement at 12–13 years. Once puberty is initiated, cyclical therapy with oestrogen and progesterone leads to menstrual cycles. Successful pregnancies have been described with ovum induction and in vitro fertilisation.

endocrinology and syndromes

82.   Phenylketonuria

Answers: A C D E

The metabolic block in phenylketonuria is the conversion of phenylalanine to tyrosine due to a deficiency of phenylalanine hydroxylase. Incidence is around 1 in 5000. Inheritance is autosomal recessive and carrier detection and prenatal diagnosis are possible. Affected infants are normal at birth. Clinical features in the untreated patient are:

- low IQ
- poor head growth
- seizures
- fair skin 'dilute pigmentation' – due to inadequate melanisation
- eczema-like rash.

Diagnosis is by measuring the plasma phenylalanine, which will be raised. The urine has a mousy, pungent odour due to the presence of phenylacetic acid, a metabolite of phenylalanine. Screening is carried out on all babies born in the UK by the Guthrie card. A drop of blood is collected on the card, and the blood is then used to measure the whole blood phenylalanine by a bacterial inhibition assay. This is done at 4–5 days, ideally after a feed. Treatment is with a diet that is selectively low in phenylalanine. The diet needs to be lifelong, particularly during pregnancy when untreated or partially treated phenylketonuria is teratogenic to the unborn child. The teratogenicity manifests as severe mental retardation with microcephaly.

83.   Bone age

Answers: B D E

The bone age defines skeletal maturation and if compared with chronological age gives an idea of growth potential. A child with a delayed bone age compared with chronological age has more growth potential than a child whose bone age equals the chronological age. The bone age, chronological age and height can be used to predict final adult height using special tables (eg Bayley–Pinneau). An X-ray of the left wrist is used to assess bone age. There are two systems in use:

- Greulich and Pyle system – comparing epiphyseal centres of the left hand and wrist to those in an atlas. The knee is sometimes used in younger children.
- TW2 system – where each epiphyseal centre is scored and the sum of the scores gives an estimate of the bone age.

endocrinology and syndromes

Causes of delayed bone age:

- constitutional short stature
- growth hormone deficiency
- androgen deficiency
- cortisol excess
- Turner's syndrome
- chronic disease, eg asthma, cystic fibrosis, chronic inflammatory bowel disease, coeliac disease
- malnutrition.

Causes of advanced bone age:

- hyperthyroidism
- androgen excess
  - congenital adrenal hyperplasia
  - precocious puberty
- oestrogen excess
- cerebral gigantism – Sotos' syndrome.

Familial short stature is a common cause of short stature in children. The parents' heights are usually on the lower centiles. Growth velocity is normal and bone age is equal to chronological age. Constitutional growth is slow with delayed puberty. Height velocity is normal but height, pubertal development and bone age are 2–4 years delayed. A family history is common and catch up does occur. Growth hormone excess has no effect on bone age, but causes an increase in linear growth.

84. Noonan's syndrome

Answers: A B D

This has an incidence of 1 in 1000–2500 live births. It occurs in both males and females. It is usually sporadic but occasionally familial (autosomal dominant with variable expressivity). The gene defect has been isolated on chromosome 12.

Clinical features of Noonan's syndrome:

- normal at birth
- neonatal feeding difficulties
- short stature and delayed puberty
- cardiac defects (pulmonary stenosis, peripheral pulmonary artery stenosis, PDA, ASD)
- broad or webbed neck
- chest defect deformity (pectus carinatum or pectus excavatum)
- cubitus valgus
- characteristic facies (hypertelorism, anti-mongoloid slant, micrognathia, high arched palate, ptosis).

The majority of females are fertile. Direct transmission from parent to child occurs in 30–70%. In males, cryptorchidism is often present which may lead to inadequate secondary sexual development. Bleeding problems occur in 20%. Mild to moderate mental retardation occurs in 30%.

85. Gynaecomastia

Answers: A B E

Breast tissue grows whenever the ratio of oestrogens to androgens is increased relative to normal adult values. This occurs in most newborn males due to maternal hormones. It also occurs in some males in early puberty when there is an increase in circulating oestrogen which occurs before the surge in masculinising hormones occurs. Differential diagnosis includes:

- physiological pubertal gynaecomastia
- familial gynaecomastia
- Klinefelter's syndrome
- hypergonadotrophic hypogonadism
- hepatic tumours and cirrhosis
- thyroid disease
- starvation
- adrenal/testicular tumours
- drugs:
  - steroids
  - tricyclics
  - cimetidine
  - spironolactone
  - cytotoxics
  - exogenous oestrogens.

86. Prader-Willi Syndrome

Answers: B C

The incidence of Prader–Willi Syndrome is 1 in 10 000. Occurrence is sporadic and associated with a micro-deletion in the long arm of chromosome 15 (70% of cases) or maternal uniparental disomy of the same area of chromosome 15. The condition goes through three main phases: an initial infantile hypotonic phase, followed by a childhood obese phase and then an adolescent phase during which behavioural problems predominate.

Clinical features of Prader–Willi syndrome:

- reduced fetal movements/infantile hypotonia
- dysmorphic features

- childhood hyperphagia and obesity
- short stature, delayed bone age, hypogonadism and infertility
- low IQ
- Diabetes mellitus.

Life expectancy is reduced as a consequence of the obesity and associated cardiac and respiratory complications.

87. Congenital adrenal hyperplasia

Answers: A C D E

The incidence of congenital adrenal hyperplasia is 1 in 5000. Inheritance is autosomal recessive. The gene defect is known and is part of the human leukocyte antigen (HLA) complex on chromosome 6. Antenatal diagnosis is possible by either chorionic villous sampling or by amniocentesis. Ninety-five per cent of defects are due to 21-hydroxylase deficiency, 75% of which are salt losers. 11-β-hydroxylase deficiency is the second commonest type and associated with hypertension after the first few years.

Presentation can be in any of the following ways:

- salt losing crises
- premature isosexual development (boys – small testes, large penis and scrotum)
- virilisation in females
- hypertension (11-β-hydroxylase deficiency).

Characteristic features of a salt-losing crisis include a low plasma sodium and chloride and a raised potassium with an elevated plasma renin and low plasma aldosterone.

Diagnosis:

- raised plasma 17-hydroxyprogesterone and raised urinary pregnanetriol (21-hydroxylase deficiency)
- raised plasma 11-deoxycortisol and 11-deoxycorticosterone (11-β-hydroxylase deficiency).

Treatment is by steroid replacement therapy. Hydrocortisone is used to replace corticosteroid activity, and fludrocortisone to replace mineralocorticoid activity. Monitoring of treatment is controversial and includes:

- measurement of growth
- bone age
- blood pressure
- plasma electrolytes
- steroid biochemistry (plasma 17-OH progesterone profiles in 21-hydroxylase deficiency).

endocrinology and syndromes

88. Growth hormone deficiency

Answers: A D

The incidence of growth hormone deficiency is 1 in 4000. The male to female ratio is 2:1. The majority of cases are idiopathic.

Causes of growth hormone deficiency:

- genetic – primary defect in growth hormone production
- congenital abnormality – associated with midline defects, eg septo-optic dysplasia, cleft lip and palate
- acquired – perinatal/postnatal infections, central nervous system infection, radiotherapy
- neoplasia – craniopharyngioma, glioma
- trauma – perinatal, basal skull fracture
- autoimmune.

Treatment of growth hormone deficiency is with growth hormone replacement therapy by injection. Growth hormone will increase the final adult height in children with proved growth hormone deficiency. It also increases the final adult height in girls with Turner's syndrome, in prepubertal children with chronic renal insufficiency and those with Prader–Willi syndrome (National Institute for Health and Clinical Excellence (NICE) guidelines 2002). It is also licensed for use in short children who are considered to be small for gestational age at birth. Growth hormone therapy has also been given for short stature due to emotional deprivation, skeletal dysplasia and familial short stature, although the results have been disappointing with no improvement in final adult height.

89. Growth hormone

Answers: A B E

Pharmacological stimuli of growth hormone secretion:

- insulin
- arginine
- glucagon
- L-dopa
- clonidine
- prostaglandin E_2
- bombesin
- galanin
- growth hormone releasing hormone
- strenuous exercise.

Provocation tests of growth hormone secretion are potentially hazardous. Insulin tolerance tests are now only performed in specialist centres because of the risk of severe hypoglycaemia. Other stimuli of growth hormone secretion such as glucagon and clonidine have important side-effects; glucagon causes vomiting and general fatigue and late hypoglycaemia, and clonidine causes drowsiness and hypotension.

90.   Precocious puberty

Answers: B C D

The commonest forms of sexual precocity are early breast development (thelarche) or the appearance of pubic or axillary hair (adrenarche). Isosexual (appropriate for sex) precocious puberty can be either true (central, gonadotrophin dependent) or false (gonadotrophin independent). True precocious puberty is 10 times commoner in girls than in boys. It is said to have occurred if the changes of puberty occur before the age of 8 years in girls and 9 years in boys.

Central (true) precocious puberty

This is gonadotrophin dependent and occurs as a consequence of the premature activation of gonadotrophin pulsatility which causes the onset of puberty. It is characterised by accelerated growth, advanced bone age and pubertal levels of LH, FSH and the sex steroids oestrogen and testosterone. It is usually idiopathic in girls (80%), an underlying aetiology being much commoner in boys. A CT head scan is indicated in all boys.

Causes:

* idiopathic
* hamartoma
* neurofibroma
* glioma
* hydrocephalus
* post trauma
* post meningitis/encephalitis
* prolonged untreated hypothyroidism.

False or gonadotrophin independent precocious puberty is characterised by a lack of consistency between different aspects of pubertal development, for example pubic hair and acne with no testicular development. Examples include congenital adrenal hyperplasia, oestrogen producing ovarian tumour, adrenal tumour and medication including anabolic steroids and the oral contraceptive pill.

endocrinology and syndromes

91. Fragile X Syndrome

Answers: A B D

Fragile X syndrome is a common disorder among mentally handicapped individuals (6% males, 0.3% females). The fragile site is on the long arm of chromosome X at Xq27.3. Inheritance is X-linked, but expression is due to the process of allelic expansion. The fragile X locus normally has 2800 trinucleotide base repeats, a small increase in the repeats makes it unstable and through successive generations there is an expansion in the repeats (female transmission increases the repeats) until the increase becomes clinically significant resulting in the fragile X syndrome.

Clinical features include: mental retardation (IQ 30–55 in males, mild mental retardation in females), prominent jaw, long face, large ears, macro-orchidism, hypotonia and joint laxity. The testicular enlargement is more prominent post puberty. Psychological features include cluttering of speech, hyperactivity, emotional instability and autistic features.

Other disorders associated with allelic expansion include:

- Huntingdon's disease (male transmission increases the repeat)
- myotonic dystrophy (maternal transmission increases the repeat).

In both disorders an increase in the repeat increases the severity of the disease with onset at an earlier age.

92. Galactosaemia

Answers: B C D E

Galactosaemia is a rare autosomal recessive disorder. The incidence is around 1 in 50 000 live births.

Three separate defects have been described:

- Galactokinase deficiency which causes cataracts only.
- Mild galactose–1-phosphate-uridyltransferase deficiency – Duarte variant in which there are no symptoms, but erythrocyte galactose–1-phosphate-uridyltransferase activity is reduced.
- Severe galactose–1-phosphate uridyltransferase deficiency – widespread, generalised disorder which produces mental retardation, failure to thrive, cataracts, jaundice, hypoglycaemia and hepatomegaly. There is a rapid progression to irreversible severe mental retardation and cirrhosis in undiagnosed patients.

Severe galactose–1-phosphate-uridyltransferase is the commonest presentation. It usually presents in the neonatal period. Reducing substances are present in the

endocrinology and syndromes

urine after the first feed. This is detectable on testing with Clinitest tablets. Urine dipstick for glucose is negative. Diagnosis is confirmed by measuring the enzymes. Treatment is with a lactose-free diet, but the outcome is variable. Some degree of mental retardation is usual. A number are severely retarded.

93. Aldosterone

Answer: A

Aldosterone is produced in the zona glomerulosa of the adrenal cortex. Secretion is regulated by activation of the renin-angiotensin system. Renin production occurs in the juxtaglomerular apparatus in response to a drop in serum sodium or a fall in blood pressure. The effect of aldosterone is on the sodium–potassium exchange pump in the distal tubules of the kidney. It acts to increase absorption of sodium from the distal tubule in exchange for potassium or hydrogen ions. Increased sodium absorption increases water absorption and blood pressure. Hypoaldosteronism results in a low serum sodium and a high serum potassium with a low aldosterone and high renin. Deficiency of aldosterone occurs in adrenal hypoplasia, inborn errors of steroidogenesis, Addison's disease, adrenoleukodystrophy, exogenous steroid withdrawal, destruction of adrenal gland (eg haemorrhage, tuberculosis) or drugs which cause increased steroid metabolism (eg rifampicin, ketoconazole, phenytoin, phenobarbital). Pseudohypoaldosteronism is due to end-organ resistance to aldosterone. It results in hyponatraemia, hyperkalaemia with a raised renin and aldosterone.

94. Normal physiological and endocrine changes of puberty

Answers: A B D

In the three years prior to puberty low levels of pulsatile LH become detectable during sleep. LH and FSH are produced in the anterior pituitary and released due to pulsatile gonadotrophin releasing hormone (GnRH) secreted by the hypothalamus. There is an increase in the amplitude and frequency of LH secretion as puberty approaches which causes enlargement of the gonads. In males, the testicles produce testosterone and in girls the ovaries produce oestradiol and ovarian androgens, which, with the adrenal androgens, produce secondary sexual characteristics.

Average age at onset of puberty is 11 years in girls/11.5 years in boys. The first sign is breast bud development, followed by the appearance of pubic hair 6–12 months later. Menarche usually occurs 2–2.5 years after breast bud development. Peak height velocity in girls occurs at breast stage 2–3 and virtually always precedes menarche. Onset of puberty in boys is at 11.5 years. The first sign is testicular enlargement (greater than 3 ml) and thinning of the scrotum. This is followed by

endocrinology and syndromes

pigmentation of the scrotum and growth of the penis, and pubic hair follows. Peak height velocity (growth spurt) is two years later in boys than in girls and occurs at testicular stage 4–5 (ie testicular volume 10–12 ml), which is around 13–14 years of age. Breast enlargement occurs in 40–60% of boys (significant enough to cause social embarrassment in 10%) and is a result of oestradiol produced by the metabolism of testosterone. It usually resolves within 3 years. During puberty, elongation of the eye often occurs causing short sightedness.

95. Type 1 (insulin dependent) diabetes

Answer: E

Type 1 diabetes (insulin dependent diabetes mellitus – IDDM) occurs as the result of destruction of pancreatic islet cells. Clinical symptoms occur when there is approximately 20% of islet cell activity remaining. Pathogenesis is thought to be autoimmune. In 80–90% of newly diagnosed diabetic patients there are islet cell antibodies. There is an association with HLA antigens: HLA-B8, HLA-BW15, HLA-DR3 and HLA-DR4 (each of these give a two- to three-fold increased risk of developing type 1 diabetes). Homozygosity to the absence of aspartic acid in the HLA-DQ beta chain confers a 100-fold increased risk.

Siblings of an affected individual are at a 1–7% risk of developing type 1 diabetes (annual UK incidence 7.7 per 100 000). There is a seasonal variation in incidence with peaks during the autumn and winter months. There is also an increased incidence after Coxsackie, mumps and rubella epidemics suggesting that an initial viral infection triggers an autoimmune response against islet cells. There is a peak incidence at age 5–7 years (when children start school and exposure to viral infection increases) and at puberty (10–14 years).

Treatment with immunosuppressive agents has been found to lengthen the honeymoon period. The risks of treatment are greater than the benefits of starting insulin later.

96. Complications of type 1 diabetes

Answers: B C D E

Complications can be acute or chronic, acute complications being hypoglycaemia, hyperglycaemia and ketoacidosis. Complications can be grouped according to systems:

- central nervous system – diabetic coma, hypoglycaemia, mood change and irritability
- peripheral nervous system – mononeuropathies (facial nerve the most common), peripheral neuropathy, sensory loss

- musculoskeletal – proximal myopathy, joint contractures
- vascular – peripheral vascular disease, ischaemic heart disease, hypertension
- eyes – cataracts, retinopathy, acute myopia with hyperglycaemia which recovers with treatment
- renal – urinary tract infection, nephropathy
- skin – lipohypertrophy, lipoatrophy, skin infections, vaginal candidiasis
- autoimmune – thyroid disease, Addison's disease, coeliac disease
- growth – pubertal delay (with poor control), excess weight gain (with poor dietary compliance), weight loss (due to poor control or inadequate intake), short stature, Mauriac's syndrome
- pregnancy – increased risk of intrauterine death, congenital anomalies, macrosomia and neonatal hypoglycaemia.

Mauriac's syndrome

This is IDDM associated with dwarfism. The dwarfism is associated with a glycogen-laden enlarged liver, osteopenia, limited joint mobility, growth failure and delayed puberty. It is due to under insulinisation.

97. Graves' disease

Answers: B C D

Graves' disease is thyrotoxicosis associated with eye manifestations. Five percent of cases present in childhood, the peak incidence being during adolescence. There is a female predominance (5:1), and a family history is common. There is an association with HLA B8, HLA DR3.

Clinical features of Graves' disease:

- emotional disturbance
- irritability
- poor attention span
- tremor
- tachycardia
- increased appetite
- weight loss
- diarrhoea
- goitre
- exophthalmus and ophthalmoplegia
- lid lag
- cardiac involvement (rare in childhood).

endocrinology and syndromes

T_3 and T_4 are elevated, TSH is low. TSH receptor stimulating antibodies are usually present at diagnosis and disappear as the condition remits. Approximately half of childhood cases will remit spontaneously within 2–4 years. Many will progress to become clinically hypothyroid. Medical treatment is with carbimazole and propranolol (the latter to control acute symptoms). Block replacement means that both carbimazole and thyroxine are used. Definitive treatment (favoured by many) is either by subtotal thyroidectomy or the use of radioactive iodine. Severe eye disease may require treatment with prednisolone.

Neonatal thyrotoxicosis is a transient condition resulting from the placental transfer of thyroid stimulating antibodies from a thyrotoxic mother.

Other diseases associated with HLA B8/DR3:

- Addison's disease
- type 1 diabetes
- coeliac disease
- chronic active hepatitis
- systemic lupus erythematosus
- dermatomyositis
- autoimmune thyroiditis
- primary sclerosing cholangitis.

98. Chromosome deletions

Answers: B C

Deletions occur when a piece of chromosome is missing and are detectable on routine chromosome preparations. Micro-deletions are smaller and require higher quality preparations to be detected and so need to be specifically requested. Examples of deletions include:

- Wolf–Hirschhorn syndrome – 4p-
- cri du chat syndrome – 5p-.

Examples of micro-deletions include:

- William's syndrome – 7q23-
- WAGR syndrome – 11p13-
- Prader–Willi syndrome –15q11–13- (paternal)
- Angelman's syndrome – 15q11–13- (maternal)
- Rubinstein–Taybi syndrome – 16p13-
- DiGeorge (CATCH 22) – 22q11-.

99.   Achondroplasia

Answers: A B C E

Achondroplasia is autosomal dominant, and 80% of cases represent new mutations. The incidence is 1:20 000. Changes present at birth and include

- large head with short extremities
- frontal bossing
- flat nasal bridge
- trunk and limbs are short, with major shortening proximally (humerus and femur)
- spinal stenosis
- small foramen magnum.

Diagnosis is by skeletal survey. Special growth charts have been developed. Development is initially delayed with hypotonia but in the absence of hydrocephalus long-term motor and mental development is normal. Complications include hydrocephalus and cervical or lumbar cord compression secondary to the small foramen magnum and narrow spinal canal. Bowing of the legs and lordosis also occur and may need orthopaedic intervention. Life span is normal.

100.   *c: acanthosis nigrans*

Type 2 diabetes in childhood has become an increasingly recognised problem over recent years. Predisposing factors include ethnicity (highest incidence in Asian and African American racial groups), obesity, a positive family history of type 2 diabetes and female sex. Intrauterine growth retardation is also known to be a risk factor. Insulin resistance and impaired glucose tolerance are seen. Presentation is rarely acute with children often having no or mild symptoms only for a considerable length of time before diagnosis although ketoacidosis can occur. Acanthosis nigricans is a marker of high insulin levels and thus helps to differentiate type 2 from type 1 diabetes in affected individuals.

Treatment is aimed at achieving good glycaemic control (to minimise risk of micro-and macro-vascular complications) and maintenance of a reasonable weight. There appears to be a greater risk of nephropathy than retinopathy. Dietary adjustments and oral hypoglycaemic agents (eg metformin) can be used, but in some cases, insulin may be required. The role of prevention is likely to assume greater significance.

endocrinology and syndromes

101. D: Long-term consequences include lowered IQ and decreased head size

Causes of hypoglycaemia:

- excessive glucose utilisation
    - hyperinsulinism (eg IDM, insulin producing tumour)
    - defects in alternative fuel production (eg medium chain acyl CoA dehydrogenase deficiency (MCAD))
    - sepsis
- glucose underproduction
    - inadequate stores (eg preterm, small for gestational age (SGA))
- abnormal hepatic glucose production (eg glycogen storage disease type I, galactosaemia, maple syrup urine disease)
- hormonal abnormalities (eg panhypopituitarism, growth hormone and cortisol deficiency)
- toxins (eg ethanol and propranolol).

Usual definition of hypoglycaemia is a blood sugar of less than 2.6 mmol/l. To aid diagnosis of possible underlying metabolic abnormality it is critical that samples (blood and urine) are taken at the time of hypoglycaemia. As hypoglycaemia can be asymptomatic, 'at risk' babies such as SGA, premature and IDM should have frequent screening for hypoglycaemia for at least the first 24 hours of life. Treatment consists of an iv bolus of 10% dextrose (2.5 ml/kg) followed by an iv infusion to match normal hepatic glucose production (typically 5–8 mg/kg/min in an otherwise normal neonate). Intramuscular glucagon is the treatment of choice within the home setting only. It is known that even asymptomatic hypoglycaemia in the neonatal period can have long-term consequences in the form of neurocognitive impairment and abnormalities apparent on neuroimaging.

102. A: Precocious puberty

Diagnosis of McCure Albright Syndrome requires at least two features of the triad of polyostotic fibrous dysplasia, café au lait pigmentation and autonomous endocrine hyperfunction to be present. The commonest endocrine abnormality is gonadotrophin-independent precocious puberty (ie autonomous ovarian or testicular function). It is far commoner in girls than boys, with breast development and vaginal bleeding being seen in some cases before a year of age. Hyperthyroidism, hypercortisolism and acromegaly can also be seen. Adrenocorticotropic hormone (ACTH)-independent Cushing's syndrome generally results in growth failure and hypertension in infancy.

Fibrous dysplasia most commonly affects long bones, ribs and skull and can be asymptomatic or cause pain and pathological fracture in more severe cases. A family history of café au lait spots raises the suspicion of neurofibromatosis (an autosomal dominant condition) whereas McCune–Albright syndrome is sporadically occurring. Non-endocrine abnormalities may include hypophosphataemia, chronic liver disease, tachycardia and cardiac arrhythmia.

Treatment is aimed at correcting the underlying endocrine abnormality, with specialist orthopaedic input if bony lesions are problematic. Potential complications include loss of final adult height potential (due to precocious puberty and/or hypophosphataemia), pathological fractures and sudden death.

103. C: Ambiguous genitalia/intersex conditions

The presence of ambiguous genitalia and intersex conditions constitute a medical and social emergency and requires diagnostic input from a team of professionals including paediatricians, surgeons, geneticists and psychologists. The commonest cause, congenital adrenal hyperplasia (CAH) may also be a life-threatening condition if associated with salt-wasting. Hence there should be no delay in performing diagnostic tests which should include chromosomal analysis, urea and electrolytes, hormonal investigation (blood and urine) and abdominal and pelvic ultrasound scans. Other causes include $5\text{-}\alpha$-reductase deficiency, androgen insensitivity syndrome and exposure to high levels of maternal androgens in the first trimester of pregnancy.

In normal embryological development, the presence or absence of a Y chromosome leads to gonadal differentiation in the sixth week. The process can be disrupted by exposure to inadequate or excessive amounts of androgens (testosterone and dihydrotestosterone) and Mullerian-inhibiting substance or by end-organ insensitivity to their actions. Caution must be exercised in the presence of incompletely descended palpable gonads. While only testicular material descends fully, ovotestes (as seen in true hermaphroditism) can sometimes be felt in labioscrotal folds. Conversely, the absence of palpable gonads in an otherwise fully virilised infant should raise the possibility of a severely virilised female with CAH.

The development of gender identity is a complex, poorly understood process, with evidence showing that it is determined not only by phenotypic appearance but by the brain's pre- and post-natal development. Parents should be given as much information as possible to enable them to make informed decisions about gender assignment and possible subsequent genital surgery.

endocrinology and syndromes

104. E: It may result in subclinical coronary artery sclerosis and atherosclerosis in childhood

An increasing problem that is difficult to treat and has implications for both physical and psychosocial health in childhood and beyond. The majority of children are obese due to their lifestyle and not any underlying medical condition. There is little evidence to support the long-term effectiveness of the currently used strategies of an improved dietary intake and increased levels of physical activity. Risk factors associated with obesity are deprivation and increasing age. There is no difference in prevalence of obesity between boys and girls. Parental obesity is a risk factor for persistence of childhood obesity into adulthood. As childhood is a period of growth, body mass index (BMI) is not a static measurement but varies with age and sex. Obesity in childhood is therefore defined as a BMI > 95th centile for age and sex.

Consequences of obesity include hypertension, an increased risk of developing or worsening asthma and abnormalities of foot structure and function. In addition, adverse lipid profiles, insulin resistance and hyperinsulinaemia are also seen, leading to atherosclerosis and coronary artery disease, which are seen with greater frequency in obese children at post mortem. Girls are more likely than boys to suffer psychological distress related to their obesity. Adults who were obese children are also more at risk of cardiovascular disease and have an increased mortality risk per se.

105. GROWTH AND DEVELOPMENT

1. B – Turner's syndrome

A karyotype is indicated in any female with short stature even if dysmorphic features are not obviously present. Some girls with Turner's syndrome may have height within the normal range up to the age of 11 years as is the case here. Presentation in adolescence and adulthood is often with issues regarding puberty and fertility as well as short stature. Adrenarche (pubic hair growth) occurs at a normal age but breast development is absent due to ovarian failure (confirmed by elevated levels of FSH and LH which excludes hypopituitarism as a cause). Thyroid functions should also be checked due to increased risk of hypothyroidism which can also affect growth. Growth hormone can be administered to increase final height, although growth hormone deficiency is not a feature of Turner's syndrome. In this case, the child has an appropriate bone age excluding constitutional delay as the cause of her short stature. The parental heights and target centile range are not suggestive of familial short stature.

endocrinology and syndromes

2. A – Russell–Silver syndrome

The primary abnormality is growth failure, presenting with intrauterine growth retardation (IUGR) (compare with Noonan's syndrome where birth weight typically normal), feeding difficulties, failure to thrive or post-natal growth retardation. Final height is typically less than or equal to −3.6 SD below the mean. Features described here that are consistent with the diagnosis of Russell–Silver syndrome include facial dysmorphism in the form of triangular facies, but normal head circumference, the head therefore appearing disproportionately large. Other features may include clinodactyly of the little finger, hypospadias or posterior urethral valves, cardiac defects (rare) and late closure of the anterior fontanelle. Approximately 10% of patients have uniparental disomy of chromosome 7, but the aetiology is not defined in the majority of cases. Babies with feeding difficulties may require nasogastric feeds. Growth hormone treatment may be used when the child is school aged but growth hormone levels are typically normal.

Infants with William's syndrome (see Question 2) are described as having 'elfin facies' and may also present with failure to thrive, but hypercalcaemia is typically present and cardiovascular involvement (most often supravalvular aortic stenosis) is commonly seen. Growth hormone deficiency typically presents in childhood with a reduced growth velocity rather than in infancy, unless it is associated with hypoglycaemia or other endocrine/midline abnormalities such as hypopituitarism or septo-optic dysplasia.

3. C – Constitutional delay of growth and puberty

This is the commonest cause of short stature and pubertal delay. It is more commonly seen in children whose height has been on a lower growth centile pre-puberty. It is a variant of normal and not a disorder, but can cause psychological trauma for some affected individuals requiring intervention. It is approximately twice as common in boys as girls. Typically affected individuals have a normal birth weight with deceleration in both height and weight velocity in the first 3–6 months of life. Bone age is typically delayed by 2–4 years. Physical examination is normal. There is typically a family history of delayed puberty in first- or second-degree relatives of either sex.

This is a diagnosis of exclusion. Random growth hormone measurements are of little value as its release from the pituitary gland is pulsatile. IGF–1 (insulin-like growth factor 1) should be measured instead as a reflection of growth hormone production. Both growth hormone and IGF–1 results may appear decreased in the context of chronological age in the presence of delayed bone age and they should therefore be interpreted with caution. Other routine blood tests may be performed to exclude systemic illness such as inflammatory bowel disease or autoimmune disorders. Magnetic resonance imaging (MRI) of the pituitary gland

endocrinology and syndromes

may be indicated in the presence of abnormal hormonal profiles or symptoms such as headache. No treatment is required for the majority although in males experiencing psychological difficulties due to their delayed development and growth, short courses of androgens can accelerate linear growth and onset of pubertal changes. This has not been shown to have a detrimental effect on adult height, but it will not increase final adult stature.

Children with Noonan's syndrome (see Question 86) do not always have any immediately obvious dysmorphic facial features but careful examination is required as the diagnosis of this condition is usually on the basis of clinical findings only. Kallmann's syndrome (hypogonadotropic hypogonadism associated with anosmia) typically presents with delayed puberty, but individuals with this condition have a normal height for age.

106. HYPOCALCAEMIA

1. B – DiGeorge syndrome (see Question 173)

Hypocalcaemia is a feature and may cause abnormal muscular activity. Characteristic facies include low-set ears and hypertelorism. Feeding difficulties are common causing failure to thrive. Cardiac abnormalities may also be present.

2. F – Pseudopseudohypoparathyroidism

Dysmorphic features described consistent with diagnosis of pseudohypoparathyroidism (see below) but normal biochemistry means the diagnosis is one of pseudopseudohypoparathyroidism.

3. E – Chronic renal failure

Hypocalcaemia can be a feature of chronic renal failure (see below and Question 266). High serum phosphate in presence of osteopenia indicative of renal pathology (NB: low serum phosphate and osteopenia suggests vitamin D deficiency or hypophosphataemic rickets.) Fanconi's syndrome is associated with a low serum phosphate (see Question 273).

endocrinology and syndromes

Hypocalcaemia

Hypocalcaemia is frequently asymptomatic. If clinical manifestations occur, they are due to disturbance in cellular membrane potential, eg tetany and arrhythmias such as heart block. A reduction in the ionised fraction of calcium can result in symptoms in the presence of a normal total plasma calcium level, eg in severe alkalosis. Hypocalcaemia is the major stimulus for parathyroid hormone secretion. Causes include:

- hypoparathyroidism – low calcium, high phosphate.
- pseudohypoparathyroidism – low calcium in the presence of normal/raised parathyroid hormone levels, ie lack of normal response to parathyroid hormone. Characteristic phenotype of short stature, rounded face, obesity, shortened fourth and fifth metacarpals, developmental delay.
  (NB: pseudopseudohypoparathyroidism presents with above phenotype but normal biochemical profile).
- vitamin D deficiency (rickets) – causes increased calcium mobilisation from bone so plasma calcium levels often within reference range. Low phosphate and elevated alkaline phosphatase with classical X-ray appearances of metaphyseal cupping and widening (splaying) and osteopenia.
- DiGeorge syndrome (see Question 173).
- chronic renal failure – due to both reduced production of $1,25(OH)_2D_3$ and hyperphosphataemia secondary to reduced renal excretion of phosphate.
- renal tubular disease – including Fanconi's syndrome.
- magnesium depletion.
- hypoproteinaemia.
- septic shock.

GASTROENTEROLOGY AND NUTRITION ANSWERS

107. Familial adenomatous polyposis coli

Answer: C

Juvenile polyps

Eighty-five per cent of polyps seen in childhood. They present at age 2–6 years with painless blood per rectum. Most polyps are solitary and located within 30 cm of the anus. They are not pre-malignant.

Peutz–Jegher syndrome

This is autosomal dominantly inherited. It consists of diffuse gastrointestinal hamartomatous polyps associated with hyperpigmentation of the buccal mucosa and lips. It is pre-malignant.

Gardner's syndrome and familial adenomatous polyposis coli

Best considered together. Both conditions are inherited as an autosomal dominant. Gardner's syndrome is familial adenomatous polyposis plus bony lesions, subcutaneous tumours and cysts. Both conditions carry a high risk of colonic carcinoma, and prophylactic colectomy at the end of the second decade is advised.

108. *Helicobacter pylori*

Answer: B

Helicobacter pylori is a Gram-negative organism. Infection is usually acquired in childhood, prevalence rates, however, are variable. Persistent infection causes a chronic gastritis which may be asymptomatic. There is a strong relation between *Helicobacter* infection and peptic ulceration in adults. *Helicobacter pylori* is also a carcinogen. There is no proved association between *Helicobacter* infection and recurrent abdominal pain. Transmission is faeco-oral and familial clustering is common. Diagnosis is by the following:

- serology
- rapid urease tests – C13 breath test, CLO test
- histology

- culture (difficult).

Treatment is indicated for gastritis or peptic ulceration. There are various regimens, the most common in children is omeprazole, amoxicillin and metronidazole for 2 weeks.

Other causes of antral gastritis and peptic ulceration
- Zollinger–Ellison syndrome
- Crohn's disease
- anti-inflammatory drugs
- auto-immune gastritis (adults).

109. Crohn's disease

Answers: A D E

Crohn's disease is a chronic inflammatory disorder of the bowel involving any region from mouth to anus. The inflammation is transmural with skip lesions. There has been an increase in incidence over the past 10 years in children across all age groups, and 10–15% of cases present in childhood, usually in the second decade. The prevalence in the childhood population is 10–20 per 100 000. The commonest presenting symptoms are abdominal pain, diarrhoea and weight loss. Growth failure with delayed bone maturation and delayed sexual development is common. The diagnosis is made on the basis of clinical symptoms, raised inflammatory indices and diagnostic tests including barium radiology and colonoscopy with biopsy. Treatment is difficult as the disease often runs a chronic relapsing course. The aim of treatment is to induce a disease remission and facilitate normal growth and development.

The most widely used treatment in children is enteral nutrition, used as an exclusion diet for up to 8 weeks followed by a period of controlled food re-introduction. The type of enteral nutrition used varies and can be either elemental (protein broken down into amino acids) or polymeric (whole protein). This induces remission in up to 90% of patients. Maintenance is with 5-aminosalicylic acid (ASA) derivatives. Unfortunately disease relapse is common and either repeated courses of enteral nutrition or corticosteroids are required. Corticosteroid dependence or resistance can occur and additional immunosuppression (eg azathioprine) or surgery is often required.

Extra-intestinal manifestations of Crohn's disease:

- joint disease in 10% – ankylosing spondylitis rarely
- skin rashes – erythema nodosum, erythema multiforme, pyoderma gangrenosum
- liver disease (rare in childhood) – sclerosing cholangitis, chronic active hepatitis, cirrhosis

- uveitis, episcleritis
- osteoporosis
- clubbing.

NB: Ankylosing spondylitis and sclerosing cholangitis are rare associations, rather than characteristic features of Crohn's disease.

110. Hydrolysed protein formulae

Answers: A D

A hydrolysed protein is one which is broken down into oligopeptides and peptides. A hydrolysed protein milk formula is therefore one which contains whole protein broken down into oligopeptides and peptides. An elemental formula is one in which the protein is broken down further into single amino acids. The following are hydrolysed protein formulae:

- Pregestimil
- Nutramigen
- Prejomin
- Pepti-Junior
- Flexical
- Neocate
- Elemental EO28.

Neocate and Elemental EO28 are elemental formulae. These formulae are indicated in conditions where the protein in milk is implicated in the pathogenesis as an antigen. Examples include:

- cows' milk protein intolerance
- enteropathies, eg post-gastroenteritis
- post-necrotising enterocolitis
- short gut
- severe eczema
- Crohn's disease.

Hydrolysed protein formulae are generally lactose free as are soya milk preparations. Wysoy and Formula S are both lactose-free soya milks. The indications for a soya milk preparation are similar to the indications for a hydrolysate. A soya preparation is cheaper. If used for cows' milk protein intolerance then cross reactivity with soya protein is common and about one-sixth of patients will also be intolerant to the soya preparation. In this circumstance it is necessary to use a hydrolysed formula. Prematil is a pre-term formula. Maxijul is a glucose polymer. Paediasure is a whole-protein nutritional supplement.

gastroenterology and nutrition

111. Meckel's diverticulum

Answers: A B D E

Meckel's diverticulum is a remnant of the vitello-intestinal duct which is present in 2% of individuals. In 50% it contains ectopic gastric, pancreatic or colonic tissue. It is located in the distal ileum on the anti-mesenteric border within 100 cm of the ileo-caecal valve and is around 5–6 cm long. It usually presents with intermittent, painless blood per rectum. Bleeding can be quite severe and may require a blood transfusion. Other presentations include intussusception (commoner in older males), perforation and peritonitis. The technetium scan is used to look for ectopic gastric mucosa. Other causes of blood per rectum in childhood include:

- anal fissure
- volvulus
- intussusception
- peptic ulcer
- polyp
- inflammatory bowel disease
- haemolytic uraemic syndrome
- infective colitis
- Henoch–Schönlein purpura
- vascular malformation
- oesophagitis/varices
- epistaxis
- necrotising enterocolitis.

112. Breast feeding

Answers: A E

This is a difficult question which recurs and is somewhat controversial. Contraindications to breast feeding are either absolute (always apply) or relative.

Absolute contraindications:

- galactosaemia
- cytotoxic (immunosuppressive) drugs, eg methotrexate, cyclophosphamide.

Relative contraindications:

- tuberculosis
- hepatitis B
- chickenpox
- maternal ill health
- amiodarone

gastroenterology and nutrition

- atenolol
- ergot alkaloids
- gold salts
- radiopharmaceuticals.

With regard to tuberculosis, infants can be immunised at birth with isoniazid-resistant bacille Calmette Guérin (BCG) and treated with a course of isoniazid. With regard to HIV, the virus has been cultured from breast milk and is transmitted in it. In the Western world this makes breast feeding a contraindication as it will increase the perinatal transmission rate. The problem is not so straightforward in the developing world where the risks associated with bottle feeding are high.

113. Abetalipoproteinaemia

Answers: A D E

Abetalipoproteinaemia is inherited as autosomally recessive. Long-chain fatty acids are transmitted as chylomicrons along the thoracic duct. Betalipoprotein is part of the chylomicron. The pathogenesis of abetalipoproteinaemia is failure of chylomicron formation with impaired absorption of long-chain fats with fat retention in the enterocyte. Fat malabsorption occurs from birth. The condition presents in early infancy with failure to thrive, abdominal distension and foul smelling, bulky stools. Symptoms of vitamin E deficiency (ataxia, peripheral neuropathy and retinitis pigmentosa) develop later. The child is normal at birth.

Laboratory diagnosis:

- low serum cholesterol
- very low plasma triglyceride level
- acanthocytes on examination of the peripheral blood film
- absence of betalipoprotein in the plasma.

Treatment is by substituting medium-chain triglycerides for long-chain triglycerides in the diet. Medium-chain triglycerides are absorbed via the portal vein rather than the thoracic duct. In addition, high doses of the fat-soluble vitamins (A, D, E and K) are required. Most of the neurological abnormalities are reversible if high doses of vitamin E are given early.

Causes of acanthocytosis:

- abetalipoproteinaemia
- chronic liver disease
- hyposplenism

Associations of retinitis pigmentosa:

- abetalipoproteinaemia
- Laurence–Moon–Biedl syndrome
- Usher's syndrome

gastroenterology and nutrition

- Refsum's disease
- Alport's syndrome
- familial
- idiopathic.

114. Acrodermatitis enteropathica

Answers: C D E

This shows autosomal recessive inheritance. The basic defect is impaired absorption of zinc in the gut. It presents with skin rash around the mouth and peri-anal area, chronic diarrhoea at the time of weaning and recurrent infections. The hair has a reddish tint, and alopecia is characteristic. Superinfection with *Candida* is common as are paronychia, dystrophic nails, poor wound healing and ocular changes (photophobia, blepharitis, corneal dystrophy). Diagnosis is by serum zinc levels and the constellation of clinical signs. This is difficult as serum zinc is low as part of the acute phase response. Measurement of white cell zinc levels is more accurate. The plasma metallothionein level can also be measured. Metallothionein is a zinc-binding protein that is decreased in zinc deficiency but not in the acute phase response. The condition responds very well to treatment with oral zinc. Zinc deficiency can cause the following:

- iron deficiency anaemia
- acrodermatitis enteropathica
- hyperpigmentation
- poor wound healing
- immunodeficiency
- growth failure
- hypogonadism.

Clinically important trace elements are:

- chromium
- copper
- cobalt
- molybdenum
- manganese
- selenium
- zinc.

115. Vitamin A

Answers: A B C D E

Vitamin A is a fat-soluble vitamin (as are D, E and K). Deficiency causes night blindness, poor growth, xerophthalmia, follicular hyperplasia and impaired resistance to infection. Excess causes carotenaemia, hyperostosis with bone pain, hepatomegaly, alopecia and desquamation of the palms. Acute intoxication causes raised intracranial pressure. Dietary sources of vitamin are:

- milk
- fat
- fruit and vegetables
- egg
- liver.

Vitamin A has an important role in the resistance to infection particularly at mucosal surfaces. In developing countries where vitamin A deficiency is endemic, vitamin A reduces the morbidity and mortality in severe measles.

116. Breast feeding

Answers: A B D

Breast feeding and infection

Ten per cent of the protein in mature breast milk is secretory IgA. Lymphocytes, macrophages, proteins with non-specific anti-bacterial activity and complement are also present. There have been many studies in the developing world to show that infants fed formula milk have a higher mortality and morbidity, particularly from gastrointestinal infection. In the UK, studies have been done which show:

- breast feeding for more than 13 weeks reduces the incidence of gastrointestinal and respiratory infections
- the response to immunisation with the Hib vaccine is higher in breast fed than in formula fed infants.

The risk of necrotising enterocolitis in low birth weight babies is lower in those who are breast fed.

Breast feeding and allergy

The incidence of atopic eczema in infants born to atopic mothers is reduced by breast feeding. Overall however there is no reduction in atopy apart from this specific circumstance.

gastroenterology and nutrition

Breast feeding and neurological development

Although there are confounding variables which make study of this subject difficult, there is work that suggests that neurological development is enhanced in breast fed infants.

Breast feeding and diabetes

Infants who are breast fed have a reduced risk of developing diabetes.

Breast feeding and infantile colic

There is no good evidence to show that breast feeding reduces the incidence of infantile colic.

117. Vitamin K

Answers: C D E

The Royal College of Paediatrics and Child Health guidelines on vitamin K prophylaxis for haemorrhagic disease of the newborn are:

- All newborn infants should be given vitamin K.
- Intramuscular vitamin K, 1 mg, ensures adequate prophylaxis in normal term infants.
- If given orally, two doses of 2 mg vitamin K should be given to term infants at birth and at 4–7 days of age respectively. Further doses should be given at monthly intervals to exclusively breast fed infants until mixed feeding is established.
- Infants with jaundice suggestive of cholestasis, and infants with unexplained bleeding, should receive further vitamin K, preferably parenterally.

Vitamin K is a fat soluble vitamin, which is contained in cows' milk, green leafy vegetables and pork. There is very little in breast milk. Deficiency in the newborn period presents as haemorrhagic disease of the newborn. This usually presents on day 2 or 3 with bleeding from the umbilical stump, haematemesis and malaena, epistaxis or excessive bleeding from puncture sites. Diagnosis is by prolongation of the prothrombin and partial thromboplastin times with the thrombin time and fibrinogen levels being normal. Treatment is with fresh frozen plasma and vitamin K. There is no proved association between intramuscular vitamin K and childhood cancer.

gastroenterology and nutrition

118. Xylose tolerance test

Answers: B D E

The xylose tolerance test is an indirect method used to assess small bowel absorption. Xylose is a carbohydrate. A load (15 mg/m^2, max 25 g) is ingested and a blood level taken at 1 hour. A level of less than 25 mg/dl is suggestive of carbohydrate malabsorption. The test is neither sensitive nor specific. False-positive results are obtained in pernicious anaemia and when there is gut oedema. Other indirect tests of gastrointestinal function are:

- serum albumin
- faecal fat
- faecal elastase
- stool pH and reducing substances
- stool α–1 antitrypsin
- hydrogen breath test.

The hydrogen breath test is for carbohydrate malabsorption. The principle is that malabsorbed carbohydrate will pass to the colon where it is metabolised by bacteria and hydrogen gas is released. The gas is then absorbed and released in the breath. If there is a peak it suggests carbohydrate malabsorption. An early peak raises the possibility of bacterial overgrowth. Lactulose which is a non-absorbable carbohydrate can be given to ensure the colonic flora can metabolise carbohydrate and to assess transit time.

Albumin

Hypoalbuminaemia can occur secondary to reduced protein intake, reduced production by the liver in chronic liver disease, gut and renal loss. α–1 antitrypsin in the stool is a sensitive marker of enteric protein loss. Gastrointestinal causes of protein loss include:

- inflammatory bowel disease
- coeliac disease
- cystic fibrosis
- Schwachman's syndrome
- infection
- intestinal lymphangiectasia
- Mentriere's disease.

gastroenterology and nutrition

119. Folic acid (folate)

Answers: A C

Dietary sources of folate include liver, green vegetables, cereals, orange, milk, yeast and mushrooms. It is destroyed by excessive cooking. It is absorbed from the proximal small bowel. Deficiency causes megaloblastic anaemia, irritability, poor weight gain and chronic diarrhoea. Thrombocytopenia can occur. The serum folate reflects recent changes in folate status and the red cell folate is an indicator of the total body stores. Treatment of deficiency is with oral folic acid. Folate levels are not affected by the acute phase response. Causes of folate deficiency include:

- reduced intake
- coeliac disease
- tropical sprue
- blind loop syndrome
- congenital folate malabsorption (autosomal recessive)
- increased requirements (infancy, pregnancy, exfoliative skin disease)
- increased loss (haemodialysis)
- methotrexate
- trimethoprim
- anticonvulsants
- oral contraceptive pill.

There is an association between folate deficiency in early pregnancy and neural tube defects in the fetus.

120. Breast milk

Answers: B C D E

The composition of human milk at term per 100 ml (Department of Health 1988) is as shown in table.

Energy	70 kcal
Protein	1.3 g
Carbohydrate	7.0 g
Fat	4.2 g
Osmolality	264 mosm/kg
Sodium	0.65 mmol
Potassium chloride	1.54 mmol
Calcium	0.88 mmol
Magnesium	0.12 mmol
Phosphate	0.48 mmol
Iron	1.36 μmol

121. Carbohydrate intolerance in childhood

Answers: B C

Disorders of disaccharide absorption

- Primary:
  - congenital alactasia
  - congenital lactose intolerance
  - sucrose–isomaltase deficiency.
- Secondary (acquired):
  - post-enteritis (rotavirus), neonatal surgery, malnutrition
  - late-onset lactose intolerance.

Disorders of monosaccharide absorption

- Primary – glucose–galactose malabsorption.
- Secondary (acquired)
  - post-enteritis
  - neonatal surgery
  - malnutrition.

Carbohydrate intolerance is usually lactose intolerance and usually acquired. The deficient enzyme is the brush border enzyme lactase which hydrolyses lactose into glucose and galactose. The intolerance will present with characteristic loose explosive stools. The diagnosis is made by looking for reducing substance in the stool following carbohydrate ingestion. The test uses Clinitest tablets (which detect reducing substance in the stool) and the detection of more than 0.5% is significant. Treatment is with a lactose-free formula in infancy and a reduced lactose intake in later childhood. Following gastroenteritis, carbohydrate intolerance can be either to disaccharides or monosaccharides. Both types of intolerance are usually transient and both respond to removal of the offending carbohydrate. Both mono- and disaccharides will result in the reducing substances in the stool being positive.

Glucose–galactose malabsorption

This is a rare autosomal recessively inherited condition characterised by rapid-onset watery diarrhoea from birth. This responds to withholding glucose (stopping feeds) and relapses on re-introduction. The diagnosis is essentially a clinical one. Reducing substances in the stool will be positive and small bowel biopsy and disaccharide estimation normal. Treatment is by using fructose as the main carbohydrate source. Fructose is absorbed by a different mechanism to glucose and galactose.

gastroenterology and nutrition

122. Pre-term and term formulae

Answers: A C D

The principal differences are that pre-term formula contains more electrolytes, calories and minerals. All of the following are higher in pre-term than term formula: Energy, protein, carbohydrate, fat, osmolality, sodium, potassium, calcium, magnesium, phosphate and iron. There are many different formula feeds on the market and it is important to be aware of the differences between mature breast milk, term and pre-term formula and cow's milk.

123. Human (breast) milk and cow's milk

Answer: None correct

The energy content is the same. Human milk contains less protein than cows' milk – the cows' milk having a much higher casein content. The fat, although different qualitatively is the same in amount. Human milk contains more carbohydrate. Cow's milk contains more of all of the minerals except iron and copper.

124. Nutritional supplements

Answers: A D

Nutritional supplements based on glucose polymer are:

- Maxijul
- Caloreen
- Polycal
- Fortical
- Hycal.

Nutritional supplements based on fat are:

- Calogen
- Liquigen
- MCT Pepdite.

A nutritional supplement based on glucose polymer and fat is Duocal.

Fat-based nutritional supplements generally contain more calories per ml. Calogen contains 450 kcal per 100 g and Maxijul between 180 and 380 kcal per 100 g depending on the preparation used. Term formula milks, either whey- or casein-based contain the same amount of calories, which is the same as mature breast milk and cow's milk (66–70 kcal per 100 ml). Breast milk fortifiers are often added to breast milk given to pre-term babies.

125. Immunoglobulin A

Answers: B D E

IgA makes up 15% of circulating immunoglobulin. In its secretory form it is the predominant immunoglobulin at respiratory and gastrointestinal surfaces.

Selective IgA deficiency

This is a common disorder, with an incidence of 1 in 600. It is associated with an increased incidence of infection, atopic disease and rheumatic disorders:

- respiratory tract infection
- gastrointestinal tract infection, particularly giardiasis
- Crohn's disease, ulcerative colitis, coeliac disease (see Question 133)
- Autoimmune/rheumatoid conditions including rheumatoid arthritis, systemic lupus erythematosus and pernicious anaemia

Immunoglobulin therapy is not worthwhile if isolated IgA deficiency is present. This is because there is only a small amount of IgA in immunoglobulin preparations and sensitisation is therefore likely. If there is coexistent IgG deficiency or IgG subclass deficiency then immunoglobulin therapy may be appropriate.

126. Failure to thrive

Answers: C D

Failure to thrive is a failure to gain weight at an adequate rate. The aetiology can be organic or non-organic (psychosocial deprivation). Low birth weight and pre-term birth are associations of failure to thrive but not causes of it. Failure to thrive occurs as a consequence of one of the following:

- failure of carer to offer adequate calories
- failure of the child to take sufficient calories
- failure of the child to retain adequate calories.

Clearly this can be organic or non-organic. Insufficient calories may be offered as a consequence of parental neglect or because of a failure of the carer to appreciate the calorie requirements of the child. Insufficient calories may be taken as a consequence of feeding difficulties (eg cerebral palsy) and calories may not be retained because of absorptive defects or lost because of vomiting or diarrhoea. The investigation of failure to thrive is generally only fruitful when specific pointers to organic problems are elucidated in the history. The management of non-organic failure to thrive requires dietary assessment often accompanied by hospital admission for evaluation and to ensure an adequate weight gain can be obtained if sufficient calories are given.

gastroenterology and nutrition

Organic causes of failure to thrive

- gastrointestinal – coeliac disease, cow's milk protein intolerance, gastro-oesophageal reflux
- renal – urinary tract infection, renal tubular acidosis
- cardiopulmonary – cardiac disease, bronchopulmonary dysplasia
- endocrine – hypothyroidism
- neurological – cerebral palsy
- infection/immunodeficiency – HIV, malignancy
- metabolic – inborn errors of metabolism
- congenital – chromosomal abnormalities
- ENT – adeno-tonsillar hypertrophy.

127. Carbohydrate digestion

Answers: A B D

Carbohydrates are consumed as monosaccharides (glucose, fructose, galactose), disaccharides (lactose, sucrose, maltose, isomaltose) and polysaccharides (starch, dextrins, glycogen). Salivary and pancreatic amylase breaks starch down into oligosaccharides and disaccharides. Pancreatic amylase aids carbohydrate digestion but carbohydrate digestion is not dependent on it. Disaccharidases (maltase, sucrase, lactase) in the microvilli hydrolyse:

- oligo- and disaccharides into monosaccharides
- maltose into glucose
- isomaltose into glucose
- sucrose into glucose and fructose
- lactose into glucose and galactose.

Monosaccharides are then absorbed, glucose and galactose by an active transport mechanism and fructose by facilitated diffusion.

128. Wilson's disease (hepatolenticular degeneration)

Answers: B D E

The incidence of Wilson's disease is 1 in 500 000 and there is autosomal recessive inheritance. The gene is known and is on chromosome 13. The pathology is a consequence of decreased biliary excretion of copper and impaired caeruloplasmin production. Caeruloplasmin is the plasma protein which transports copper. Effects of Wilson's disease are:

- liver – chronic active hepatitis, portal hypertension and fulminant hepatic failure
- brain – progressive lenticular degeneration due to copper deposition

- cornea – Kayser-Fleischer rings
- lens – sunflower cataract
- kidney – renal tubular disorders
- blood – haemolysis.

The hepatic presentation can be as asymptomatic hepatomegaly, acute hepatitis, chronic active hepatitis, portal hypertension (ascites, oedema, variceal haemorrhage) or fulminant hepatic failure. The lenticular degeneration usually presents with tremor. Diagnosis is by a low plasma caeruloplasmin level and high urinary copper excretion. The latter can occur in other forms of hepatitis and a liver biopsy is often required. In equivocal cases the increased copper excretion after chelation with D-penicillamine is of diagnostic importance. Serum copper levels are not helpful. If untreated the condition is fatal, usually by the age of 30 years. If treated the prognosis is good. Treatment is with oral penicillamine as a copper binding agent in conjunction with a low copper diet. Patients on penicillamine require vitamin B_6 supplements as it is an anti-metabolite. The condition does not usually present under the age of 5 years.

129. Neonatal jaundice

Answers: B C E

Neonatal jaundice is classified as either early (<14 days) or late (>14 days). Jaundice can either be conjugated (direct) or unconjugated (indirect). Unconjugated is fat soluble and does not spill over into the urine. Conjugated is water soluble and is present in the urine as bilirubinuria. Up to 50% of normal newborns become clinically jaundiced in the early neonatal period. Causes of unconjugated hyperbilirubinaemia in the neonatal period include:

- physiological
- breast milk
- sepsis
- haemolysis
  - rhesus incompatibility
  - ABO incompatibility
  - hereditary spherocytosis
  - glucose 6-phosphate dehydrogenase deficiency
  - pyruvate kinase deficiency
- polycythaemia/bruising
- hypothyroidism
- galactosaemia
- cystic fibrosis including meconium ileus
- Crigler–Najjar syndrome.

gastroenterology and nutrition

130. Flat small intestinal mucosa

Answers: A C E

Causes:

- coeliac disease
- transient gluten intolerance
- cows' milk sensitive enteropathy
- soy protein intolerance
- gastroenteritis and post gastroenteritis syndromes
- giardiasis
- auto-immune enteropathy
- acquired hypogammaglobulinaemia
- tropical sprue
- protein energy malnutrition
- severe combined immunodeficiency
- anti-neoplastic therapy.

131. Coeliac disease

Answer: D E

The prevalence of coeliac disease is 1 in 2000. It has associations with HLA B8, DR7, DR3 and DQw2. There is an increased incidence in first-degree relatives. There is intolerance to gluten which is present in wheat, rye, barley and oats. Coeliac disease presents after 6 months of age (ie after gluten has been introduced into the diet). Chronic diarrhoea and poor weight gain (short stature in older children) generally occur. Other features include anorexia, lethargy, generalised irritability, abdominal distension and pallor. Diagnosis is by small bowel biopsy (endoscopic duodenal or jejunal). The characteristic features on biopsy are of sub-total villous atrophy, crypt hypertrophy, intracellular lymphocytes and a lamina propria plasma cell infiltrate. It is of crucial importance that the child's gluten intake is adequate at the time of the biopsy.

Treatment is with a gluten-free diet for life. There is a long-term risk of small bowel lymphoma if the diet is not adhered to. The gluten-free diet itself has no long-term complications. The standards for the diagnosis of coeliac disease are set out by the European Society of Paediatric Gastroenterology. Diagnosis is confirmed by characteristic histology and a clinical remission on a gluten-free diet. There are indications for a subsequent gluten challenge and these include initial diagnostic uncertainty and when the diagnosis is made under the age of 2 years. The latter being because at that age there are other causes of a flat jejunal biopsy and these are listed above. A gluten challenge involves an initial control biopsy on a gluten-free diet followed by a period on gluten with a repeat biopsy after 3–6 months and then again after 2 years, sooner if symptoms develop. There are reports of late relapse following gluten challenge. Antibody testing in the screening of children with failure to thrive and in the ongoing management of children with coeliac disease is helpful. The biopsy remains the gold standard for diagnosis. Antibody tests available are:

- IgG anti-gliadin
- IgA anti-gliadin
- IgA anti-reticulin
- IgA anti-endomysial
- Anti-tissue transglutaminase

The IgA antiendomysial antibody is the most sensitive and specific and the most widely used. However false-negatives occur in children who are IgA deficient. This means IgA levels should be done routinely alongside the endomysial antibody test.

Associations of coeliac disease include:

- increased incidence of small bowel malignancy, especially lymphoma
- increased incidence of IgA deficiency
- increased incidence of autoimmune thyroid disease, pernicious anaemia and diabetes mellitus (HLA B8 associations)
- dermatitis herpetiformis.

132. Hepatitis

Answer: A

Hepatitis B is a DNA virus. Diagnosis is by detection of the HBsAg. HBeAg positive patients carry a larger virus load and are more infectious. Acute and ongoing chronic infection is associated with anti-HBcIgM. Anti-HBe and anti-HBs antibodies appear as an effective immune response develops. All HBsAg-positive subjects are infective. The route of transmission is parenteral, and peri-natal transmission rate is dependent on the maternal serology. If the mother is HBsAg positive and HBeAg negative the risk is 12–25%. If the mother is both HBsAg positive and HBeAg positive the risk is 90%. The younger the age at infection the less the likelihood of symptomatic liver disease but the greater the risk of prolonged viral carriage. Ninety per cent of infants infected in the first year of life become chronic carriers.

Clinically the disease is often asymptomatic but an acute hepatic picture can develop. Acute liver failure occurs in less than 1%. The risk of fulminant hepatitis is increased by co-infection with hepatitis D. In those with a typical hepatic picture the chronic carrier rate is low. Chronicity results in an increased risk of cirrhosis and hepatocellular carcinoma. Males are more likely to become chronic carriers than females. Chronically infected children have a 25% lifetime risk of cirrhosis or hepatocellular carcinoma. Prevention is by both active and passive immunisation. Interferon alfa is a recognised treatment of chronic infection.

gastroenterology and nutrition

Hepatitis D is an RNA virus which requires the hepatitis B surface antigen for its assembly and virulence. It is transmitted like hepatitis B. The severity of the liver damage increases if there is co-existent hepatitis B infection. Diagnosis is by serology. Hepatitis B vaccine or immunity following infection offers protection.

133. Hepatitis

Answers: B D

Hepatitis A is an RNA virus. Diagnosis is by detection of the hepatitis A virus IgM. The route of transmission is faeco-oral. There is no carrier state and fulminant hepatic failure is rare (<0.1%). Liver function, however, may be abnormal for up to 1 year. Prevention is by either passive or active immunisation. Passive immunisation is with immunoglobulin and lasts for 3–6 months. Active immunisation is with a live attenuated virus, with booster immunisation being required after 12–18 months. Clinical symptoms are initially non-specific and include anorexia, nausea, fatigue and fever associated with epigastric pain and tender hepatomegaly. The icteric phase then develops with jaundice, pale stools and dark urine. Sometimes there is pruritus, depression and persistent jaundice with raised transaminases for a prolonged period. The prothrombin time should be monitored. A raised prothrombin time raises the possibility of severe hepatic necrosis or decompensation of underlying liver disease.

Hepatitis E is an RNA virus. Epidemics occur in developing countries. In the UK infection is usually seen in travellers from endemic areas. The route of transmission is faeco-oral. The clinical course of hepatitis E infection is similar to hepatitis A. Complete recovery from acute infection occurs. Chronic infection has not been described although acute fulminant hepatic failure can occur and is commoner during pregnancy. Diagnosis is by serology. No vaccine or prophylactic treatment is available.

134. Hepatitis

Answers: A B D E

Hepatitis C is an RNA virus. The route of transmission is either perinatal or parenteral. The vertical transmission rate is 9%, higher in HIV positive mothers. Diagnosis is usually by serology with the detection of the anti-HCV antibody. Blood and blood products for transfusion have been screened for hepatitis C virus since 1990. Infection is usually asymptomatic or an acute hepatitis can occur. Fulminant hepatitis is uncommon but can occur. HCV RNA detection establishes the presence of viraemia confirming infection and infectivity. Persistence of HCV RNA indicates continuing infection. Chronic infection is common (prevalence 0.2–0.7% in northern Europe, 1–2% in Southern Europe and Japan) with the development of cirrhosis and hepatocellular carcinoma in a number of cases after an interval of 10–15 years. Treatment with interferon-alfa has been given. No vaccine is available. Breast feeding is not contraindicated for HCV sero-positive mothers but if nipples are cracked and bleeding, caution is advised.

135. Colitis

Answers: B C

Abdominal pain associated with bloody diarrhoea is indicative of colitis. Colitis can be infective or non-infective.

Causes of infective colitis:

- *Salmonella* species
- *Shigella* species
- *Campylobacter pylori*
- *Escherichia coli* 0157 (and other *E. coli*)
- *Clostridium difficile* (pseudomembranous colitis)
- *Yersinia*
- tuberculosis
- cytomegalovirus
- *Entamoeba histolytica*
- *Enterobius vermicularis.*

Causes of non-infective colitis:

- ulcerative colitis
- Crohn's disease
- necrotising enterocolitis
- microscopic colitis
- Behçet's disease
- food allergic colitis.

136. *Giardia lamblia*

Answers: B C E

This is a protozoal parasite which is infective in the cyst form. It also exists in the trophozoite form. It is found in contaminated food and water. Clinical manifestations may be:

- asymptomatic
- acute diarrhoeal disease
- chronic diarrhoea.

The latter may be associated with malabsorption and an abnormal small bowel mucosa. Diagnosis is by stool examination for cysts or examination of the duodenal aspirate at small bowel biopsy. It is treated with metronidazole.

137. Intussusception

Answers: A D E

The peak incidence of intussusception is at 6–9 months and there are 1–4 per 1000 live births. The male to female ratio is 4:1. It is commoner in the spring and autumn. Usually presents with spasmodic pain, pallor and irritability. Vomiting is an early feature and rapidly progresses to being bile stained. Passage of blood-stained stools often occurs and a mass is frequently palpable. The presentation, however, is often atypical. The intussusception is usually ileo-caecal, the origin being either the ileo-caecal valve or the terminal ileum. An identifiable cause is commoner in those who present later – Meckel's diverticulum, polyp, reduplication, lymphosarcoma and Henoch–Schönlein purpura being examples. Diagnosis is usually on clinical grounds. Confirmation is by plain abdominal X-ray, ultrasound or air or barium enema examination. Treatment is either with air or barium enema reduction if the history is short or surgically at laparotomy. Resuscitation with albumin is usually required. Contraindications to air or barium enema include peritonitis or signs of perforation.

138. Gilbert's syndrome

Answers: A D E

Gilbert's syndrome is defined as unconjugated hyperbilirubinaemia with no evidence of haemolysis and normal liver function tests. Liver biopsy is normal. The prevalence is 6%, and it is commoner in males than females. Inheritance is autosomal dominant with incomplete expression. The pathogenesis is unclear but probably represents a mild functional deficiency of the enzyme UDP glucuronyl transferase. The clinical picture is of mild fluctuating jaundice (serum bilirubin 30–50 µmol/l) aggravated by infection, exertion and fasting. Of some diagnostic use is the fact that the condition improves with phenobarbital and worsens with nicotinic acid.

Other inherited causes of hyperbilirubinaemia include:

- Crigler–Najjar syndrome – type 1 (autosomal recessive) is due to complete absence of UDP glucuronyl transferase in the liver. Jaundice (unconjugated) presents soon after birth and rapidly progresses to toxic levels (kernicterus). Untreated, death usually occurs by the end of the first year. Diagnosis is by estimation of hepatic UDP glucuronyl transferase activity in a specimen obtained by needle liver biopsy. Repeated exchange transfusions and phototherapy aid short-term survival. The only long-term therapeutic option is liver transplantation. Type 2 (autosomal dominant) is less severe and responds to treatment with phenobarbital. There is usually less than 10% of normal levels of UDP glucuronyl transferase activity present. Kernicterus is unusual.

- Dubin–Johnson syndrome – autosomal recessive. Presents with conjugated hyperbilirubinaemia and bilirubinuria. It is due to a reduced ability to transport organic anions such as bilirubin glucuronide into the biliary tree. There is black pigmentation of the liver on biopsy. Life expectancy is normal, and the jaundice is exacerbated by alcohol, infection and pregnancy. It may not present until early adulthood.
- Rotor syndrome – autosomal recessive. It presents with conjugated hyperbilirubinaemia. It is due to a deficiency in organic anion uptake as well as excretion. No black pigment is present in the liver. There is normal life expectancy, and the jaundice exacerbated by alcohol, infection and pregnancy. Sulphobromophthalein excretion test is abnormal.

139. Ulcerative colitis

Answers: A C D E

Ulcerative colitis is an inflammatory disease limited to the colonic and rectal mucosa. It is the more distal bowel that is the most involved. Inflammation is neither pan-enteric or transmural as is seen in Crohn's disease. A backwash ileitis into the terminal ileum is often seen. The characteristic histology in the colon is of mucosal and submucosal inflammation with goblet cell depletion, cryptitis and crypt abscesses but no granulomas. The inflammatory change is usually diffuse rather than patchy. The aetiology is unknown. The disease is commoner in females than in males. Childhood prevalence is around 4 per 100 000, and 10–15% present in childhood. Although unusual, the disease can present with predominantly extra-intestinal manifestations including growth failure, arthropathy, erythema nodosum, occult blood loss, non-specific abdominal pain, cholangitis and raised inflammatory indices. The gut disease can be mild, moderate or severe. The symptoms of colitis are diarrhoea, blood per rectum and abdominal pain. Systemic disturbances may accompany more severe disease: tachycardia, fever, weight loss, anaemia, hypoalbuminaemia and leucocytosis. Complications of ulcerative colitis are:

- toxic megacolon
- growth failure
- cholangitis
- cancer

gastroenterology and nutrition

- non-malignant stricture.

The cancer risk reflects the disease severity and duration of disease. Regular screening is carried out in adult life. Diagnosis is by endoscopy and biopsy with classic histological features seen. A small number of children have an indeterminate or unclassified colitis. The differential diagnosis of colitis is wide and a list of the causes of non-infective and infective colitis are listed in Answer 137.

Treatment of ulcerative colitis:

- 5-ASA derivatives
- local or systemic steroids
- azathioprine to reduce steroid toxicity in steroid-dependent patients
- surgery.

Differences between Crohn's disease and ulcerative colitis:

Crohn's disease	Ulcerative colitis
Pan-enteric	Colon only
Skip lesions	Diffuse
Transmural	Mucosal
Granulomas	Crypt abscesses
Peri-anal disease	

140. Recurrent abdominal pain

Answers: A C

Recurrent abdominal pain is common in childhood, affecting up to 10% of the school age population. In the majority of cases the aetiology is non-organic. The condition is commoner in girls than in boys and a family history is common. The pain is usually peri-umbilical and rarely associated with other gastrointestinal symptoms such as diarrhoea, blood per rectum or weight loss. Abdominal pain accompanied by other symptoms is suggestive of organic pathology. Night pain is suggestive of oesophagitis or peptic ulceration. Diarrhoea with blood per rectum suggests colitis and diarrhoea associated with weight loss suggests malabsorption syndrome.

141. Portal hypertension

Answer: D

Aetiology

Pre-hepatic causes:

- portal vein thrombosis
- sepsis
- pancreatitis
- umbilical catheterisation (artery or vein)
- omphalitis.

Intra-hepatic causes:

- pre-sinusoidal
  - neoplasia
  - schistosomiasis
  - hepatic cyst
- sinusoidal
  - cirrhosis
  - biliary atresia
  - neonatal hepatitis
  - α 1 antitrypsin deficiency
- post-sinusoidal
  - veno-occlusive disease.

Post-hepatic causes:

- Budd–Chiari syndrome
- right ventricular failure
- constrictive pericarditis.

Clinical features of portal hypertension:

- splenomegaly
- ascites
- prominent abdominal vessels (caput medusa)
- oesophageal varices
- haemorrhoids
- rectal varices.

Complications of portal hypertension

- ascites – compromising respiration, infection, hypoalbuminaemia
- variceal bleeding
- porto-systemic encephalopathy
- splenomegaly with hypersplenism.

gastroenterology and nutrition

142. Vitamin A

Answers: A B E

Other properties include enhancing night vision through the *cis* retinal variant of retinol. Vitamin A deficiency causes supression of both humoval and cell mediated immunity. Clinical signs include loss of night vision and keratomalacia the early signs of which are called Bitot's spots.

143. D: Commonest in the pre-school age group

Rectal prolapse is commonest between the ages of 1 and 5 years and can involve protrusion of the mucosal layer alone or all layers (procidentia).

Causes of RP:

- idiopathic
- increased abdominal pressure
  - constipation
  - chronic cough
- diarrhoeal disorders
  - acute infection
  - malabsorption
- cystic fibrosis (25% of patients with CF have rectal prolapse and CF accounts for 10% of all cases of rectal prolapse)
- neuromuscular syndromes
- child abuse (anal sex).

It is usually painless, although failure to reduce the prolapsed tissue can result in the formation of oedema and ulceration. Parents can be taught to reduce a prolapse at home. Surgery is occasionally required but is associated with complications.

144. C: Precipitated by a child's refusal to use school toilets

Constipation is defined as painful or infrequent defecation. An extremely common problem in childhood including the pre-school age group, it is rarely associated with any underlying medical problem. A vicious cycle usually develops whereby a child associates pain with defecation and then withholds stool in an attempt to avoid such discomfort. This retention of stool causes enlargement of the rectum and distal colon (megacolon) to accommodate the faeces and the normal urge to defecate is lost. Eventually, faecal incontinence (soiling) may ensue. Parents may be able to identify a trigger to the start of the problem, eg a change in milk, toilet training, after an illness or starting a new school. Abdominal X-rays can be helpful in assessing the degree of faecal loading but are not required

gastroenterology and nutrition

routinely. Other investigation is rarely indicated. Treatment involves clearing the colon (ideally via the oral route but sometimes enemas or even disimpaction under general anaesthesia is required), followed by establishing a regular bowel habit (often requires both behavioural and therapeutic interventions). Treatment is usually required for many weeks or months, with education and reassurance of parents in all cases.

145. B: Treatment with sodium valproate

Pancreatitis is uncommon in childhood. Unlike in adults, the commonest causes are abdominal trauma, viral infection (mumps, rubella, Coxsackie B, cytomegalovirus), medication (sodium valproate) and congenital anomalies of the pancreato-biliary system. It typically presents with epigastric pain (which can radiate through to the back), nausea and vomiting and low grade fever. Elevated serum amylase levels are seen in the majority of cases of acute pancreatitis but can take up to 48 hours to reach peak levels. Other abdominal pathologies can cause a rise in serum amylase but rarely to the degree seen in pancreatitis.

Medical management consists of rehydration and analgesia, and may also include a period of being 'nil by mouth', sometimes sufficient to require total parenteral nutrition. Antibiotics may also be indicated in some cases. The length of the illness is variable. Ultrasound and computed tomography (CT) are the most commonly used imaging modalities, but magnetic resonance imaging (MRI) and endoscopic retrograde cholangiopancreatography (ERCP) can also be helpful. Findings are variable and include a normal-looking pancreas in some cases. Surgical involvement may be required if necrosis, abscess or pseudocyst formation occurs.

146. A: Addition of an acid suppressant

Prevalence of gastro-oesophageal reflux (GOR) varies with age, but nearly all infants have some degree of reflux. However, it is frequently transient and causes no morbidity. Peak incidence (from pH studies) is at approximately 4 months of age. In symptomatic individuals, resolution of symptoms is usually seen by the age of 2 years, correlating with developmental maturity including a more upright posture and intake of solids. Premature infants and children with neurological impairment have a higher incidence of GOR than the general population.

There is no clear relationship between the severity of GOR on pH study and symptom severity. In addition to irritability and vomiting, affected individuals may present with feeding difficulties, apnoeas, failure to thrive, aspiration, stridor or haematemesis. Oesophagitis and oesophageal strictures may result from more severe cases of GOR. GOR is caused in part by more frequent and prolonged relaxation of the lower oesophageal sphincter than would be considered normal.

gastroenterology and nutrition

Oesophagitis itself can cause further impairment of lower oesophageal sphincter function. When needed, investigation is ideally done in the form of 24-hour pH probe. Upper gastrointestinal contrast studies are useful in delineating the anatomy but not for diagnosing reflux in itself. Similarly endoscopy can tell you about the presence or otherwise of oesophagitis and strictures but not about intraluminal pH.

Treatment involves parental reassurance and advice regarding lifestyle measures such as type, timing and size of feeds and positioning of baby. Medical treatments include alginates (infant Gaviscon), acid suppression (no direct studies have been done in children to compare H_2 blockers with proton-pump inhibitors) and prokinetic agents, including metoclopramide and domperidone. Cisapride is not recommended due to potential cardiotoxic side-effects. Drug treatment is not indicated in all cases, but should be used when growth is affected or when symptoms occur with sufficient frequency or severity to cause distress to the infant and/or caregivers. GOR may be associated with cow's milk protein intolerance in which case a hydrolysed formula should be substituted. In those cases where medical management is deemed to have failed, surgical intervention in the form of a fundoplication may be beneficial. Potential operative complications and failure rates mean that this option should be reserved for only the most severe cases.

147. D: Advice about dietary intake

There are numerous causes of diarrhoea in childhood including:

- infection – viral, bacterial, parasitic
- malabsorption –transient or long term, primary or secondary, fat, protein or carbohydrate
- Toddler's diarrhoea
- inflammatory bowel disease.

Rotavirus is the commonest cause of diarrhoea worldwide, followed by adenovirus. *Salmonella*, *Shigella* and *Campylobacter* are the next most common infecting organisms. Carbohydrate malabsorption is most frequently seen secondary to infective diarrhoea (see Question 123). Liver and pancreatic diseases resulting in bile salt and pancreatic enzyme deficiency cause fat and protein malabsorption.

Loose stool with undigested food particles (often described as peas and carrots by parents) are seen with toddler diarrhoea, which is thought to be caused by reduced gut transit time in children, exacerbated by excessive fruit juice intake, with possible influences of low dietary fat intake and emotional stress. It is self-limiting. It sometimes presents as alternating constipation and diarrhoea. Failure to thrive is never a feature of this condition. It is primarily a disease of exclusion and any evidence of atypical features should prompt further investigation.

gastroenterology and nutrition

Parental reassurance is imperative as well as advice on type and amount of fluid intake (approximate daily requirement for a preschool child is 100 ml/kg/day, to include water contained within food). Loperamide can be given for symptomatic benefit but only in selected cases and short periods due to potential side effects including constipation.

This scenario is typical of toddler's diarrhoea. As the child is thriving there is no indication for immediate invasive investigations. Stool testing could be arranged but is unnecessary at this stage. It would be more appropriate to offer the parent's reassurance and dietary advice and offer to see the child again to ensure symptoms are improving and growth maintained. If growth or symptoms deteriorate or the child fails to respond to the dietary measures advised, further appropriate investigations could be arranged.

148. Prolonged jaundice

1. H – Glucose 6-phosphate dehydrogenase deficiency

This is an X-linked disorder, commonest in those of African, Asian and Mediterranean origin. Haemolysis can be precipitated by oxidative drugs or chemicals, infection or fava bean ingestion. Heterozygote females can develop haemolytic attacks. Deficiency can vary from mild (>60% normal enzyme activity detected) to severe (<10%). In neonates, phototherapy and exchange transfusion may be required. Advice regarding avoidance of known precipitants is important for future management. (See also Question 156).

2. A – Biliary atresia

Biliary atresia is characterised by obliteration of the extrahepatic biliary system and should be considered in all neonates with conjugated (direct) hyperbilirubinaemia. Incidence is higher in Asian and black races than in Caucasians, and more females are affected than males. Stools may be pigmented normally at birth and become gradually paler over the first few weeks of life. Appetite, growth and weight gain may be normal. Hepatomegaly may be present early and an enlarging spleen can suggest cirrhosis and portal hypertension. Surgical treatment in the form of portoenterostomy (Kasai's procedure) before the age of 2 months has been shown to reduce the likelihood of the development of irreversible biliary cirrhosis and need for transplant. Complications following Kasai's procedure include cholangitis, portal hypertension and cirrhosis.

3. G – Congenital cytomegalovirus infection

If primary infection with cytomegalovirus occurs during pregnancy, there is a 40% risk of transmission to the fetus. As only approximately 50% of women of childbearing age in the developed world are seropositive for cytomegalovirus (compared with nearly 100% in developing countries), there is a substantial risk of congenital infection in this population. Congenital cytomegalovirus infection may be symptomatic or asymptomatic, although the latter are still at risk of neurological sequelae (especially sensorineural deafness). Symptomatic congenital cytomegalovirus infection is characterised by intra-uterine growth retardation, hepatosplenomegaly, thrombocytopenia, microcephaly, ventriculomegaly, chorioretinitis and sensorineural deafness. Over 90% of survivors have neurological or neurodevelopmental sequelae.

Infection occurs via contact with infected body secretions and hence infection can also occur parentally (during birth or via breast milk). Prenatal acquisition may lead to lymphadenopathy, hepatitis and pneumonitis. Viral culture for cytomegalovirus can be performed on most body fluids including blood, urine, saliva and cerebrospinal fluid . CT brain imaging is imperative for all infants with suspected congenital cytomegalovirus as presence of calcification has a positive predictive value of identifying those at risk of neurological sequelae.

149. Rectal bleeding

1. H – Henoch Schönlein purpura

As well as renal complications, this IgA mediated small vessel vasculitis of unknown aetiology can also cause purpura, arthralgia/arthritis (most commonly affecting knees and ankles), abdominal pain and gastrointestinal bleeding, testicular swelling and central nervous system involvement including seizures and mononeuropathies. The median age of onset is 4–5 years, with approximately 75% of cases occurring between 2 and 14 years of age. Gastrointestinal complications include intussusception, bowel wall perforation or infarction. Pain is secondary to vasculitic involvement of small mesenteric or bowel mucosa vessels. Systemic symptoms may precede the onset of the rash, which typically appears on buttocks, thighs, feet and ankles. The appearances of this rash vary from erythematous, macular or urticarial, through to blanching papules, palpable purpura or bullae, necrotic and ulcerating lesions. (See also Question 267.)

2. E – Hirschsprung's disease

Hirschsprung's disease is due to congenital agangliosus of the bowel, always involving the anus and extending proximally to a variable degree. Although 90% of cases of Hirschsprung's disease are diagnosed in the neonatal period with failure to pass meconium, it can also be a cause of chronic constipation if a very short aganglionic segment is involved. In these instances, a history of difficulty with passage of stools which has been present since birth should be obtained. It is up to four times commoner in males. Associated abnormalities include cardiac (2–5%) and trisomy 21 (5–15%). Diagnosis is confirmed by demonstrating absence of ganglion cells in the rectum. Suction biopsy can be performed at the bedside without need for anaesthetic although the sections can be more difficult to interpret than full thickness biopsies taken under general anaesthetic.

Medical management in the neonate includes close attention to fluid balance and hydration along with colonic lavage. Surgical care includes identifying the transition zone at laparotomy and formation of a colostomy proximal to this (with presence of ganglion cells being confirmed during the procedure with frozen sections). Definitive repair usually occurs when the child is older. Complications of Hirschsprung's disease include enterocolitis (in 10–30%) where the patient is at risk of bowel perforation. Other complications post surgery include anastomotic leak and stricture formation.

3. I – Meconium ileus

Up to 15% of cases of cystic fibrosis (see also Questions 352 and 353) present as meconium ileus. Other surgical presentations of cystic fibrosis include rectal prolapse and nasal polyps. Meconium ileus is caused by production of abnormally viscid and adherent meconium. Characteristically the proximal ileum is greatly dilated and contains thick sticky meconium while distal ileum and colon are collapsed and obstructed by thickly packed round meconium pellets. Infants are often small for dates but associated malformations are rare. In complicated meconium ileus, the dilated bowel may volve and subsequently perforate, causing meconium peritonitis. Abdominal X-rays in these cases typically shows areas of calcification. Up to 20% will have a history of maternal polyhydramnios. Treatment of meconium ileus includes contrast enemas to 'wash out' the inspissated meconium pellets. If this is unsuccessful, and in cases where perforation has occurred, laparotomy will be required. Differential diagnosis includes Hirschsprung's disease and neonatal small left colon syndrome (seen with increased frequency in infants of diabetic mothers).

gastroenterology and nutrition

HAEMATOLOGY, ONCOLOGY AND POISONING ANSWERS

150. Iron deficiency anaemia

Answer: B

The commonest cause of iron deficiency anaemia in childhood is dietary. Iron is absorbed in the proximal small intestine. It is usually the case that about 10% of the ingested load is absorbed. This can be increased by the simultaneous administration of vitamin C. Iron deficiency anaemia is particularly common in the first year of life. Both breast and cow's milk are low in iron and iron-rich foods such as fortified cereals and infant formula milks need to be taken. The symptoms and signs of iron deficiency include pallor, fatigue, pica and poor appetite, the latter exacerbating the problem. Splenomegaly is present in 10–15%. There is much recent evidence which suggests that iron deficiency even in the absence of anaemia is a cause of reduced intellectual performance and that this responds well to therapy.

Laboratory features:

- microcytosis
- hypochromia
- low serum iron
- increased total iron binding capacity
- low serum ferritin
- thrombocytosis (occasional thrombocytopenia).

Treatment is with oral iron. A reticulocyte response should be seen within a few days, and 6 mg/kg/day of elemental iron is required. Chronic blood loss needs to be considered as an alternative cause of iron deficient anaemia particularly if stools are positive to blood or there are suggestive features in the history. β-Thalassaemia trait is an important differential diagnosis.

β-Thalassaemia trait

- HbA_2 3.4–7% (normal adult 1.5–3.5%)
- HbF   2–6% (normal adult < 2%).

HbA_2 levels are low in iron deficiency anaemia.

Iron absorption

Iron is absorbed in its ferrous form (approximately 10% of intake) according to body needs. This process is aided by gastric juice and vitamin C and inhibited by fibre and steatorrhoea. Iron is transported in plasma in the ferric state bound to transferrin. It is stored in liver, spleen bone marrow and kidney as ferritin. Following breakdown of haemoglobin the iron is conserved and reused.

151. Acute idiopathic thrombocytopenic purpura (ITP)

Answer: E

The incidence is 4 per 100 000 children per year. Peak age is 2–4 years, and incidence in boys and girls is equal. It is commonest in the winter and spring, and often preceded by an upper respiratory tract infection. It is probably immune mediated although the precise mechanism is not known. Differential diagnosis includes:

- infection
- drugs
- collagen disorders
- familial thrombocytopenia
- leukaemia
- aplastic anaemia
- portal hypertension with hypersplenism.

In general ITP is a benign self-limiting illness. Management is controversial with US/UK differences in approach. Investigations are determined by the clinical history and physical examination. A full blood count and blood film is essential in all cases. Other investigations are as appropriate. A bone marrow is required if there is doubt about the diagnosis and leukaemic infiltration is a possibility. Bed rest is not helpful. Treatment options include steroids, intravenous immunoglobulin (IVIG) or nothing. Steroids and IVIG will increase the platelet count in about 12 hours if treatment is required. Currently IVIG is the preferred option the dosage is variable but generally it is 0.8 g/kg as a one off dose, 400 mg/kg for 5 days or 1 g/kg for 2 days. Chronic idiopathic thrombocytopenia occurs more commonly in girls and is defined as the persistence of the thrombocytopenia beyond 6 months. Treatment options include steroids, regular IVIG and splenectomy. Intracranial haemorrhage is a rare complication of ITP.

152. Glanzmann's thrombasthenia

Answers: B C

This is autosomally recessively inherited, with the gene locus on chromosome 7. Pathogenesis is a failure of platelet aggregation in response to ADP, collagen and thrombin. This is due to a defect in glycoprotein IIb and IIIa both being part of the platelet membrane and deficiency resulting in a failure of the platelet to bind fibrinogen. It is a rare condition and presents in early childhood with recurrent bleeding. Platelet count and morphology are normal. The only possible long-term treatment is bone marrow transplantation. In the short term tranexamic acid can be used to control acute bleeding.

Bernard–Soulier syndrome

This is an autosomal recessive condition. The characteristic features are giant platelets with a reduced life span and hence thrombocytopenia and a prolonged bleeding time. Platelet aggregation is normal.

153. Hereditary spherocytosis

Answers: A C

The incidence of hereditary spherocytosis is 1 in 5000 people of northern European extraction. It is inherited as an autosomal dominant with variable penetrance. It usually presents in childhood with the classic triad of anaemia, jaundice and splenomegaly. The jaundice is unconjugated and worsens with viral infections. Pigmented gallstones are present in 85% by the second decade. Neonatal jaundice is common. Aplastic crises can occur. The diagnosis is made on clinical grounds, by observing the spheroidal cells on a blood film and by the increased osmotic fragility of red cells when tested. Treatment is symptomatic or by splenectomy. The spleen is the site of red cell destruction. Removal of the spleen will reduce haemolysis and reduce the incidence of gallstones. There is, however, an increased risk of pneumococcal and other infection with splenectomy and pneumococcal vaccine and life-long prophylactic penicillin needs to be given.

haematology, oncology and poisoning

154. Glucose 6-phosphate dehydrogenase deficiency

Answers: B C E

This has X-linked inheritance. It is commoner and more severe in males but females are affected. The enzyme protects the red cell membrane from oxidant stress keeping glutathione in its reduced state. Can either present with an acute haemolytic crisis or as a chronic haemolytic anaemia. Infection, eg hepatitis A and diabetic ketoacidosis may also provoke a crisis. Neonatal jaundice is common. Diagnosis is by estimation of the glucose 6-phosphate dehydrogenase level (can be normal during a crisis). Its management includes avoidance of precipitating factors and substances/drugs to avoid include:

- fava beans
- aspirin
- antimalarials
- sulphonamides
- dapsone
- nitrofurantoin
- nalidixic acid
- methylene blue
- naphthalene.

155. Wiskott–Aldrich syndrome

Answers: C D E

This has an X-linked inheritance. The gene has been localised to the short arm of the X chromosome. Prenatal diagnosis and carrier detection is possible in 98%. Clinical features of Wiskott–Aldrich syndrome are:

- recurrent infections secondary to immunodeficiency
- eczema
- thrombocytopenia with reduced platelet size
- malignant potential
- laboratory investigations
- reduced platelet number and reduced platelet size
- low serum IgM, normal IgG and raised IgA and IgE
- T cell defect.

Acute haemorrhage is a significant cause of death (20%), other causes being infection and malignancy. Survival beyond the teenage years is rare. Bone marrow transplant offers a potential cure.

TAR (thrombocytopenia, absent radii) syndrome

- Autosomal recessive
- Absent radii
- Thrombocytopenia
- Variable other manifestations including cardiac, renal, gastrointestinal, and skeletal.

156. Vitamin B$_{12}$ deficiency

Answer: A

To be absorbed vitamin B$_{12}$ must combine with intrinsic factor which is secreted by the parietal cells of the stomach. The complex is then absorbed in the terminal ileum. Symptoms and signs of B$_{12}$ deficiency are:

- megaloblastic anaemia
- smooth tongue
- ataxia
- hyporeflexia
- up-going plantars.

Pernicious anaemia is the commonest cause of B$_{12}$ deficiency in adults. It is due to deficiency of intrinsic factor and is associated with either parietal cell or intrinsic factor antibodies. These are not detected in children with juvenile pernicious anaemia. Schilling's test is used to assess the absorption of vitamin B$_{12}$ from the gut. Other causes of B$_{12}$ deficiency include:

- nutritional, eg vegans
- infants of vegan mothers particularly if breast fed
- inflammatory bowel disease
- tuberculosis affecting the terminal ileum
- surgical resection of the terminal ileum, eg necrotising enterocolitis
- bacterial overgrowth (blind loop syndrome)

The mean corpuscular volume is raised in vitamin B$_{12}$ deficiency.

B$_{12}$ deficiency is rare in coeliac disease at presentation.

haematology, oncology and poisoning

157. Sickle cell disease

Answers: A B C D E

Sickle cell disease is due to synthesis of an abnormal haemoglobin. There are various forms, Hb SS is the commonest and the most severe. Sickling occurs during hypoxia which causes the abnormal haemoglobin to crystallise making the red cell stiff. This then blocks the microcirculation causing infarction. Clinical expression is varied, some patients leading an almost normal life. In utero diagnosis can be made by chorionic villus sampling at 10 weeks. Diagnosis at birth can be made on heel prick or cord blood. This allows early follow-up and treatment.

Crises due to sickling are precipitated by anoxia, cold, infection and dehydration. Painful vascular occlusive crises occur in bone, the common sites being hips, shoulders, vertebrae and the bones of the hands and feet. Sickling can also result in pulmonary infarction, splenic infarction (causing hyposplenism), gut infarction and cerebrovascular accidents. Treatment of a crisis involves intravenous antibiotics, intravenous fluid, oxygen, analgesia and sometimes blood transfusion. Acute sequestration of blood may occur in the spleen or lung (acute chest syndrome) causing an acute anaemia. An aplastic crisis can occur secondary to infection with parvovirus B19.

There is functional hyposplenism. Prophylactic penicillin and pneumococcal immunisation (after the third birthday) need to be given. Although often large in the first few years the spleen reduces in size throughout childhood as a consequence of autoinfarction. Nocturnal enuresis is common (45% of 8-year-olds). Growth rate is reduced but puberty delayed resulting in a reasonable final height in most cases. Mortality is low in the first 6 months, peaks between 6 and 12 months and falls after first year. In Jamaica, mortality is 5% by first year, 25% by 20 years. The commonest cause of death is infection.

158. Rhesus haemolytic disease

Answers: C D E

Haemolytic disease of the newborn occurs as a consequence of the transplacental passage of anti-D antibodies (IgG) from the rhesus negative mother to the rhesus positive fetus. This can only occur if the mother has been sensitised. Other rhesus antibodies (eg anti C and E) can occur and produce less severe disease. The use of anti-D passive immunisation in mothers within 72 hours of delivery has reduced the incidence of the disease. Sensitisation in the mother (rhesus negative) can occur following miscarriages, abortions and previous deliveries of rhesus positive fetuses.

Haemolytic disease can occur in utero and may produce hepatosplenomegaly, ascites and hydrops (which can be detected on ultrasound). Screening is done on rhesus positive mothers at booking, 28 weeks, 34 weeks and at time of delivery.

If anti-D antibodies are found the tests are repeated every 2 weeks. If titres are high (greater than 10 IU/ml) referral to a specialist centre is indicated. Titres above 100 IU/ml indicate severe disease. If the anti-D antibody titres are high then in utero monitoring of the fetus is carried out by amniocentesis to measure bilirubin levels in the amniotic fluid. If amniotic bilirubin levels indicate a high degree of haemolysis is present then cord blood sampling is performed. Fetal anaemia will be the consequence of severe haemolysis and can be treated with in utero blood transfusions. Severe disease is an indication for premature delivery (at 34–36 weeks), the infant being likely to require exchange transfusion after birth. The severity of disease will increase with successive pregnancies.

ABO haemolytic disease

This usually occurs in mothers with blood group O who have IgG anti-A or anti-B antibodies which will cross the placenta and react if the baby is blood group A or B and cause haemolysis. The degree of haemolysis is generally only mild. It occurs in 3% of births. Phototherapy usually controls the jaundice. Diagnosis is by measuring anti-A or anti-B antibodies in a blood group O mother with a blood group A, B or AB neonate with a positive direct Coombs' test.

159. Anaemia secondary to chronic disease

Answers: C D

Anaemia can occur in any disease with chronic inflammation. Characteristic features include:

- normal MCV
- normochromia
- normal or low reticulocyte count
- low serum iron
- low iron binding capacity and transferrin saturation
- normal or raised ferritin
- increased reticuloendothelial stores of iron.

Several factors are thought to contribute to the anaemia including decreased red cell survival, inflammatory mediators suppressing erythrocyte production, a blunting of the erythropoietin response to anaemia and trapping of iron by macrophages reducing utilisation for new red cells. Anaemia is usually not less than 9 g/dl. Although most cases will not respond to iron, supplements are given if serum ferritin is less than 50 µg/ml and may improve anaemia if there is co-existent iron deficiency. Anaemia secondary to chronic renal failure is due to absence of erythropoietin production and responds to treatment with recombinant erythropoietin.

haematology, oncology and poisoning

160. Neonatal thrombocytopenia

Answers: A C D E

Causes of neonatal thrombocytopenia are:

- congenital
  - TAR (thrombocytopenia, absent radii) syndrome
  - Fanconi's anaemia
  - Bernard–Soulier syndrome
  - Wiskott–Aldrich syndrome
- immune-mediated platelet destruction
  - maternal ITP
  - neonatal isoimmune thrombocytopenia
  - maternal systemic lupus erythematosus
- due to congenital infection
  - TORCH
  - congenital syphilis
- sepsis
- polycythaemia
- drugs, eg tolazoline.

Neonatal isoimmune thrombocytopenia

This occurs in neonates who are platelet antigen (PL A1) positive born to PL A1 negative mothers. Sensitisation occurs in utero and first pregnancies can be affected. Two per cent of the population are PL A1 negative, 98% are PL A1 positive but only 6% of PL A1 negative mothers with positive fetuses will develop antibodies, and 10% of affected fetuses will have intraventricular haemorrhage with a high associated morbidity and mortality. Maternal antibodies can be monitered during pregnancy, and platelet transfusion of PL A1 negative platelets given to infants at risk.

161. Blood transfusion

Answers: B C D E

Transfusion reactions can be immediate or delayed. Immediate reactions occur in:

- haemolysis
- reaction to infected blood
- allergic reactions to platelets or white cells (causing urticaria)
- pyrogenic reactions to plasma proteins or transfused antibodies
- clotting abnormalities after large transfusions
- circulatory overload
- citrate toxicity
- hyperkalaemia.

Late reactions:

- transmission of infection, eg hepatitis A, B and C, HIV, cytomegalovirus, brucella, salmonella, toxoplasma, malaria
- iron overload
- immune sensitisation.

Reactions can be mild with pyrexia normally due to reactions to white cells, platelets or transfused plasma proteins and usually occurring in patients receiving multiple transfusions. Treatment is with iv hydrocortisone and antihistamines. If the reaction is more severe the transfusion should be stopped. Adrenaline may occasionally be required. Transfusion reactions can be reduced by using white cell depleted blood or using white cell filters. Clinical features of severe reactions include abdominal pain, back pain, flushing, headache, shortness of breath, pyrexia, rigors, chest pain, vomiting and shock.

162. Neutropenia

Answers: A B D E

Neutropenia is classified as either $< 1.0 \times 10^9/l$ or $< 0.5 \times 10^9/l$ neutrophils. Causes of neutropenia are:

congenital:

- reticular dysgenesis – failure of development of stem cells
- X-linked hypogammaglobulinaemia – neutropenia in a third of cases
- Kostmann's syndrome – severe neutropenia ($< 0.2 \times 10^9/l$)
- Schwachmann's syndrome
- cartilage-hair hypoplasia
- Fanconi's anaemia

neutropenia associated with metabolic disorders:

- propionic acidaemia
- isovaleric acidaemia
- methylmalonic acidaemia
- hyperglycinaemia

immune-mediated:

- neonatal isoimmune
- autoimmune neutropenia, eg systemic lupus erythematosus
- drugs

others:

- infection

haematology, oncology and poisoning

- drugs – chemotherapy
- Felty's syndrome (neutropenia, leukopenia, rheumatoid arthritis and splenomegaly)
- cyclical neutropenia.

Fanconi's anaemia

Autosomal recessive disorder presenting between 3 and 10 years of age with thrombocytopenia and variable pancytopenia. There are many associated features which include abnormal pigmentation, short stature, renal anomalies and mental retardation. There is an increased risk of leukaemia.

163. Causes of bone pain and anaemia

Answers: A B C D E

Vitamin C deficiency (scurvy)

The majority of cases occur between 6 and 24 months of age. Deficiency results in impairment of the formation of collagen. Symptoms are of irritability, loss of appetite, tachypnoea and generalised bone tenderness due to sub-periosteal haemorrhages. Haemorrhage may also occur in the skin, bone, subdural space and gut. Other features include poor wound healing, bluish purple spongy swelling of the gums and haematuria. X-ray changes may be seen in the long bones around the knee with white lines seen on the ends of the shafts of the femur and tibia. Areas of bone destruction may also be seen.

Neuroblastoma

This accounts for 8% of childhood cancer, and the incidence is 1 per 100 000. Median age at onset is 20 months. The tumour arises from primitive neural crest cells and can arise anywhere in the sympathetic nervous system. The commonest site is the adrenal medulla. Other sites include the cervical and thoracic sympathetic chains. Metastasis can occur anywhere with bone pain, cord compression, mediastinal mass, metastasis to skin, liver and bone marrow with bone marrow suppression and pancytopenia. Production of catecholamines may produce hypertension and products detected on urine testing include vanillylmandelic acid (VMA) and homovanillic acid (HVA). Prognosis is dependent upon staging, and the age at presentation.

Langerhans' cell histiocytosis

Langerhans' cell histiocytosis is the previously described histiocytosis X which encompasses Letterer–Siwe disease, Hand–Schüller–Christian disease and eosinophilic granuloma. Syndromes are identified according to the degree or number of organ systems involved, for example Langerhans' cell histiocytosis, solitary skull lesion instead of eosinophilic granuloma. In children presenting with generalised Langerhans' cell histiocytosis many organ systems can be involved.

164. Acute lymphoblastic leukaemia

Answers: A B C E

Acute lymphoblastic leukaemia (ALL) accounts for one-third of childhood malignancies in the UK. The overall risk of ALL is 1 in 3500 in the first 10 years of life. There is a peak incidence between 2 and 6 years of age with boys affected more than girls (ratio 1.2:1.0). There seems to be a genetic factor. In affected individuals the risk of an identical twin developing ALL is 14–20%, the risk of a sibling developing ALL is 1 in 900. Clinical symptoms at presentation include fever (60%), lethargy, bone pain, bruising, abdominal pain, anorexia and central nervous system involvement (2.5%). Signs include pallor and bruising, lymphadenopathy and hepatosplenomegaly. An anterior mediastinal mass is present in 5–10%.

Investigations show anaemia (70%), thrombocytopenia (70%), neutropenia in nearly all patients and a high white count (>50 x 10^9/l in 20%). Chest X-ray may show mediastinal mass, pleural effusions or cardiomegaly. Cerebrospinal fluid (CSF) examination shows leukaemic cells in 5% and implies central nervous system involvement. The white count at diagnosis is the most important prognostic indicator, with white count > 50 x 10^9/l indicating a worse prognosis. Other poor prognostic features include age less than 2 years at diagnosis, central nervous system involvement, presence of a mediastinal mass and being a boy. Long-term survival has improved hugely over the last two decades and is now on average 70%.

165. Thrombocytosis

Answers: B C E

Thrombocytosis may be:

physiological (premature infants):

- primary
  - Downs syndrome (transient)
  - myeloproliferative disorders
- secondary
  - infection
  - malignancy
  - post-splenectomy (absent splenic pooling)
  - chronic inflammatory disease (juvenile chronic arthritis, ulcerative colitis, Crohn's disease)
  - Kawasaki's disease, platelet count raised in second to third week of illness
  - iron deficiency
  - vitamin E deficiency.

or rebound thrombocytosis after thrombocytopenia (eg due to disseminated intravascular coagulation, chemotherapy).

haematology, oncology and poisoning

166. Aplastic anaemia

Answers: A B C D E

Aplastic anaemia is pancytopenia resulting from aplasia of the bone marrow with no evidence of extramedullary disease. Causes of aplastic anaemia are:

- congenital
  - Schwachman diamond syndrome
  - dyskeratosis congenita
- acquired
  - idiopathic (majority)
  - drugs (chloramphenicol, sulphonamides, gold, cytotoxics)
  - ionising radiation, chemicals and toxins (eg benzene, organic solvents, insecticides)
  - viral infections (eg hepatitis A and C, parvovirus, human immunodeficiency virus (HIV), Epstein–Barr virus)
  - pre-leukaemic states
  - pregnancy.

Acquired aplastic anaemia has an incidence of 1 per 100 000 with a male to female ratio of 2:1. Onset is often acute and prognosis can be poor.

167. Diseases with an increased risk of malignancy

Answers: A B C D E

- Ataxia telangiectasia – leukaemia or lymphoma in 10%
- Bloom's syndrome – risk of leukaemia or other malignancy in 25%
- Down's syndrome – risk of leukaemia in 1 in 74
- Fanconi's anaemia – leukaemia in 1 in 12
- Hemihypertrophy and Beckwith–Wiedemann syndrome – adrenal carcinoma, Wilms' tumour, hepatoblastoma
- Chédiak-Higashi syndrome – risk of lymphoma
- Gardner syndrome/familial adenomatous polyposis coli – carcinoma of colon
- Xeroderma pigmentosum – increased risk of skin cancer
- Neurofibromatosis – central nervous system tumours in 5–10%
- Tuberous sclerosis – rhabdomyoma of heart, astrocytomas
- von Hippel–Lindau syndrome – phaeochromocytoma, cerebellar haemangioblastoma and retinal angiomata
- Klinefelter's syndrome – breast cancer

168. von Willebrand's disease

Answers: A C D

Type I – classic von Willebrand's disease

This has autosomal dominant inheritance; chromosome 12 carries the defect. The pathogenesis is under-production of von Willebrand's protein, the role of which is platelet aggregation and carriage of factor VIII. Laboratory features include prolonged bleeding time, normal platelet count, normal prothrombin time and prolonged partial thromboplastin time. Diagnostic features include a reduced level of von Willebrand's protein, von Willebrand's activity and factor VIII activity. Platelet adhesion is reduced and platelets do not aggregate when the antibiotic ristocetin is added to platelet rich plasma. Clinical features reflect the bleeding tendency and include bruising, nose bleeds, bleeding from the gums, menorrhagia and prolonged bleeding after injury. Haemarthrosis is rare but can occur in severe disease. Treatment of bleeding episodes is with fresh frozen plasma or cryoprecipitate; the latter being more effective. DDAVP can be used for mild episodes.

Other types of von Willebrand's disease (types II and III) are less common.

Haemophilia

- haemophilia A – factor VIII deficiency (X-linked)
- haemophilia B – factor IX deficiency (X-linked), Christmas disease
- haemophilia C – factor XI deficiency (autosomal recessive).

Platelet function and bleeding time are normal. The level of von Willebrand's factor is normal as well.

169. Bleeding time

Answers: A D E

The bleeding time assesses platelet function, platelet number and vascular integrity. It is extremely sensitive to platelet number. Normal bleeding time is between 4 and 8 minutes. The technique is very precise and the commonest cause of a prolonged bleeding time is that this has been done incorrectly, for example too deep a cut has been made or the cuff pressure is too high. Causes of a prolonged bleeding time include:

- poor technique
- aspirin
- platelet function disorders
  - Glanzmann's thrombasthenia
  - Bernard–Soulier disease

haematology, oncology and poisoning

- thrombocytopenia from any cause
- von Willebrand's disease.

If the prolonged bleeding time is not due to a low platelet count then a defect of platelet function should be suspected. Platelet counts of more than $50 \times 10^9/l$ are usually associated with normal bleeding times.

170. X-linked agammaglobulinaemia

Answers: A C D E

This is also known as Bruton's disease. It is commoner in males. The gene is localised to the long arm of chromosome X. Prenatal diagnosis is possible. The disorder is characterised by absent or low IgA, G and M. T cell function is normal. It presents after 3–6 months as the fall in transplacentally acquired IgG occurs. Presentation is with recurrent bacterial infection. There is an increased risk of malignancy as with most other immunodeficiencies. Screening is by doing the serum immunoglobulins in children with recurrent infection. Blood group antibodies and the antibody response to immunisations given will also be absent. Regular intravenous immunoglobulin is indicated in addition to prompt treatment of infections with appropriate antibiotics. In some patients prophylactic antibiotics are indicated. Bone marrow transplantation is the treatment of choice.

171. DiGeorge syndrome (22q deletion syndrome)

Answers: B C E

This is usually sporadic although familial clustering has been reported. The gene has been localised to chromosome 22. Clinical features of DiGeorge syndrome are:

- thymic aplasia/hypoplasia (hypoplasia is commoner than aplasia)
- hypoparathyroidism
  - presents with hypocalcaemic seizures (neonatal tetany)
  - absent parathyroid hormone
- congenital heart disease
  - right-sided aortic arch
  - truncus arteriosus
  - interrupted aortic arch
  - atrioventricular septal defect
  - ventricular septal defect
  - hypoplastic pulmonary artery
  - pulmonary atresia
- facial abnormalities
  - hypertelorism
  - cleft lip or palate

haematology, oncology and poisoning

- low set ears
- anti-mongoloid slant
- others
  - imperforate anus, oesophageal atresia
  - failure to thrive
  - chronic infection (otitis media, pneumonia, diarrhoea)
  - deafness.

The total lymphocyte count can be low, normal or raised. Assessment needs to be made of the percentage of circulating mature lymphocytes by assessing their response to phytohaemoglutinin (PHA). Treatment first aims to deal with manifestations of the syndrome (hypocalcaemia, cardiac defects). In the long term, bone marrow transplantation is the treatment of choice. Graft-versus-host disease can occur following cardiac bypass and irradiated blood products need to be given to try avoiding this.

172. Osteosarcoma

Answer: C

The male to female ratio of osteosarcoma is 1.5:1 with a peak incidence in the second decade. There is an increased risk associated with retinoblastoma, previous chemotherapy and radiotherapy. Tumours occur in the metaphyseal region of long bones with the distal femur being the commonest site followed by proximal tibia and the proximal humerus. It usually presents with pain, and metastases (lung and bone) are present at presentation in 20%. Diagnosis is by radiology and biopsy, with bone appearing sclerotic on a plain radiograph. Treatment is with chemotherapy and surgery. Prognosis is 60% cure if metastases are not present at diagnosis and 20% if they are. The differential diagnosis includes Ewing's sarcoma and osteomyelitis.

Ewing's sarcoma

This has a male to female ratio of 1.5:1. It usually presents in the second decade and there are no known risk factors. Tumours may arise in any bone but are found most often in flat bones (pelvis, chest wall vertebrae) and the diaphyseal region of long bones. The presentation is with local pain and swelling. Fever and a raised erythrocyte sedimentation rate (ESR) are common. The appearance on X-ray is of a lytic lesion affecting the medullary cavity and cortical bone. The tumour elevates the periosteum giving an 'onion skin' appearance. Metastases are present in 25% at presentation. Treatment is with radiotherapy and chemotherapy, surgery is not always required. Survival depends on whether metastases are present at diagnosis and is 20% cure if they are and 70% if they are not.

haematology, oncology and poisoning

Differential diagnosis of a lytic bone lesion

- Ewing's sarcoma
- Langerhans' cell histiocytosis
- Osteomyelitis
- Lymphoma
- Neuroblastoma
- Metastatic sarcoma

173. Iron poisoning

Answers: A C D E

Ingestion of 60 mg/kg or more of iron may result in systemic iron toxicity. An abdominal X-ray may be useful to confirm iron ingestion as the tablets are radio-opaque. The effects of iron toxicity are dependent on the time after ingestion:

- Stage 1 (30 min–2 h) – local effects of gastrointestinal irritation including diarrhoea and vomiting. Haematemesis and hypotension may occur.
- Stage 2 (2–6 h) – apparent recovery during which iron absorption and accumulation of iron in tissues and mitochondria occur.
- Stage 3 (12 h) – cellular and mitochondrial damage occurs with hypoglycaemia and lactic acidosis.
- Stage 4 (2–4 days) – severe hepatic necrosis with raised aspartate aminotransferase, alanine aminotransferase, bilirubin and abnormal prothrombin time.
- Stage 5 (2–4 weeks) – late effects with scarring and stenosis of the pylorus.

Investigation of iron poisoning includes free iron levels in serum and an abdominal X-ray. Although investigations are useful, it is important to consider the child's symptoms as a guide to toxicity. The treatment is general and specific. Emesis and gastric lavage are not useful. Desferrioxamine (iron chelator) is the main therapeutic agent available. Supportive treatment needs to be given for hypotension or shock. If free iron is greater than 50 mg/dl or total iron is greater then 350 mg/dl then parenteral desferrioxamine is indicated. Desferrioxamine can cause anaphylaxis. It causes the urine to turn red while chelated iron is being excreted. Oral desferrioxamine may actually promote iron absorption and should not be used.

haematology, oncology and poisoning

174. Carbon monoxide poisoning

Answers: A B D

Carbon monoxide is a tasteless, odourless, colourless and non-irritant gas. It binds to haemoglobin to form carboxyhaemoglobin which reduces the oxygen carrying capacity of the blood and shifts the oxygen dissociation curve to the left. The affinity of haemoglobin for carbon monoxide is 250 times greater than that for oxygen. Endogenous production occurs and maintains a resting carboxyhaemoglobin level of 1–3%. Smoking increases carboxyhaemoglobin levels. Other sources of raised levels include car exhaust fumes, poorly maintained heating systems and smoke from fires.

Clinical features of carbon monoxide poisoning occur as a result of tissue hypoxia. $P_a(O_2)$ is normal but the oxygen content of the blood is reduced. Toxicity relates loosely to the maximum carboxyhaemoglobin concentration. Other factors include duration of exposure and age of the patient. Maximum carboxyhaemoglobin concentration:

- 10% – not normally associated with symptoms
- 10–30% – headache and dyspnoea
- 60% – coma, convulsions and death.

Neuropsychiatric problems can occur with chronic exposure. Treatment of carbon monoxide poisoning is with 100% oxygen which will reduce the carboxyhaemoglobin concentration. Hyperbaric oxygen is said to reduce the carboxyhaemoglobin level quicker.

175. Tricyclic poisoning

Answers: A C D

Mortality of deliberate tricyclic antidepressant overdose is 7–12%. Effects of tricyclic antidepressants include:

- anticholinergic – causing tachycardia, pupil dilatation, dry mucous membranes, urinary retention, hallucinations and flushing
- adrenergic (early) – causing hypertension and tachycardia
- α-adrenergic receptor blocking, causing prolonged hypotension
- central inhibition of neuronal re-uptake of noradrenaline, 5-hydroxytryptamine, serotonin and dopamine – leading to convulsions and coma
- cardiac – mainly ventricular tachycardia and fibrillation, a Arrhythmias are the main cause of death.

Treatment of overdose

Initial treatment is aimed at preventing absorption of the drug. Emetics should only be used if there is no central nervous system depression. Activated charcoal should be given every 2–4 hours. Arrhythmias may respond to correction of hypoxia and correction of acidosis with sodium bicarbonate aiming for a pH of 7.45–7.55. Anti-arrhythmics are best avoided. Convulsions should be treated with intravenous diazepam. Diazepam can also be used to treat delirium and agitation during recovery. Hypotension may respond to treatment with iv fluids and colloid. In overdosage, tissue concentrations quickly rise giving tissue to plasma ratios of between 10:1 and 30:1. The drug in plasma is extensively bound to plasma proteins and removal by dialysis is ineffective.

176. Aspirin poisoning

Answers: A D E

Clinical features

In young children there is dehydration and tachypnoea. Older children and adults have tachypnoea and vomiting with progressive lethargy. There is tinnitus and deafness, and hypoglycaemia or hyperglycaemia can occur. There are three phases:

- phase 1
  - may last up to 12 hours.
  - salicylates directly stimulate the respiratory centre resulting in a respiratory alkalosis with a compensatory alkaline urine with bicarbonate sodium and potassium loss.
- phase 2
  - may begin straight away particularly in a young child and last 12–24 hours.
  - hypokalaemia with as a consequence a paradoxical aciduria despite the alkalosis.
- phase 3
  - after 6–24 hours.
  - dehydration, hypokalaemia and progressive lactic acidosis. The acidosis now predominating.
  - can progress to pulmonary oedema with respiratory failure, disorientation and coma.

Management

- Gastric lavage up to 4 hours. Activated charcoal for sustained release preparations.
- Level at 6 hours plotted on a nomogram.
- Alkalisation of the urine to aid drug excretion, adequate fluids including bicarbonate sodium and potassium with close monitoring of acid base and electrolytes.
- Discuss with poisons centre.

177. Lead poisoning

Answers: A B C D E

Lead poisoning is uncommon but potentially very serious. It often results from pica (persistent eating of non-nutritive substances, eg soil) and is therefore commoner in pre-school age children. Other causes include sucking/ingesting lead paint, lead pipes, discharge from lead batteries and substance abuse of leaded petrol. Lead intoxication can be divided into acute and chronic effects, and results from its combination with and disruption of vital physiological enzymes. In acute intoxication there is a reversible renal Fanconi-like syndrome. In chronic intoxication:

- failure to thrive
- abdominal upset: pain/anorexia/vomiting/constipation
- lead encephalopathy: behavioural and cognitive disturbance drowsiness, seizures, neuropathies, coma
- glomerulonephritis and renal failure
- anaemia – microcytic/hypochromic, basophilic stippling of red cells.

Haematemesis occurs in iron poisoning; skin and hair changes are very common in arsenic intoxication. (See Question 177.)

178. Sickle cell anaemia

Answer: B

Sickle cell disease causes chronic anaemia with multisystem manifestations aside from the typical 'crises' (sequestration, aplastic, haemolytic). First presentation is usually a sequestration crisis in the pharyngeal bones at about 6 months, a dactylitis. The continual ischaemic insults to the spleen results in 'auto infarction' (and hyposplenism) in the first few years and a palpable spleen beyond this age suggest another diagnosis. The hyposplenism increases susceptibility to polysaccharide capsulated organisms particularly pneumococcus requiring vaccination and penicillin prophylaxis. It is thought that the relative deformability of the cell membrane protects against malaria.

179. Population screening programmes

Answers: C E

Minimal criteria for a screening programme are:

- of reasonable prevalence/incidence
- cheap and readily available test
- test is both specific (few false positives) and sensitive (few false negatives)
- early treatment improves long term outcomes.

Because of the above, any screening is to an extent setting specific with the yield depending on local prevalence of the problem to be screened. It is also important that the screening can tie in with pre-existing programmes/systems (eg Guthrie). Only thalassaemia and sickle cell disease are of sufficient prevalence and severity to warrant screening and in many areas all babies are tested routinely. Interventions include monitoring of growth and haemoglobin with transfusion when needed for thalassaemia and folic acid and pneumococcal prophylaxis for sickle cell disease.

180. Acute lymphoblastic leukaemia

Answer: D

Good prognostic signs are:

- female sex
- age > 2 years at presentation
- normal white cell count
- common cell type
- normal chest X-ray.

haematology, oncology and poisoning

181. E: Dietary review

Although this could be the picture of small bowel gastrointestinal loss (eg though a Meckel's diverticulum), the likeliest (and still surprisingly common) cause is over consumption of cow's milk. Iron bioavailability is poor, there is often a subclinical colitis with gastrointestinal blood loss and it 'fills children up' reducing their appetite for more appropriate iron-containing foods. Transfusion is contraindicated as by definition it is long-standing and well-compensated. Treatment is a change in diet with oral iron supplements at least until the haemoglobin starts to rise to reasonable levels. Untreated iron deficiency has adverse developmental consequences.

182. B: Single supraclavicular node

Isolated lymphadenopathy is generally benign in children. It may be related to infection in the area of local drainage. If multiple areas are involved the illness is likely to be systemic, eg a mononucleosis-like illness but it is rare even in these cases for diagnosis to require histology. The main exception to this rule is enlargement of a supraclavicular node (due to its regional drainage), which cannot be ignored and is much more likely to herald serious (especially malignant) pathology.

183. E: Delayed developmental milestones

Lead poisoning is rarely seen nowadays due to house paints being lead free. Above a certain concentration it is neurotoxic and the developmental effect is only partially reversible by chelation. Classic features of lead poisoning are:

- microcytic anaemia
- developmental delay
- constipation
- vomiting.

Treatment is by removal of the source (such as paint) and chelation therapy using dimercaprol.

A co-existing iron deficiency is common which firstly further exacerbates the anaemia and secondly contributes to increased lead absorption. Basophilic stippling is due to inhibition of pyrimidine 5' nucleotidase and results in accumulation of denatured RNA. Treatment involves:

- removing source
- chelation:
    - mild   oral D-penicillamine
    - severe   iv sodium calcium edetate (EDTA)
    - very severe   im injections of dimercaprol to increase
                            effect of EDTA.

haematology, oncology
and poisoning

184. PRESENTING SYMPTOMS OF PAEDIATRIC MALIGNANCIES

1. C – ALL

An acute limp is a classic presentation of ALL and is due to small vessel obstruction in bones or bony metastases. A good rule of thumb is to always take a full blood count and film in a child presenting with an acute painful limp.

2. E – Rhabdomyosarcoma

The orbital muscles are a common primary site for this tumour.

3. H – Histiocytosis X

Protean symptoms but a hard-to-define rash with bone pain, lytic lesions (skull particularly) and lymphadenopathy are very suspicious. Skin biopsy can help make the diagnosis.

As for the others malignancies:

- hepatoblastoma and Wilms' tumour tend to present with an abdominal mass/pain
- medulloblastoma with signs of raised intracranial pressure and cerebellar signs (infratentorial)
- Osteosarcoma with bone pain (long bones).

185. SIGNS OF POISONING

1. C – Haematemesis

Iron poisoning goes through several phases if sufficient (> 60 mg/kg elemental iron) has been ingested. In the first (< 2 hours) there is abdominal pain, hypotension and haematemesis followed by a 'purple patch'. If untreated liver function progressively deteriorates thereafter. Treatment is by resuscitation and parenteral desferrioxamine. (See also Question 175.)

2. F – Hypoventilation

Often forgotten but the **first** phase of salicylate poisoning is a respiratory alkalosis. Caused by a direct effect of the salicylate on the respiratory centre resulting in tachypnoea. Tinnitus and metabolic acidosis (later) are additional features. (See also Question 178).

3. A – Mydriasis

This is a classic anti-cholinergic effect. Other signs include:

- dry mouth
- retention of urine
- tachycardia
- abdominal cramps
- flushing
- hallucinations.

(See also Question 177.)

256

INFECTIOUS DISEASES AND IMMUNOLOGY ANSWERS

186. Polymerase chain reaction

Answers: B C E

The PCR is a means of amplifying nucleic acids. The nucleic acid being analysed (usually DNA) is known as the template, of which only a very small amount is required. This template DNA may be extracted from many sources such as:

- peripheral blood lymphocytes
- tissue/samples from infected patient
- biopsies
- amniocentesis/chorionic villus sampling.

PCR involves various steps before analysis of the final product is possible:

Extraction and denaturation – DNA is extracted from the specimen by denaturing it. This is done by heating it to 95 °C. This yields single-stranded DNA.

Annealing to primers – two or more pre-determined primers are then added to the single-stranded DNA. Primers are oligonucleotide sequences, approximately 16 nucleotides long, specific to the gene/disease being investigated. If these sequences are present in the DNA, therefore reflecting the presence of the gene/disease, the primers will bind. For annealing to occur, the overall temperature is lowered to approximately 60 °C.

Primer extension – a DNA polymerase enzyme, Taq polymerase, is then added, which will catalyse extension of the primers in a 5'–3' direction. This results in a doubling of the amount of DNA present at the start of the reaction. For this to occur the overall temperature is increased again.

Proliferation of amplified DNA – by repeating the heating cycle in step 3 a set number of times (normally 30), an exponential increase in the number of copies of amplified DNA occurs. This renders the PCR product available in sufficient amount for analysis.

Analysis of PCR product – the amplified product can now be analysed for the gene or disease being investigated. There are various techniques for analysis:

- Gel electrophoresis (normal technique) – the product will have an estimated molecular weight, and is compared with markers of pre-determined molecular weight
- Southern blotting, following digestion with an endonuclease (same method on RNA is northern blotting)
- Hybridisation with a specific labelled nucleic acid probe.

Reverse transcriptase PCR (Rt PCR)

The phenotype of an individual or cell is dependent on which genes from the overall genome are expressed. Therefore, to analyse the phenotype, analysis of only the genes being expressed is required. These genes are those that are transcribed into mRNA (messenger RNA). In order to analyse mRNA, it requires conversion to complementary DNA (cDNA) using reverse transcriptase, as RNA is not stable enough to be used in PCR. PCR performed on cDNA will reflect the content of mRNA and therefore gene expression in individual tissues.

Clinical applications of PCR

- Genetic mutations, eg DF508 in cystic fibrosis
  - pre-natal diagnosis – amniocentesis
  - chorionic villus sampling
- Viruses, eg HIV
- Bacteria, eg PCR for *Neisseria meningitidis*
- Prognostic oncogenes in tumours.

187. Tumour necrosis factor

Answers: B C D E

Tumour necrosis factor (TNF) is one of a number of cytokines involved in the inflammatory process, having a wide range of functions, many in combination with other cytokines especially interleukin (IL)–1. Its name originates from early studies of its cytotoxic effect on tumours, although it can, in fact, encourage tumour growth. It exists in two forms – TNF α and TNF β. TNF α is synthesised by many cells including macrophages, T and B lymphocytes, eosinophils, natural killer cells, astrocytes and Kupffer cells. It plays a key role in immune responses to bacteria, viruses, immune complexes, C5a, other cytokines, oxygen intermediates and in diseases such as Crohn's disease, rheumatoid arthritis and multiple sclerosis. Together with interferon γ it is cytotoxic to many tumours and has been used as chemotherapy in melanomas. It also plays a part in the processes of septic shock, multi-organ failure and cerebral malaria. TNF β is synthesised by activated T and B lymphocytes. It has a wide range of functions including actions on lymphocytes, endothelial, neuronal and bone cells.

188. IMMUNOGLOBULINS

Answer: C

The broad functions of immunoglobulins are to bind antigens and set about series of reactions to destroy antigen. They consist of two heavy and two light polypeptide chains, divided into the antigen binding fragment (Fab) and the complement binding fragment (Fc). It is the structure of the latter which varies between different immunoglobulin classes. The Fc portion binds to cell-based Fc receptors on complement, basophils, phagocytes, etc.

Immunoglobulins in descending order of serum concentration

IgG:

- most abundant Ig (70–80%)
- involved in secondary immune response
- crosses placenta by active transport
- Fc receptors bind to and activate complement via classic pathway and also bind to phagocytic cells
- four subgroups:
  - IgG1 and 3 – responses to protein antigens
  - IgG2 – responses to bacterial polysaccharides
  - IgG4.

IgA:

- present in secretions – protects mucosal surfaces
- produced in lymphoid tissue
- exists as monomer in plasma; dimer in secretions(joined by J-chain)
- activates complement via alternative pathway
- IgA deficiency is associated with:
  - autoimmune disorders, eg coeliac disease
  - infections of mucosal surfaces, eg gastroenteritis, lower respiratory tract.
  - food allergy

IgM:

- involved in primary immune response
- exists as pentamer (joined via J-chain)
- does not cross the placenta
- activates complement via classical pathway
- extremely effective against bacteria
- antibodies to ABO blood group antigens are usually IgM.

infectious diseases and immunology

IgD:

- expressed on B cells
- involved in regulating B cell activation together with IgM.

IgE:

- present in very low concentration in normal individuals
- binds to and activates basophils/mast cells via Fc receptor, and once bound causes the release of histamine and other mediators
- levels rise in:
  - atopic patients, eg asthma, eczema
  - type I hypersensitivity responses, eg anaphylaxis, acute asthma
  - parasitic infections.

Hypersensitivity reactions

- Type I – immediate
- Type II – cell-bound antigen and extracellular matrix(eg basement membrane)
- Type III – immune complexes (eg systemic lupus erythematosus)
- Type IV – delayed (eg contact dermatitis)

189. Chronic granulomatous disease

Answers: B D E

Neutrophil defects

Neutrophil defects may be congenital (see below) or acquired (due to bone marrow dysfunction). Defects may occur in any of the various steps: recognition, chemotaxis, adherence, ingestion, degranulation, killing.

Chronic granulomatous disease

The incidence 1 in 1,000,000, and it is X-linked in 50–70% and autosomal recessive (chromasome 7) in 30–40%. Neutrophils ingest but not are able to kill bacteria. Due to abnormalities in NADPH (nicotinamide adenosine dinucleotide phosphate) oxidase (reduced form), cells are unable to generate the respiratory burst (which normally produces oxygen radicals for bacterial killing). It presents in the first 3 years of life with skin infections/pneumonias/osteomyelitis/abscesses/persistent lymphadenopathy and hepatosplenomegaly/uncommon organisms. Investigation is with NBT test (yellow dye fails to turn blue when added to neutrophils due to failure of respiratory burst). The actual neutrophil numbers may be normal or increased. Management is with prophylactic antibiotics and antifungals with aggressive treatment of infections. Bone marrow transplant is an option.

Leukocyte adhesion deficiency

This is autosomal recessive with defects in adherence, chemotaxis, phagocytosis, T cell cytotoxicity. There is delayed separation and infection of umbilical cord. The affected individual has recurrent infections such as chronic granulomatous disease.

Chédiak-Higashi syndrome

This is an autosomal recessive condition. Polymorphs contain huge granules that disable chemotaxis and bactericidal properties. It may affect

- platelets – coagulation defects
- leucocytes – immunodeficiency
- melanosomes – albinism
- Schwann cells – neuropathy.

Myeloperoxidase deficiency

This is an autosomal recessive condition with defects in activity against bacteria and fungi. There is persistent candidiasis.

190. *Chlamydia*

Answers: A C D E

Chlamydia spp. are Gram-negative obligate intracellular bacteria. There are four species: *C. trachomatis*, *C. pneumoniae*, *C. psittaci* and *C. pecorum*. Infections caused by *Chlamydia trachomatis* include trachoma, the most important preventable cause of blindness worldwide. It is endemic in the Middle East and South-East Asia. Starts as aconjunctivitis and spreads from eye to eye. Flies are a frequent vector. Other manifestations of infection with *Chlamydia trachomatis* include:

- Conjunctivitis
- Pneumonia
- Non-specific urethritis
- Epididymo-orchitis
- Procto-colitis
- Reactive arthritis (Reiter's syndrome)
- Pelvic inflammatory disease (endometritis, salpingitis)
- Lymphogranuloma venereum.

infectious diseases and immunology

Vertical transmission from a mother with an infected genital tract occurs in up to 50% of cases. The majority of infants will present with conjunctivitis at 1–2 weeks. A smaller proportion (10–20%) may present with pneumonia (age 1–3 months). Treatment is with erythromycin or tetracyclines (older children and adults). *C. pneumoniae* is a cause of bronchitis and pneumonia in children and young adults. *C. psittaci* causes psittacosis, an influenza-like illness in humans. It mainly infects parrots and birds. *C. pecorum* primarily infects cattle and sheep. There is no evidence of human infection.

191. Toxoplasmosis

Answers: B D E

Toxoplasmosis is caused by the protozoan *Toxoplasma gondii*. The primary hosts are members of the cat family. Transmission to man is by ingestion of oocytes from the faeces of infected cats and the consumption of extra-intestinal forms of the parasite from undercooked meats. Toxoplasmosis usually causes a latent infection, recognised on serological testing. Overt infection is rare. Features include:

- generalised fatigue and myalgia
- lymphadenopathy (most commonly cervical)
- arthralgia
- transient maculopapular rash (rare)
- hepatosplenomegaly (rare)
- pneumonia/myocarditis (rare).

More serious manifestations can occur in the immunocompromised host and include ocular manifestation (uveitis, choroidoretinitis), pseudotumour cerebri and encephalitis. Laboratory features include atypical lymphocytosis, inversion of the CD4:CD8 ratio and eosinophilia. Diagnosis is serological, IgM antibodies appear within a few days and IgG antibodies within a few weeks. Isolation of *T. gondii* from blood, cerebrospinal fluid (CSF) or body secretions is difficult but is also diagnostic. Treatment, if required, is with a combination of pyrimethamine and sulfadiazine. The former is a folate antagonist and so folinic acid supplementation is required.

Congenital toxoplasmosis

There is a 40% risk of transmission if the mother is infected during pregnancy. The risk of infection is higher the more advanced the pregnancy. However, manifestations are more serious the earlier infection occurs. 90% of congenitally infected infants are asymptomatic in the neonatal period. The classic triad of retinochoroiditis, hydrocephalus and intracerebral calcification is uncommon and the clinical manifestations are usually non-specific. If infection is diagnosed during pregnancy then termination is an option, alternatively spiramycin has been given. Neither pyrimethamine or sulfadiazine can be given during the first trimester of pregnancy as both are teratogenic. They are used later in pregnancy.

192. *Streptococcus pneumoniae*

Answers: A C

Pneumococci (*Streptococcus pneumoniae*) are Gram-positive diplococci. There are more than 80 distinct serotypes. More than 60% of the population carry pneumococci in their nasopharynx, most of these being strains of low virulence. Diseases caused by *S. pneumoniae* are:

- otitis media
- sinusitis
- scarlet fever
- impetigo
- pneumonia
- septicaemia
- peritonitis
- septic arthritis
- osteomyelitis
- meningitis
- brain abscess.

Risk factors for pneumococcal infection:

- extremes of age
- sickle cell disease
- immunodeficiency
  - antibody deficiency – hypogammaglobulinaemia, subclass deficiency
  - phagocyte abnormalities – neutropenia, hyposplenism, asplenia
  - complement deficiencies
  - human immunodeficiency virus (HIV)
- leukaemia.

Two pneumococcal vaccines are available – Pneumovax and Prevenar (polysaccharide conjugated vaccine). The dosage schedule for each vaccine varies according to the age of the child, but Prevenar is the only one of the two licensed for administration to children under 2 years of age. Diseases for which Pneumovax is recommended in children over 2 years are:

- asplenia, splenic dysfunction, post splenectomy
- sickle cell disease
- diabetes mellitus
- immunodeficiency
- chronic respiratory disease
- congenital heart disease
- chronic renal disease – nephrotic syndrome
- chronic liver disease
- presence of cerebrospinal fluid (CSF) shunt
- presence of cochlear implant.
- child under 5 years with history of invasive pneumococcal disease.

There are 23 serotypes which cause 80% of severe infections, and it is these that are covered by the pneumococcal vaccine. Protection is not complete. Pneumovax vaccine lasts for approximately 5 years although the duration of efficacy is not clear. Antibiotic prophylaxis is indicated in at-risk groups.

Lyme disease is caused by the spirochaete *Borrelia burgdorferi*. The UK immunisation schedule is due to change to include immunisation against pnuemococcus with Prevenar for all infants from 2006/7 (see website www.immunisation.nhs.uk).

193. Atypical mycobacterial infection

Answer: C

Non-tuberculous or atypical mycobacterial infections are seen at the extremes of age. The infective agents are acid-fast bacilli found in the environment. Unlike tuberculous infection, atypical mycobacterial infection is acquired from the environment and not from person-to-person contact and hence contact tracing is not helpful. There are 13 strains of non-tuberculous mycobacteria which can potentially infect man. Common strains include *Mycobacterium avium-intracellulare*, *M. marinum* and *M. scrofulaceum*. The number of cases per year is increasing possibly due to better case recognition.

Lymphadenitis is the commonest presentation in childhood. This is usually anterior cervical or submandibular. The child usually presents between age 2 and 5 years. The lymphadenopathy is usually unilateral and systemic symptoms are rare. Spontaneous resolution may occur but often not for many months. If the lymphadenitis ruptures then a discharging sinus will develop. Pulmonary disease is rare in childhood but common in adults. There is an increased incidence in older children with cystic fibrosis. Cutaneous disease is also rare in childhood. The usual agent if it occurs is *M. marinum*. Skeletal involvement can occur and usually manifests as infected bursae, tendons and sheaths. Disseminated disease is rare but can occur in children who are immunosuppressed.

infectious diseases and
immunology

Diagnosis requires a high index of clinical suspicion. Intradermal skin tests can be helpful in distinguishing non-tuberculous from tuberculous mycobacterial infection. Incisional biopsy of infected glands is often performed in order to exclude malignancy. However, although reassuring, this often results in sinus formation which can become chronically infected. Excision biopsy is the preferred method of obtaining a histological specimen. Non-caseating granulomas are often seen. Definitive diagnosis is by culture which often takes up to three months. Complete surgical excision is the treatment of choice. If excision is not possible or incomplete then chemotherapy is required. Conventional antituberculous therapy is usually ineffective. First-line therapy is with clarithromycin and rifabutin. Second-line therapy includes ethambutol and ciprofloxacin.

Differential diagnosis of cervical lymphadenopathy:

- cervical abscess
- tuberculosis
- cat scratch fever
- mumps
- salivary stone
- malignancy
- infectious mononucleosis
- toxoplasmosis
- brucellosis.

194. Familial Mediterranean fever

Answers: B C E

This shows autosomal recessive inheritance with male predominance. The gene is carried on chromosome 16. Onset is usually in the first or second decade. Acute attacks of fever and abdominal pain (peritonitis) are characteristic. Pleuritis and arthritis can occur and 25% have skin lesions. The episodes usually occur once or twice a month. Attacks tend to remit during pregnancy but return afterwards. Colchicine can be used to suppress an attack and should be used at the first sign of prodromal symptoms. Its use as a prophylactic agent can reduce the number of attacks. Amyloidosis can complicate familial Mediterranean fever, and amyloid is deposited in the adrenals, spleen, glomeruli, alveoli and in arterioles and veins. The liver and heart are usually spared. Colchicine will reduce the incidence of amyloidosis. There are no diagnostic tests. The underlying pathology is hyperaemia and non-bacterial inflammation. It is thought to be due to deficiency of a protease which normally inhibits the chemotactic activity of C5a and IL8.

infectious diseases and immunology

195. Viruses

Answers: B C

RNA-containing viruses

- arenavirus – Lassa fever
- orthomyxovirus/paramyxovirus
    - influenza
    - parainfluenza
    - measles
    - mumps
    - respiratory syncytial virus
- picornavirus
    - enterovirus
    - rhinovirus
- reovirus – rotavirus
- retrovirus – HIV
- rhabdovirus – rabies
- rubivirus – rubella
- togavirus – hepatitis C
- torovirus – ebola fever

DNA viruses

- adenovirus
- hepadnavirus – hepatitis B

Herpes virus

- cytomegalovirus
- Epstein–Barr virus
- herpes simplex virus
- varicella zoster virus

196. Cerebrospinal fluid

Answers: C D

The normal values for CSF cell count, protein, glucose and pressure at different ages should be known and can be found in any standard reference text. CSF protein is higher in pre-term than in term infants and higher in term infants than in children or adults. Red cells are not a normal finding in the CSF of older children although they may be present as a consequence of the tap being traumatic. CSF pressure rises with age. There are many causes of a raised CSF white cell count including tumours. The CSF white cell count and glucose can be normal in bacterial meningitis.

infectious diseases and immunology

197. Impetigo

Answers: A C E

Impetigo can be classified as simple (non-bullous) or bullous. Bullae are usually flaccid, rupture easily and contain pus. The usual infecting agent is *Staphylococcus aureus*. The lesions occur in clusters, are usually found at the extremities and are highly infectious. Non-bullous impetigo is due to either *S. aureus* or group A *β-haemolytic Streptococcus*. Lesions are painless and not usually associated with systemic symptoms. Regional adenitis can occur. Topical antibiotics are not generally helpful and systemic antibiotics are the treatment of choice. Erythromycin or penicillin and flucloxacillin should be used.

198. Infectious mononucleosis

Answers: A B D E

Infectious mononucleosis (glandular fever) is caused by infection with the Epstein–Barr virus. An infectious mononucleosis-like illness can be caused by other agents including cytomegalovirus, adenovirus and toxoplasmosis. Epstein–Barr infection is often subclinical. Clinical infection is rare in the pre-school group. Spread is by transmission of oral secretions ('kissing disease'). The clinical features are of fever, pharyngitis and lymphadenopathy. The syndrome often persists for some weeks and a post-viral fatigue syndrome can occur. The appearance of a maculo-papular rash following the administration of ampicillin is quite characteristic. Splenomegaly is seen in 50%. A smaller number of patients develop mild jaundice and hepatomegaly. Laboratory features include an atypical lymphocytosis, mild thrombocytopenia and a transient elevation of the transaminases. Confirmation is by the Paul Bunnell test or Epstein–Barr virus serology. It is important to realise that (particularly in children under 5 years) the Paul Bunnell test can be negative in glandular fever due to Epstein–Barr virus infection. In such cases the presence of IgM antibody to viral capsid antigen is diagnostic. Complications are rarely seen but include splenic rupture, airway obstruction, Guillain–Barré syndrome, VII nerve palsy, agranulocytosis and pancarditis. Treatment is supportive.

Infections commonly associated with an atypical lymphocytosis are:

- cytomegalovirus
- malaria
- toxoplasmosis
- tuberculosis
- mumps.

Epstein–Barr virus is associated with:

- nasopharyngeal carcinoma
- Burkitt's lymphoma
- B cell driven lymphomas.

199. Schistosomiasis

Answers: A B C D

Schistosomes are trematodes that have a mammal as the definitive host and a snail as an intermediate host. The main schistosomes affecting man are *S. haematobium*, *S. japonicum*, *S. mansoni*, *S. intercalatum* and *S. mekongi*. Schistosomiasis is a very common infection worldwide which particularly affects children and young adults in endemic areas. Humans are infected through contact with water contaminated with cercariae, the free-living infective stage of the parasite. Infection is usually asymptomatic. The manifestations of acute infection are fever, arthralgia, lymphadenopathy, hepatosplenomegaly and a rash. This is immune complex mediated. More serious is chronic infection with retention of eggs in the host and chronic granulomatous injury. The organs affected are the urinary tract and intestine (directly) and liver, lungs and central nervous system by haematogenous spread. Granulomas surround the eggs. Cell mediated responses play a role. Chronic renal failure and bladder carcinoma can result.

S. haematobium usually affects the renal tract and can cause haematuria, frequency and dysuria and obstructive uropathy. *S. japonicum*, *S. mansoni*, *S. intercalatum* and *S. mekongi* usually cause intestinal symptoms, the most common being abdominal pain and bloody diarrhoea. Other manifestations include chronic liver disease and cirrhosis, chronic lung disease and cor pulmonale and spinal cord lesions such as transverse myelitis. Seizures can occur secondary to central nervous system disease. Diagnosis is by the identification of the eggs in excreta. Eosinophilia is common. Treatment is by eradication of the parasite using praziquantel.

200. Notifiable diseases

Answers: B C D E

Notifiable diseases are:

- acute encephalitis
- acute poliomyelitis
- acute viral hepatitis
- anthrax
- cholera
- diphtheria

infectious diseases and immunology

- dysentery (amoebic or bacillary)
- food poisoning (all sources)
- leprosy
- leptospirosis
- malaria
- measles
- meningitis (viral, bacterial, other or unspecified)
- meningococcal septicaemia without meningitis
- mumps
- ophthalmia neonatorum
- paratyphoid
- plague
- rabies
- relapsing fever (borrelia infection)
- rubella
- scarlet fever
- smallpox
- tetanus
- tuberculosis
- typhoid fever
- typhus
- viral haemorrhagic fever
- whooping cough
- yellow fever.

201. Measles

Answers: B C D

Worldwide, measles infection is very common and is associated with significant morbidity and mortality. Measles is caused by an RNA virus. Transmission is person-to-person and by droplet infection. Humans are the only host. It is a notifiable disease. Infection is rare under the age of 6 months due to the presence of maternal antibodies. Second attacks can occur. Incubation is 14 days from exposure to the appearance of the rash. Infectivity is greatest during the prodromal period and persists for 5 days after the appearance of the rash. The initial symptoms are fever, cough and coryza. The rash is an erythematous maculopapular one. It is widespread and classically starts behind the ears. Koplik's spots in the mouth are pathognomonic. Diagnosis is clinical and by serology. Complications of measles can be divided into:

- early
  - otitis media
  - laryngotracheobronchitis
  - myocarditis/pericarditis
  - encephalitis

- primary or secondary (bacterial) pneumonia
- late – subacute sclerosing panencephalitis.

Prevention of measles is by vaccination. Measles vaccination is given as part of the MMR at around 14 months of age. Since October 1996 a pre-school booster is also given because a single dose of vaccine does not confer life-long immunity.

202. Lyme disease

Answers: A C

Lyme disease is a multisystem disease caused by the spirochaete *Borrelia burgdorferi*. Transmission is by infected ticks. Vector hosts include deer and mice. Apart from transplacentally, person-to-person transmission does not occur. The most common clinical finding is a skin rash (erythema migrans) which begins 4–20 days after the tick bite. Lesions can occur at any site – most cases involve the thigh, buttocks or axilla. Associated with the rash are fever, lymphadenopathy, conjunctivitis, pharyngitis and anicteric hepatitis. Later problems (after weeks or months) include neurological, cardiac and joint involvement. Neurological involvement includes aseptic meningitis, cranial nerve involvement (facial nerve palsy being the commonest), peripheral radiculopathy, chorea, cerebella ataxia and Guillain-Barré syndrome. Cardiac involvement is rare, problems seen include atrio-ventricular block, myocarditis and left ventricular dysfunction. Arthritis occurs more commonly. It is usually of sudden onset and can be a mono-, oligo- or polyarthritis. Arthritis is generally a late manifestation.

The diagnosis is essentially a clinical one. Spirochaetes grow poorly on culture and the frequency of isolation from infected patients is low. Serological techniques include western blotting and enzyme-linked immunosorbent assay (ELISA). Fifty per cent of early stage and 80% of late stage patients are seropositive. Treatment is with antibiotics, which include penicillin, amoxicillin, erythromycin and ceftriaxone. The response to antibiotic therapy is generally good. Prognosis is excellent. About 3–4% of children develop chronic arthritis and a small number have chronic neurological or cardiac sequelae. Re-infection may occur as antibodies are not protective against future exposures.

203. Parvovirus B19 infection

Answers: A B C E

Parvovirus B19 is a DNA virus. Humans are the only host, and it is spread by droplets. Infectivity is high (particularly before the rash appears). Infection is commonest in school-age children but can occur at any age. Infection with parvovirus B19 can be asymptomatic. More commonly it presents as erythema infectiosum, initially with mild fever and upper respiratory tract symptoms with the later appearance of a facial rash (slapped cheek syndrome or fifth disease). The rash usually spreads to the trunk and can persist for several days. Other manifestations of parvovirus B19 infection include purpura, lymphadenopathy and aplastic anaemia. The aplastic anaemia is usually temporary and is commoner in children with either sickle cell disease or hereditary spherocytosis. Arthralgia/arthropathy is common in older patients, especially females. In-utero infection is associated with spontaneous abortion, hydrops fetalis and neonatal thrombocytopenia. The diagnosis of parvovirus infection is essentially a clinical one. The patient may be anaemic with a low reticulocyte count. The platelet count and white cell count may also be reduced. Anti-parvovirus IgM is the best marker of acute infection and is usually positive within two weeks of the onset of infection. Treatment is essentially symptomatic. Intravenous immunoglobulin has been used in children with immunodeficiency and those with aplastic anaemia. Differential diagnosis of parvovirus B19 infection includes:

- rubella
- measles
- enterovirus infection
- drugs
- rash and arthropathy
  - juvenile chronic arthritis
  - systemic lupus erythematosus
  - other connective tissue disease.

204. Vertical transmission of hepatitis B

Answers: A B D E

Vertical transmission is thought to account for 40% of hepatitis B worldwide. The hallmark of ongoing infection is the presence of HBsAg. The presence of antibody to HBsAg alone suggests successful immunisation; its presence along with anti-HBcAg suggests resolved infection. This is mainly thought to occur around the time of birth. The risk of transmission is increased to > 90% if the mother is hepatitis B 'e' antigen positive. Hepatitis B immunoglobulin given at birth alone reduces the risk of vertical transmission. The effect of giving active immunisation (hepatitis B vaccine at birth, 1, 2 and 12 months) and passive immunisation with hepatitis B immunoglobulin is additive. Protection is achieved in 93% of neonates. Active immunisation does not seem to be affected by transmitted maternal IgG.

205. Irritable hip

Answer: B

Transient synovitis of the hip occurs most commonly between the ages of 2 and 10 years. It affects boys more frequently than girls. The cause is uncertain; active or recent viral infection (70%), trauma and allergic hypersensitivity may play a role. Investigations should include a full blood count, ESR and X-ray of the hip joint. The ultrasound may demonstrate a small effusion. Transient synovitis of the hip resolves with bedrest, with or without traction within 7–10 days.

Septic arthritis

This can occur at any age, but it is commoner under 10 years. Children are usually pyrexial, toxic and unwell with a neutrophilia and raised ESR. X-rays can be normal initially. Aspiration of the joint is almost always necessary. Organisms responsible include *Staphylococcus aureus*, *Haemophilus influenzae*, *Escherichia coli*, *Streptococcus*, *Salmonella* and *Meningococcus*. Blood cultures are positive in 50–70%. Management is with antibiotics for at least three weeks, pain relief and rehabilitative physiotherapy. Surgical drainage is often required.

206. Vertical transmission of HIV

Answers: A C E

HIV mother to baby transmission can occur during pregnancy, during childbirth or through breast feeding. Current data show that HIV is passed on to 25% of babies born to untreated HIV–infected mothers but only 4% of treated HIV–infected individuals in the USA. Internationally, the risk of transmission is up to 48% in breastfed infants, but 24% if no breastfeeding occurs. Of children with AIDS in the UK, 85% acquire the disease vertically. Risk factors for vertical transmission of HIV are:

- advanced maternal disease
  - symptomatic AIDS
  - low CD4 count
  - presence of other sexually transmitted diseases
  - higher viral load.

- in the peri-natal period:
  - amnionitis
  - vaginal delivery
  - pre-term and post-term delivery
  - low birth weight
  - prolonged rupture of membranes
  - invasive procedures
  - breast feeding

infectious diseases and immunology

- maternal immunity
  - cigarette smoking
  - neutralising antibody.

Factors that reduce the transmission rate:
- delivery by caesarean section
- avoidance of breast feeding
- anti-retroviral therapy

- zidovudine (nucleoside reverse transcriptase inhibitor)
  - orally from second trimester onwards
  - intravenously during delivery
  - orally to newborn for 6 weeks

combination anti-retroviral therapy to women with more advanced disease or higher viral load (zidovudine plus second nucleoside reverse transcriptase inhibitor plus non-nucleoside reverse transcriptase inhibitor or protease inhibitor). Other anti-retroviral therapy is undergoing evaluation

- avoid rupturing of membranes if possible
- avoid invasive procedures, eg fetal scalp blood sampling
- passive immunisation of mother and child with HIV hyperimmune immunoglobulin
- vitamin A supplementation to mother.

207. Erythema nodosum

Answers: A B C D E

Causes of erythema nodosum:

- idiopathic
- streptococcal infection
- tuberculosis
- leptospirosis
- histoplasmosis
- Epstein–Barr virus infection
- herpes simplex virus
- yersinia
- sulphonamides
- oral contraceptive pill
- systemic lupus erythematosus
- Crohn's disease
- ulcerative colitis
- Behçet's syndrome
- sarcoidosis
- Hodgkin's disease.

infectious diseases and immunology

208. Systemic lupus erythematosus

Answers: A C D E

Twenty percent of systemic lupus erythematosus begins in childhood. There is a higher incidence in dark-skinned racial groups. The female to male ratio is 8:1. HLA (human leucocyte antigen) associations are B8, DW2/DR3 and DW2/DR2. The onset can be insidious or acute. Early features usually include fever, malaise, arthralgia and a rash. There are many other manifestations and many organ systems can be involved. Treatment is with immunosuppression and anti-inflammatory agents. Clinical features are:

- butterfly rash
- discoid rash
- erythematous macules
- nail changes
- erythema nodosum
- erythema multiforme
- arthritis and arthralgia
- polyserositis (pleuritis, pericarditis, peritonitis)
- cardiac including thrombosis and myocardial infarction
- pulmonary fibrosis
- renal (nephrotic syndrome, nephritis, chronic renal failure)
- gastrointestinal (hepatosplenomegaly)
- seizures
- psychosis

Laboratory features are:

- anaemia of chronic disease
- leucopenia
- thrombocytopenia
- Coomb's positive haemolytic anaemia
- serology:
  - ANA is positive in 95% of cases of active systemic lupus erythematosus, although there are other causes of ANA positivity (see later). There are different types of ANA which are more specific
  - anti-Ro antibodies present in neonatal lupus
  - anti-DNA antibody which is specific for systemic lupus erythematosus and associated with renal involvement
  - anti-Sm (soluble nuclear protein) antigen
  - C3 is low in severe lupus and is a marker of disease activity
  - anti-cardiolipin antibody is often present and reflects a thrombotic tendency.

Drug-induced systemic lupus erythematosus

Certain drugs can induce systemic lupus erythematosus and ANA positivity and these include anticonvulsants, hydralazine, sulphonamides and procainamide. The disease tends to run a milder course. Central nervous system and renal involvement are unusual.

Causes of ANA positivity in children

- Juvenile chronic arthritis (particularly the pauciarticular type, ANA positivity associated with eye disease)
- Chronic active hepatitis
- Scleroderma
- Mixed connective tissue disease
- Drugs
- Epstein–Barr virus infection
- Chronic active hepatitis

Causes of anti-neutrophil cytoplasmic antibodies (ANCA)

- Ulcerative colitis
- Crescentic glomerulonephritis
- Cholangitis

209. Perthes' Disease

Answers: A D

The pathology is of ischaemic necrosis of the femoral head involving the epiphysis and adjacent metaphysis. The process is initially a destructive one followed by regeneration. The incidence is 1 in 2000. Age at presentation is between 2 and 10 years. The male to female ratio is 4:1. It usually occurs in isolation but can occur in association with congenital dislocation of the hip, mucopolysaccharidosis, achondroplasia and rickets. Ten per cent of cases are bilateral. Diagnosis is by lateral X-ray of the appropriate hip joint.

Slipped upper femoral epiphysis

This is associated with obesity and micro-genitalia. Twenty per cent are bilateral. It usually presents with knee and hip pain. Lateral X-ray of the hip is diagnostic. Complications include premature epiphyseal fusion and avascular necrosis.

210. Immunisations

Answers: B D

infectious diseases and immunology

211. Immunisations

Answers: A B C E

212. Immunisations

Answer: A

A thorough knowledge of immunisation is required and the reader is referred to the 1996 DoH's *Immunisation Against Infectious Disease* (Green book) Contraindications and indications to vaccination depend on the vaccine used and the medical condition of the child. Immunocompromised individuals (eg congenital immune disorders, children on high dose corticosteroids or immunosuppressive therapy and children with malignancy or other tumours of the reticuloendothelial system) should not receive live vaccines. Live polio vaccine should not be given to siblings of immunocompromised individuals due to the risk of viral transmission. Salk (killed poliovirus vaccine) became the routine polio immunisation in the UK in August 2004.

HIV-positive individuals with or without symptoms can receive MMR and the live polio vaccine if required. They should not receive BCG, yellow fever or oral typhoid vaccines. DTP/Hib/IPV vaccination is contraindicated only if on previous exposure to a dose of a pertussis containing vaccine, confirmed anaphylaxis occurred, or if there is a known anaphylactic reaction to neomycin, streptomycin or polymyxin B. Reactions to pertussis vaccination are reduced in studies using the acellular pertussis vaccines rather than cellular pertussis vaccines.

MMR, influenza and yellow fever vaccines produced in chick embryos are contraindicated in children with a history of having had an anaphylactic reaction to egg. The most recent *Immunisation Against Infectious Disease* suggests that the MMR is probably safe even if the child has had an anaphylactic reaction to egg. Cases in which there is any concern should be immunised in hospital. The most common side-effects after MMR vaccination are fever and rash a week after vaccination. Parotid swelling occasionally occurs in the third week. The incidence of meningoencephalitis (rare, with complete recovery) has fallen since the change in the mumps vaccine component of MMR. Live vaccines are ineffective up to 3–12 months after immunoglobulin infusions, they are also less effective if given within 3 weeks of a previous live vaccine.

Common side-effects of BCG vaccination include localised skin ulceration, sterile abscess at injection site and regional adenitis. BCG vaccine should only be given after testing for hypersensitivity to tuberculoprotein, except in neonates in whom testing is not necessary before vaccine is given.

Influenza vaccines are recommended only for children at high risk, eg chronic respiratory disease (including asthma, bronchopulmonary dysplasia and cystic fibrosis), chronic heart disease, chronic renal disease, diabetes mellitus and other endocrine disorders. Pneumococcal vaccine is indicated in those at increased risk of pneumococcal infection, eg sickle cell disease, asplenic patients, immunocompromised children (including HIV). (See Question 194.) Routine immunisation against pneumococcus is to be introduced in the UK to all children in the first year of life.

213. Meningococcal infection

Answers: B D E

Meningococci are Gram-negative diplococci. Group B is the commonest cause of infection since introduction of the vaccination against group C in 1999. Group C strains used to account for 40% of infection in the UK prior to the vaccine introduction, but is now responsible for < 10% of cases. Group A accounts for 1–2% of cases in UK but is common in other parts of the world. Peak age are 0–5 and 15–19 years. Meningococcal carriage rate is 5–15%. Transmission is by droplet spread, and incubation period is 2–7 days. Symptoms vary from fulminant disease to insidious with mild prodromal symptoms. Mortality around 10% (higher in septicaemia). Early on the rash may be non-specific, later the rash may be petechial or purpuric and does not blanch with pressure.

Vaccination

- No vaccine available against group B organisms.
- Meningococcal Plain Polysaccharide A and C vaccine is effective against A and C. Young infants respond less well than older children. Immunity lasts 3–5 years. Immunity to C group is only transitory.
- Meningococcal Conjugate Group C vaccine is effective against group C. Is protective in younger children. It was introduced as part of the routine child immunisation programme in autumn 1999.

Schedule

See website www.immunisation.nhs.uk for up-to-date immunisation schedule in the UK.

214. HLA B27

Answers: A C

Conditions associated with HLA B27 positivity

- Ankylosing spondylitis
- Reiter's syndrome

infectious diseases and immunology

277

- Arthritis of inflammatory bowel disease and psoriasis
- Acute iridocyclitis
- Pauciarticular arthritis of older children
- Reactive arthritis following infection with *Salmonella, Shigella, Yersinia enterocolitica, Campylobacter*

Ankylosing spondylitis

Ninety five per cent of cases of ankylosing spondylitis are associated with HLA B27 positivity. Ankylosing spondylitis occurs predominantly in adolescents with an onset usually over the age of 8 years. The classic arthritis is of the sacroiliac joint and lower lumbar spine although other joints are involved, particularly in the early stages. Twenty-five per cent develop an acute iridocyclitis.

Reiter's syndrome

Reiter's syndrome classically comprises the triad of sterile urethritis, arthritis and ocular inflammation. Gastrointestinal symptoms and skin rashes also occur. Reiter's syndrome is commoner in males than in females. The arthritis is usually pauciarticular. It can occur following infection with *Shigella, Yersinia, Campylobacter* and *Chlamydia*.

Inflammatory bowel disease

Ten per cent of children with inflammatory bowel disease develop an arthritis. A number develop ankylosing spondylitis and this is associated with HLA B27 positivity.

Reactive arthritis

Reactive arthritis can occur following infection with *Salmonella, Shigella, Yersinia enterocolitica* and *Campylobacter pylori*. There is an HLA B27 association. The relation between Reiter's syndrome and reactive arthritis is unclear.

Psoriatic arthritis

Psoriatic arthritis has a weak HLA B27 association. The arthritis itself is commoner in girls. It is asymmetrical. Nail pitting and distal interphalangeal joint involvement is common.

Neither Marfan's syndrome nor diabetes mellitus have an association with HLA B27 positivity. Dermatomyositis is associated with HLA B8/DR3.

infectious diseases and
immunology

216. Kawasaki's disease

Answers: C D

Kawasaki's disease is an acute, self-limiting, systemic vasculitis of unknown aetiology that affects infants and young children. The vasculitis involves medium and small vessels. Clinical and epidemiological characteristics suggest toxin-induced superantigen stimulation. Person-to-person transmission has not been documented. Diagnostic criteria for Kawasaki's disease are:

- fever persisting for 5 days or more
- four of the following:
  - bilateral non-suppurative conjunctivitis
  - polymorphous exanthema
  - cervical lymphadenopathy
  - inflammation of the tongue, lips and oral mucosa
  - oedema and erythema of the hands and feet
- illness not explained by a known disease process.

Atypical Kawasaki's disease implies that not all the diagnostic criteria are met but clinically the child is felt to have Kawasaki's disease and later coronary artery dilatation or other pathognomonic criteria develop. Atypical Kawasaki's disease is commoner in infants than in older children. Infants have a higher incidence of coronary artery aneurysms. There are three stages of the disease: acute, subacute and convalescent. The acute stage lasts 0–2 weeks and comprises fever, conjunctivitis, oral changes, irritability, rash and lymphadenopathy. The subacute stage lasts for 21 days and is when skin peeling, thrombocytosis and coronary artery aneurysms occur. Symptoms resolve during the convalescent phase. There is usually a leukocytosis, raised C-reactive protein (CRP), raised ESR and a transient disturbance of liver function in the acute stage. Thrombocytosis occurs later. These abnormalities resolve during the convalescent phase. The major complications are cardiac with the development of coronary artery aneurysms which occur in 10–40% of untreated patients. The majority of patients do well, however, 1–2% die of cardiac complications, eg myocardial ischaemia.

Treatment is with intravenous immunoglobulin administered within the first 10 days of the illness at a dose of 2 g/kg. This is associated with a reduction in symptoms and the incidence of coronary artery aneurysms. Aspirin is also used for its anti-inflammatory and anti-platelet effects. A high dose of 100 mg/kg/day is used in the acute phase with a maintenance dose of 5 mg/kg/day in the convalescent phase. All children in whom the diagnosis of Kawasaki's disease is suspected should be referred for an echocardiogram.

infectious diseases and immunology

216. Rubella

Answers: B C D E

Transmission of rubella is by droplet spread. The incubation period is 14–21 days. The infection can be asymptomatic, however, rubella infection is now rare as a consequence of the immunisation programme. Prodromal symptoms may or may not be present and precede the rash by 1–5 days. These include fever, coryza, conjunctivitis and lymphadenopathy (sub-occipital, post auricular and cervical). The rash is macular and lasts for 3–5 days. Complications include persistent lymphadenopathy, arthritis, neuritis, thrombocytopenic purpura and encephalitis (associated with a CSF lymphocytosis). Differential diagnosis of rubella includes:

- infectious mononucleosis
- toxoplasmosis
- enteroviral infection
- roseola, scarlet fever
- mycoplasma
- parvovirus infection.

Viral isolation is difficult and diagnosis is by serology. Treatment is supportive. Prevention is by immunisation with the MMR vaccine. Congenital rubella occurs secondary to maternal infection in the first trimester. Clinical manifestations are variable and include:

- jaundice
- thrombocytopenia
- growth retardation
- cardiac abnormalities
- eye problems (cataracts, blindness, microphthalmia)
- deafness
- microcephaly
- fetal death
- stillbirth.

217. Humoral immunodeficiency

Answer: D

Defects in humoral immunity/B cell immunity results in susceptibility to bacterial infection and are the result of an absolute or qualitative deficit in B lymphocytes. Cell mediated/T cell immune deficiency renders the 'host' susceptible to viral and fungal pathogens. Classic defects of acquired cell-mediated immunity problems are HIV and tuberculosis. Inherited defects reduce T cell mobility, phagocyte function and cytokine production. Candidiasis, chronic diarhhoea and failure to thrive all suggest a serious cell-mediated immune problem. Urinary tract infections and hepatitis simplex virus 1 cold sores usually have no immune implications. Recurrent abscesses are an indication to check immunoglobulins as well as of course fasting glucose.

218. Live vaccines

Answer: E

All the others in the question are killed or attenuated. Live vaccines include:

- measles
- mumps
- rubella
- BCG
- varicella zoster
- yellow fever
- oral polio.

Killed/attenuated vaccines include:

- pertussis
- injected polio
- hepatitis A and B
- haemophilus influenza B
- toxins
- diphtheria
- tetanus.

infectious diseases and immunology

219. Contraindications to pertussis vaccination

Answer: E

The only absolute contraindications with the previously used whole cell pertussis vaccine were a severe local or generalised reaction such as erythema of the whole injected leg, temperature > 40 °C or post-vaccination seizure. Reactions with the new acellular vaccine are much rarer and these contraindications no longer apply. In short, there are NO absolute contraindications any longer though a lot of folklore persists surrounding pertussis vaccination. In the past vaccination has been deferred/avoided for family history of fits, developmental delay or febrile fits.

220. D: Thick film for malarial parasite

This child has malaria until proved otherwise. Malaria prophylaxis reduces risk but is by no means a guarantee of protection particularly if doses have been forgotten or possibly not absorbed (simultaneous diarrhoea and vomiting) or where there is early resistance. The gold standard is a thick film as it screens a greater quantity of blood than a thin film. The latter is essentially a monolayer of blood on a slide and is better for species identification. The film should be repeated if there is any doubt. It is entirely appropriate to do blood cultures as well because the malaria screen may prove negative.

221. E: Mantoux test

Tuberculosis tends to be a harder diagnosis in children than adults as sputum is harder to obtain. Often treatment has to be started empirically and the child watched for response, eg defervescence. The best test however, is Mantoux test. Heaf test uses purified protein derivative (PPD) but at such high concentrations that it is prone to false-positive results and only suited for population screening in low-exposure settings (now being phased out even in the UK). A positive (> 10 mm) reaction in a Mantoux even with a previous BCG is diagnostic though there may be false *negatives* in immunosuppressed children, such as those with severe malnutrition or advanced HIV.

infectious diseases and immunology

222. A: Zoster immunoglobulin

The immunosuppressed children need protection as this child is infectious. Infectivity is from 5 days before the rash appears until the last crop. Aciclovir is only indicated once there are signs of infection. ZIG given intramuscularly is the appropriate measure as well, of course, as keeping the child from visiting until non-infectious.

223. INVESTIGATIONS

1.   E – Immunoglobulins

Though this could be primarily respiratory, a likelier diagnosis is a hypogammaglobulinaemia. Ig levels are confirmatory. The commonest type (Bruton's) is X-linked. Treatment is regular (approximately 6-weekly) immunoglobulin transfusion and antibiotic prophylaxis.

2.   B – Bone marrow aspirate

This is visceral leishmaniasis or kala azar, a protozoan systemic illness caused by *Leishmania donovani*. The vector is the phlebotomine sandfly. The amastigote forms invade multiple organs. Presentation includes visceromegaly, weight loss, lymphadenopathy and severe susceptibility to infection (tuberculosis especially) Untreated, the mortality is high and usually due to opportunistic infections. Diagnosis is best made by marrow or splenic biopsy. Treatment is by prolonged parenteral sodium stibogluconate (Pentostam) or pentamidine, and if the regimen is adhered to it is usually successful.

3.   H – None of the above

This scenario is typical of hepatitis A rather than hepatitis B. Hepatitis A is common in young children, spreads by the oro-faecal route and is self-limiting. Typically the systemic symptoms and rise in LFTs (transaminases especially) precede the jaundice. Serology is confirmatory. An oral vaccine is recommended for some tropical areas.

infectious diseases and immunology

224. DIAGNOSIS

1. G – Cytomegalovirus infection

This is most likely to be a mononucleosis type illness. Monospot is confirmatory (though the younger the child the more likely to be false negative). The presence of atypical lymphocytes and the clinical picture are effectively as good.

2. I – None of the above

This child fulfils the diagnostic criteria for Kawasaki's disease, a clinical diagnosis (See Chapter 1). Prompt treatment with high-dose aspirin and immunoglobulin with referral for echocardiography is required.

3. E – Lyme disease

This is caused by *Borrelia burgdorferi* and carried by ticks. There may well be a history of a tick bite or recent travel to areas rich in deer or other tick vectors. The disease was first described in Lyme, Connecticut, USA. Symptoms include:

- erythema migrans
- arthritis
- encephalopathy

Serology becomes positive in the second week. Treatment involves a prolonged (2 week) course of appropriate antibiotics, amoxicillin being the most widely used.

NEONATOLOGY
ANSWERS

225. α-Fetoprotein

Answers: B C D E

In the UK, at 16 weeks' gestation (second trimester), screening for Down's syndrome and neural tube defects is carried out by maternal blood tests. Risk calculation is estimated from maternal age together with levels of α-fetoprotein (AFP), α-human chorionic gonadotrophin (hCG) and unconjugated oestriol; the so-called triple blood test. AFP is produced from embryonic endodermal tissues, in particular the yolk sac and fetal liver. It is excreted via fetal urine into the amniotic fluid and thence crosses into the maternal circulation. In open neural tube defects, AFP leaks out of neurological tissue directly into the amniotic fluid. Conditions associated with elevation of AFP include:

- anencephaly
- spina bifida, myelomeningocele
- twins
- abdominal wall defects (gastroschisis, exomphalos)
- blighted ova, intra-uterine death, threatened abortion
- Turner's syndrome
- Patau's syndrome
- teratoma
- congenital nephrotic syndrome
- posterior urethral valves
- Meckel–Gruber syndrome
- haemangioma of cord/placenta
- oligohydramnios
- conditions associated with decreased AFP levels
- Down's syndrome (plus elevation of hCG)
- other chromosomal abnormalities.

Diabetic mothers

Following detection of raised AFP, a detailed ultrasound of the fetus is performed and amniocentesis is offered to allow measurement of amniotic fluid AFP and cytogenetic studies. Pregnancies carrying normal fetuses with raised AFP levels have an increased risk of pre-term labour and intrauterine growth retardation (IUGR).

neonatology

226. Amniotic fluid

Answers: B C D

The fetus normally swallows 200–500 ml/day of amniotic fluid and passes 300–800 ml/day of urine. Polyhydramnios (> 2000 ml) is associated with an increased risk of pre-term labour, prolonged rupture of membranes, cord prolapse and placental abruption. It occurs in 1 in 250 pregnancies, and 50% are associated with a fetal abnormality, 20% with maternal diabetes and in 30% the cause is unknown. Causes include:

- maternal diabetes
- fetal anaemia
- anencephaly
- hydrocephalus
- tracheo-oesophageal fistula
- duodenal atresia
- spinal bifida
- cleft lip and palate
- neuromuscular disease (poor swallowing) –, eg myotonic dystrophy
- syndromes – achondroplasia, trisomies, congenital infection.

Oligohydramnios (< 200 ml) is associated with an increased risk of pulmonary hypoplasia and postural deformities. Causes include:

- amniotic fluid leak (prolonged rupture of membranes)
- in-uterine growth retardation (placental insufficiency)
- renal agenesis (Potter's syndrome)
- urethral valves
- prune belly syndrome.

227. Nitric oxide

Answers: A C

Nitric oxide has a wide range of physiological functions including neurotransmission, vascular tone modulation (relaxation), platelet inhibition, endocrine actions and activity against bacteria. In neonates, its action of smooth muscle relaxation is used as therapy for conditions associated with increased pulmonary vascular resistance, such as persistent pulmonary hypertension of the newborn (PPHN), respiratory distress syndrome, meconium aspiration and pneumonia. Nitric oxide is synthesised in vascular endothelium from L-arginine and oxygen, catalysed by nitric oxide synthase. Vascular smooth muscle relaxation is mediated via cyclic guanylate monophosphate (cGMP), itself produced in abundance in the presence of nitric oxide. At birth nitric oxide is involved in the conversion to normal postnatal respiration produced by lowering of pulmonary vascular resistance. Inhibition or failure of synthesis of endogenous nitric oxide

neonatology

leads to development of PPHN, characterised by hypoxia and hypertension which inhibits further nitric oxide production. Inhaled nitric oxide acts to:

- relax smooth muscle and vasodilate pulmonary vasculature
- reverse hypoxaemia
- improve ventilation–perfusion mismatching.

Nitric oxide diffuses rapidly through alveoli and the response is practically immediate (less than 15 minutes). It appears more effective when administered with high-frequency oscillatory ventilation (HFOV). Due to the therapy being inhaled, vasodilation is largely selective and systemic hypotension is rarely a problem. An added advantage over other vasodilators is its very short half-life (~5 seconds). It is however rapidly metabolised to toxic metabolites (NO^-, NO_2^-, NO_3^-) and together with haemoglobin forms methaemoglobin. Therefore monitoring levels of such products is essential. Units must also scavenge nitric oxide and nitrous oxide from exhaust gases and monitor levels due to health hazards to staff.

228. Assessment of gestational age

Answers: B D E

Gestational age assessment is usually done by calculation from the first day of the mother's last menstrual period or an early ultrasound. Gestational age can be estimated after birth by careful physical and neurological examination. This needs to be done on the first day as some signs change rapidly after birth. Physical signs used include:

- skin colour, texture and opacity
- lanugo hair
- plantar creases
- oedema of the feet and hands
- ear form and firmness
- breast size
- nipple formation
- genital appearance.

Neurological criteria depend on muscle tone (decreased in pre-terms) and joint mobility (increases with gestational age). The scarf sign refers to when the arm is pulled across the supine infant to wrap it around the opposite shoulder. The elbow reaches the opposite axilla in very pre-term infants but does not reach the midline in term infants.

neonatology

229. Persistent fetal circulation

Answers: A B E

Persistent fetal circulation (persistent pulmonary hypertension of the newborn) is characterised by hypoxia which is out of proportion to the severity of lung disease, a structurally normal heart and evidence of right-to-left shunting either at the ductus or through the foramen ovale. Echocardiography is the investigation of choice to confirm the diagnosis. Risk factors include birth asphyxia, group B streptococcal sepsis, pulmonary hypoplasia (diaphragmatic hernia, oligohydramnios, pleural effusion), meconium aspiration syndrome, hyaline membrane disease, maternal indometacin and high-pressure ventilation. Management includes minimal handling, maintenance of a normal arterial blood pressure, normalisation of acid base status and broad spectrum antibiotics. Hyperventilation, by driving down the P_aCO_2 causes vasodilation and a rise in P_aO_2. Tolazoline dilates both the pulmonary and systemic circulation. It is best infused through a central line direct into the right atrium. The systemic vasodilation means that colloid support often needs to be given concurrently. Other pulmonary vasodilators include magnesium sulphate, prostacyclin and nitric oxide. Other therapeutic approaches include high frequency oscillatory ventilation and extracorporeal membrane oxygenation (ECMO).

Extracorporeal membrane oxygenation

ECMO is a form of cardiopulmonary bypass that allows gas exchange outside the body and increases systemic perfusion. It is commonly performed as veno-arterial ECMO (right internal jugular to carotid). Blood pumped into the circuit is oxygenated by a membrane oxygenator and returned. Veno-venous ECMO allows gas exchange but does not support the cardiac output.

230. Air leak syndrome in the newborn

Answer: E

A pneumothorax is present in approximately 1% of newborns (the quoted figure is variable) and is usually asymptomatic. Risk factors for pneumothorax include:

- respiratory distress syndrome
- active resuscitation
- meconium aspiration
- pulmonary hypoplasia (primary or secondary to renal disorders, diaphragmatic hernia, etc.)

Risk factors in ventilated babies are:

- high peak pressure and mean airway pressure
- high positive end expiratory pressure
- prolonged inspiratory time

neonatology

- increased I:E ratios
- inadequate sedation (controversial)

Asymptomatic pneumothoraces or pneumothoraces causing only minor symptoms in term babies can be treated with 100% oxygen to hasten absorption by decreasing the partial pressure of nitrogen in the blood which increases the absorption of nitrogen from the pneumothorax. Insertion of an underwater seal drain is indicated in all infants with moderate or severe symptoms and in virtually all ventilated babies with a pneumothorax regardless of whether or not the pneumothorax is under tension. Pneumomediastinum, pneumopericardium and pneumoperitoneum can all be asymptomatic. However all can be responsible for an acute deterioration in the clinical state of a ventilated baby. A pneumopericardium can cause acute cardiac tamponade.

231. Small for gestational age neonates

Answers: A B C D

An neonate is considered small for dates or small for gestational age if its birth weight is less than two standard deviations below the mean for its gestational age. There are many causes of this: maternal, fetal and placental (see below). Small for gestational age neonates can be symmetrically or asymmetrically growth retarded. Asymmetric growth retardation (head growth spared) is the commonest. Symmetrical growth retardation occurs secondary to an insult early in pregnancy such as an intrauterine infection in the first trimester.

Causes of infants being born small for gestational age

- Maternal:
  - physiological – maternal height, age <20 or >35, multiparity
  - pathological – toxaemia, hypertension, smoking, alcoholism, malnutrition, chronic disease.
- Fetal:
  - physiological – genetic potential, multiple pregnancy, female sex
  - pathological – chromosomal, infection, syndromal.
- Placental
  - infarction, tumour, abruption, feto-fetal transfusion.

Problems of small for gestational age infants

- Perinatal asphyxia
- Meconium aspiration syndrome
- Hypothermia
- Hypoglycaemia
- Polycythaemia
- Heart failure

neonatology

- Persistent fetal circulation
- Pulmonary haemorrhage
- Increased risk of infection
- Necrotising enterocolitis
- Dysmorphology.

Retrolental fibroplasia is a sequela of retinopathy of prematurity which occurs in pre-term infants, usually only those born under 32 weeks' gestation.

232. Steroid therapy in the neonate

Answers: C D E

Steroids were frequently used in the past for babies with chronic lung disease particularly those who were ventilator dependent and they undoubtedly are useful (mechanisms below). Recent evidence from individual trials and meta-analyses has shown unequivocal associations between use of steroids (particularly repeat courses) and adverse long term neurological outcomes. Steroids are now used therefore only as a last resort where all other means have been tried. Proposed mechanisms of action are:

- stabilisation of membranes
- reduction in pulmonary oedema
- increased surfactant synthesis
- reduction of airway inflammation
- relief of bronchospasm.

Side-effects of steroids in neonates are:

- hypertension
- gastrointestinal bleeding
- gastric perforation
- hyperglycaemia
- sepsis
- cataracts
- cardiomyopathy
- leucocytosis.

neonatology

233. Necrotising enterocolitis

Answers: A C E

Necrotising enterocolitis is a condition of unknown aetiology commonest in infants below 1500 g and characterised by transmural intestinal necrosis. Predisposing factors are:

*   hypoxia
*   hypotension
*   prematurity
*   small for dates
*   birth asphyxia
*   hypothermia
*   fluid overload
*   exchange transfusion/umbilical catheterisation
*   anaemia
*   polycythaemia
*   formula feeding/hypertonic feeds
*   rapidly increasing enteral feeding in pre-terms.

Necrotising enterocolitis can occur in outbreaks. In less than 50% is an organism isolated. Organisms isolated include *Escherichia coli*, *Staphylococcus epidermidis*, rotavirus and *Clostridium perfringens*. *Clostridium welchii* causes gas gangrene. Medical treatment consists of nil by mouth with nasogastric decompression, total parenteral nutrition and intravenous antibiotics. Ventilatory support is often required. Patients require regular monitoring (clinical, haematological, biochemical and radiological). Babies with necrotising enterocolitis who fail to respond to medical therapy need to be assessed by a paediatric surgeon. The indications for surgery include perforation of the bowel, persistent bowel obstruction, presence of a fixed mass and continued deterioration despite medical therapy. Late complications of necrotising enterocolitis include:

*   stricture formation
*   short bowel syndrome
*   blind loop syndrome
*   cholestasis
*   fistula
*   cyst formation
*   polyposis.

neonatology

234. Birth injuries

Answers: A C E

Fractures are said to occur in up to 1% of infants at the time of their birth with clavicular fractures being the commonest. Risk factors include shoulder dystocia and breech delivery. Injury to the cervical spine is rare but can occur (with or without X-ray changes). Excessive rotation during cephalic deliveries results in injury at C1–2 level and breech deliveries with excessive traction result in damage at C6–T1. Hypotonia, hyporeflexia and hypoventilation ensue. Magnetic resonance imaging (MRI) is useful for diagnosis. Brachial plexus injuries usually result from traction injury during the delivery of babies with shoulder dystocia.

- Upper brachial plexus, Erb–Duchenne paralysis (C5–6). Affected arm is held in the waiter's tip position. Biceps and supinator reflexes are absent. Hand grasp is preserved. Diaphragmatic involvement can cause paradoxical movement of the chest wall on the affected side.
- Lower brachial plexus injury, Klumpke's paralysis (C8–T1), claw hand deformity, absent triceps jerk and palmar grasp with sometimes an ipsilateral Horner's syndrome.
- Total brachial plexus injury, Erb–Duchenne–Klumpke, combines features of both.

There are important differences between caput succedaneum (oedema over the presenting part of the scalp) and cephalohaematoma (haematoma between the skull and periosteum).

Caput succedaneum	Cephalohaematoma
Diffuse, ecchymotic, oedematous overlying skin	Normal overlying skin
Present at birth	Not present until a few hours after birth
Disappears over a few days	Reabsorbed over 2 weeks to 3 months Can calcify
May extend over suture lines	Limited by suture lines
No treatment needed	May require phototherapy for jaundice

neonatology

235. Recurrent apnoea in pre-terms

Answers: A B C D E

Apnoea is a common symptom in pre-term babies. It can be primary (recurrent apnoea of prematurity) or secondary to other phenomena. Causes of secondary apnoea are:

- infection
- gastrointestinal tract – overfeeding, passage of stool, gastro-oesophageal reflux
- metabolic – hypoglycaemia, hypernatraemia, hyponatraemia
- cardiovascular – hypotension, fluid overload, heart failure
- respiratory – hypoxia, pneumonia, respiratory distress syndrome
- nervous system – haemorrhage, birth asphyxia, drugs.

Apnoea with no underlying cause is apnoea of prematurity. This usually presents in pre-terms within a few days of birth and disappears by about 34 weeks' gestation. Many factors are thought to have a role in the pathogenesis including immaturity of the respiratory centre, upper airway collapse, environmental temperature and sleep state. Apnoea of prematurity is usually treated with a respiratory stimulant such as caffeine or theophylline.

236. Respiratory distress syndrome

Answers: A B C

Respiratory distress syndrome (hyaline membrane disease) accounts for 30% of all neonatal deaths. The incidence is directly proportional to gestation. It is due to immaturity of the enzyme systems required to synthesise surfactant in the type 2 alveolar cells. Deficient surfactant on the alveolar surface results in high surface tension and atelectasis. This results in decreased lung compliance and a failure to establish a functional residual capacity. The major components of surfactant are dipalmitoyl phosphatidyl choline (lecithin), phosphatidyl glycerol, apolipoproteins (surfactant proteins SP-A, B,C,D) and cholesterol. Factors that increase the risk of respiratory distress syndrome are:

- prematurity
- male sex
- twin pregnancy
- caesarean section
- hypothermia
- hypoglycaemia
- birth asphyxia
- maternal diabetes.

cardiology

Antenatal steroids administered to the mother 48–72 hours before delivery will reduce the incidence of respiratory distress syndrome. Surfactant, which can be natural (Survanta, Curosurf) or synthetic (Exosurf, ALEC) is administered to ventilated pre-term infants either prophylactically (soon after birth) or as rescue when symptoms develop. A meta-analysis suggests that at > 30 weeks' gestation, prophylaxis is worthwhile. Surfactant reduces the severity and the mortality from respiratory distress syndrome. Other causes of respiratory distress in pre-terms include:

- transient tachypnoea of the newborn
- meconium aspiration syndrome
- birth asphyxia
- pulmonary haemorrhage
- sepsis including congenital pneumonia
- pneumothorax
- congenital abnormality – diaphragmatic hernia, tracheo-oesophageal fistula
- persistent fetal circulation
- congenital heart disease
- congenital lung cyst/congenital lobar emphysema
- pulmonary hypoplasia.

237. Phototherapy

Answers: A D E

Phototherapy reduces serum unconjugated bilirubin levels. It uses light at a wavelength of 420–550 nm in the blue green spectrum and causes bilirubin to become water soluble which allows excretion without conjugation. It is indicated for the treatment of infants with pathological unconjugated hyperbilirubinaemia and is sometimes used prophylactically in very low birth weight babies. It reduces the need for exchange transfusion in infants with hyperbilirubinaemia, but when the indications for exchange exist it is not a substitute. There is no absolute consensus as to the level at which phototherapy should be started although there are a number of charts which are widely used. Phototherapy is continued until the unconjugated bilirubin drops to safe levels. Colour of the skin does not alter its efficacy. Rebound hyperbilirubinaemia usually occurs after stopping phototherapy. Skin colour is inaccurate as a method of assessment of the bilirubin level of infants who are under phototherapy. Infants' eyes should be covered while they are under phototherapy. Complications of phototherapy include loose stools, rash, dehydration, hypothermia, reduced mother infant bonding.

neonatology

238. Infants of diabetic mothers

Answers: C D E

Clinical features of babies of diabetic mothers include:

- general:
  - macrosomia – but also can be small for gestational age secondary to placental insufficiency
  - normal head size
  - increased subcutaneous fat
  - birth trauma.
- central nervous system:
  - jitteriness
  - hyperexcitability
  - hypotonia
  - lethargy
  - convulsions
- respiratory distress syndrome
- cardiovascular:
  - cardiomegaly (30%)
  - transient hypertrophic cardiomyopathy
  - persistent fetal circulation
- renal vein thrombosis
- metabolic:
  - hypoglycaemia (usually within the first few hours)
  - hypocalcaemia
  - hypomagnesaemia
  - hyperbilirubinaemia
- haemotological:
  - polycythaemia
- Congenital malformations (three-fold increase):
  - cardiac (ventricular septal defect, atrio-ventricular septal defect, transposition of the great arteries, coarctation of the aorta)
  - neural tube defects including anencephaly
  - holoprosencephaly
  - sacral agenesis
  - hydronephrosis
  - renal agenesis
  - duodenal atresia
  - anorectal malformations
  - microcolon
  - increased risk of diabetes mellitus.

neonatology

239. Neonatal polycythaemia

Answers: B C

Polycythaemia refers to a raised haematocrit (packed cell volume). Neonatal polycythaemia is usually said to be present if the venous packed cell volume is greater than 65%. Predisposing factors are:

- post-maturity
- small for gestational age
- delayed cord clamping (maternal-fetal transfusion)
- feto-fetal transfusion
- Beckwith–Wiedemann syndrome
- Infant of a diabetic mother
- 13/18/21 trisomy
- adrenogenital syndrome
- hypothyroidism
- high altitude.

Clinical features/complications are as follows:

- respiratory – tachypnoea, respiratory distress, persistent fetal circulation
- cardiovascular system – heart failure, acrocyanosis
- gastrointestinal – feeding problems, vomiting, necrotising enterocolitis
- renal – renal vein thrombosis
- nervous system – lethargy, hypotonia, seizures, irritability
- skin – plethora
- haematological – thrombocytopenia
- biochemical – hypoglycaemia, hypocalcaemia, hyperbilirubinaemia.

Treatment of polycythaemia includes ensuring an adequate fluid intake and attention to predisposing factors. Symptomatic infants may require a partial exchange transfusion of blood for either fresh frozen plasma or human albumin. The indications for this are controversial. Consideration of exchange should be in those infants who are symptomatic with a packed cell volume greater than 65% or those who have a packed cell volume greater than 70%. Late neurological sequelae are seen in some infants with symptomatic polycythaemia.

neonatology

240. Perinatal asphyxia

Answers: A C E

Risk factors for perinatal asphyxia can be maternal, fetal or placental. Examples include:

- maternal – amnionitis, toxaemia, diabetes, smoking
- fetal – multiple gestation, small for dates, pre-term gestation, congenital abnormalities
- placental – insufficiency, abruption.

Effects of asphyxia are as follows:

- respiratory – persistent fetal circulation, pulmonary haemorrhage, surfactant deficiency
- cardiovascular – myocardial ischaemia and heart failure, hypotension
- central nervous system – hypoxic ischaemic encephalopathy, intracranial haemorrhage, cerebral oedema, cerebral infarction (periventricular leukomalacia)
- renal – acute tubular necrosis, adrenal haemorrhage
- gastrointestinal – perforation, ulceration, necrotising enterocolitis
- metabolic – hyponatraemia (inappropriate antidiuretic hormone secretion), hypoglycaemia, hypocalcaemia
- haematological – disseminated intravascular coagulation, haemorrhage.

Hypoxic ischaemic encephalopathy is graded as follows:

- grade I – irritability, hypotonia, poor suck, no seizures
- grade II – lethargy, abnormal tone, requirement for tube feeds, seizures
- grade III – comatose, severe hypotonia, failure to maintain respiration without respiratory support, prolonged seizures.

Less than 10% of cerebral palsy is as a consequence of perinatal asphyxia.

241. Bile stained vomiting

Answer: E

Duodenal atresia

This accounts for 25–40% of all intestinal atresias. Half are pre-term and 20–30% have Down's syndrome. Malrotation, oesophageal atresia, anorectal malformations and congenital heart disease are associated abnormalities. Bilious vomiting with abdominal distension on day one is common. Visible gastric peristalsis can occur.

neonatology

Pyloric stenosis

This has multifactorial inheritance. There is projectile non-bilious vomiting, with onset between 3 weeks and 5 months. The baby presents hungry and with weight loss. First born males are more commonly affected. Palpable pyloric tumour and visible gastric peristalsis are present. Mild unconjugated hyperbilirubinaemia and hypochloraemic, hypokalaemic metabolic alkalosis also occur. Ultrasound confirms the diagnosis. Treatment is by pyloromyotomy (Ramstedt's procedure) after correction of the electrolyte and acid–base disturbance.

Malrotation

This refers to incomplete rotation of the mid gut during fetal development. This results in the small bowel occupying the right side of the abdomen and the large bowel the left. The caecum is often sub-hepatic. The mesentery along with the superior mesenteric artery is attached by a narrow stalk which can twist around itself producing a mid gut volvulus. Infants can present with bile stained vomiting and abdominal distension in the first few weeks or later with episodes of abdominal colic and vomiting. Diagnosis is by barium meal and follow through. Barium enema may show a malpositioned caecum but is not the investigation of choice.

Meconium can still be passed with obstruction of the upper small bowel. Meconium ileus occurs in cystic fibrosis and is the presenting feature in 20%. Presentation is in the neonatal period with failure to pass meconium and abdominal distension. It is treated with Gastrografin enemas, and up to 50% require surgery.

242. Neonatal haematology

Answers: C E

Cord haemoglobin levels in term infants range from 14–20 g/dl. The levels in pre-terms are lower. Over the first few months a physiological anaemia occurs. This is due to reduced red cell survival, relative hyperoxia and increasing blood volume due to increasing weight. Anaemia at birth is most commonly due to immune haemolysis. The other main cause is acute blood loss. Anaemia due to reduced red cell production is not usually noticed till 3–4 weeks of age. Fetal haemoglobin constitutes 70% of the haemoglobin at birth. It contains two alpha and two gamma chains. α-thalassaemia may present in the neonatal period, β-thalassaemia does not. Fetal haemoglobin is resistant to alkaline denaturation unlike adult haemoglobin; this is the basis of the Apt test used to differentiate fetal blood from swallowed maternal blood in the gut (for example on a gastric aspirate).

neonatology

Causes of anaemia in the neonate are:

- blood loss:
  - placental abruption
  - feto-fetal haemorrhage
  - feto-maternal bleed
  - cephalhaematoma
  - intraventricular haemorrhage
  - iatrogenic – surgical, frequent sampling, snapped cord at delivery

- haemolysis
  - ABO incompatibility
  - rhesus disease
  - hereditary spherocytosis
  - glucose 6-phosphate dehydrogenase deficiency
  - impaired production
  - pure red cell aplasia – Diamond–Blackfan syndrome.

243. Problems associated with pre-term gestation

Answers: A B C D E

Many problems are associated with pre-term gestation. A number are listed below:

- respiratory distress syndrome
- pneumothorax
- chronic lung disease
- hypotension
- patent ductus arteriosus
- hyponatraemia
- hypernatraemia
- glycosuria
- hypoglycaemia
- hyperglycaemia
- hyperbilirubinaemia
- intraventricular haemorrhage
- periventricular leukomalacia
- retinopathy of prematurity
- anaemia
- infection
- necrotising enterocolitis
- apnoea of prematurity.

Details of these problems should be learnt and can be found in any of the pocket books of neonatal intensive care.

neonatology

244. Neonatal fits

Answers: B C E

Causes of neonatal fits include:

- hypoxic ischaemic encephalopathy
- intraventricular haemorrhage
- meningitis
- hypoglycaemia
- hypocalcaemia
- hyponatraemia
- hypernatraemia
- inborn error of metabolism
- kernicterus
- fifth day fits
- drug withdrawal
- congenital malformation
- idiopathic.

Both Wilson's disease and lead poisoning present outside the neonatal period, but DiGeorge's syndrome can present with hypocalcaemia. Other causes of hypocalcaemia in the neonatal period include maternal vitamin D deficiency, high phosphate milks, renal failure, primary hypoparathyroidism, maternal hyperparathyroidism and hypomagnesaemia.

245. Congenital dislocation of the hip

Answers: A B D E

Risk factors for congenital dislocation of the hip are as follows:

- family history (positive in 20%)
- female sex (female:male 6:1)
- breech delivery (factor in 30%)
- spina bifida
- being first born
- oligohydramnios.

The left hip is more likely to be dislocated than the right. Ultrasound is the best test for diagnosis. The clinical tests of hip instability are Ortolani's and Barlow's.

246. Conjugated hyperbilirubinaemia in the neonatal period

Answers: C D E

Causes of conjugated hyperbilirubinaemia in the neonatal period are as follows:

- infectious – hepatitis A, B, C, cytomegalovirus, rubella, herpes simplex
- metabolic – cystic fibrosis, tyrosinaemia, galactosaemia, fructosaemia
- intrahepatic – Alagille's syndrome, congenital hepatic fibrosis
- extrahepatic – biliary atresia, choledochal cyst, inspissated bile syndrome
- toxic – total parenteral nutrition related, sepsis, urinary tract infection, drugs
- endocrine – hypopituitarism, hypothyroidism
- miscellaneous – intestinal obstruction.

All neonates with prolonged neonatal jaundice (greater than 2 weeks) need investigation. Neonates with a predominantly conjugated hyperbilirubinaemia require more extensive investigation including radiology particularly to exclude biliary atresia which has a much better outcome if surgery (Kasai procedure) is performed within the first 8 weeks. A liver unit may need to be involved early.

247. Chickenpox

Answers: B C

Children born to mothers who develop chickenpox during the period from 7 days before delivery to 7 days after should be given varicella zoster immunoglobulin (ZIG). Breast feeding should be encouraged and any baby who develops chickenpox lesions should be treated with iv aciclovir. Untreated the mortality is around 30%. ZIG should probably be offered to infants exposed to chickenpox during the neonatal period (ie up to 4 weeks of age). This is not always possible as ZIG is in short supply. If a mother develops chickenpox during the first trimester then the infant is at risk of developing congenital varicella syndrome; the risk being 1–2%. The congenital varicella syndrome includes limb hypoplasia, microcephaly, cataract, growth retardation, and skin scarring.

neonatology

248. Cataracts

Answers: A B C

Cataract describes a total or partial opacity of the lens. The following are causes of cataracts:

- hereditary — autosomal dominant
- idiopathic/sporadic
- congenital infection
  - cytomegalovirus
  - toxoplasmosis
  - herpes simplex
  - infectious mononucleosis
- metabolic
- galactosaemia
- Wilson's disease
- diabetes mellitus
- vitamin D deficiency
- neonatal hypoglycaemia
- hypoparathyroidism
- syndromes
  - Lowe's syndrome
  - Marfan's syndrome
  - Down's syndrome
  - Conradi's syndrome
  - Rothmund–Thomson syndrome
  - dystrophia myotonica
- other:
  - atopic cataract (as part of atopic dermatitis)
  - retinopathy of prematurity
  - corticosteroid induced.

Coloboma

Coloboma result from failure of closure of the fetal fissure. Coloboma may affect the iris (resulting in it being key-shaped), lens, retina, choroid and optic nerve. Causes include:

- sporadic
- familial — autosomal dominant
- chromosomal abnormalities
- syndromes
  - CHARGE syndrome
  - Meckel–Gruber syndrome.

neonatology

The CHARGE syndrome consists of:

- coloboma
- heart defects
- atresia of choanae
- retarded growth
- genital hypoplasia
- ear anomalies.

Corneal clouding

The cornea is a clear structure lining the front of the eye. Clouding of the cornea results in reduced visual acuity and an inability to see structures within the eye clearly on examination. Causes include:

- infections
  - bacterial, fungal and protozoan
  - herpes type I
  - rubella
  - measles
- trauma
  - direct blow
  - birth trauma
- metabolic
  - mucopolysaccharidoses type I (Hurler's syndrome)
  - cystinosis
  - tyrosinaemia
  - mucolipidoses type IV
- infantile congenital glaucoma
- corneal dystrophies
- corneal dysgenesis, eg sclerocornea
- exposure – any condition leading to excessive dry eyes
- familial dysautonomia
- pre-term

NB: Clouding of the cornea is present in fetuses until approximately 27 weeks gestation.

Retinopathy of prematurity

Retinopathy of prematurity is a condition affecting low birth weight premature infants particularly less than 1000 g. It is a disorder in which normal development of retinal vessels is interrupted. Progression of retinal vasculogenesis starts at the optic nerve and grows into the retina throughout fetal life. Premature infants are born with avascular peripheral retina. After birth, aggressive ventilation leads to hyperoxia which down regulates vascular endothelial growth factor (VEFG). The avascular retina itself then becomes hypoxic, which leads to excess production of

neonatology

VEGF which stimulates neovascularisation. This may then regress (as is the case in over 90%) or lead to scarring, retinal detachment and blindness. Sequelae include:

- visual impairment
- myopia
- astigmatism
- strabismus
- amblyopia
- glaucoma
- cataract.

249. Sudden infant death syndrome

Answers: A B C D

Maternal and paternal smoking, lower parental age and prone sleeping position are all risk factors. Any household smoking is associated even after adjustment for confounders. Supine sleeping position is unequivocally protective. Other risk factors include:

- over-heating
- family history of sudden infant death syndrome
- antecedent respiratory infection
- antecedent weight loss

250. Prolonged neonatal jaundice

Answer: E

Prolonged jaundice by definition is that which persists beyond 2 weeks in a term baby. Even without any tests, this baby almost certainly has breast milk jaundice. Arguably, it needs no investigation at all, but a split bilirubin to confirm that all is unconjugated can be reassuring rendering other test superfluous and is therefore widely advocated and done. Breastfeeding should not be stopped. Should however, the baby have any other signs including pale stools poor weight gain or worsening and conjugated jaundice much more extensive investigation is required.

251. Oxygen transfer from the placenta to fetus

Answer: A

The left shift of the dissociation curve enables haemoglobin F to pick up oxygen transplacentally. None of the other factors are true or have any bearing on this. Fetal haemoglobin (HbF) is composed of alpha2gamma2 globin chains while adult Hb is mainly alpha2beta2. HbF has reduced 2, 3 DPG causing a left shift in the

neonatology

oxygen dissociation curve in other words for a given pO2 the saturation increases. HbF therefore has a high avidity for oxygen which helps transplacental transfer. This does, however, mean that unloading to the tissues is slower. 2, 3 DPG levels rise rapidly in the first few days to cope with metabolic demand. Other causes of a left shift in the curve are:

- Alkalosis
- Hypocapnia
- Hypothermia

252. E: *Listeria*

L. monocytogenes is a ubiquitous Gram positive rod with a number of animal vectors. Transmission is often put down to a food-borne route (soft cheeses, uncooked meats etc). In pregnant women, infection gives a 'flu-like' illness, and infectivity to the fetus is unpredictable. In neonates there are a number of features:

- early
  - pre-term delivery
  - septicaemia
- late (> 5 days)
  - meningitis.

Late intrauterine infection with *Listeria* typically causes pre-term delivery with meconium which is unusual as prematurity tends to be associated with delayed passage of meconium due to neuromuscular immaturity. If considered/cultured, additional cover is needed, and ampicillin is the usual choice in addition to broad spectrum cover with cefotaxine or penicillin and gentamicin.

253. C: Muscle biopsy

This is the picture of congenital/severe spinal muscular atrophy (SMA), also called (eponymously) Werdnig–Hoffman syndrome. Babies are alert but floppy with absent reflexes and tongue fasciculation. Diagnosis is made by muscle biopsy. Creatine kinase (CK) is only mildly raised. There is no curative treatment and even with supportive treatment most babies die of respiratory failure at less than 12 months.

254. E: Review on the following day

Day 1 murmurs are extremely common and the vast majority due to (physiological) closure of the ductus. In the absence of other signs review on the following day is all that is required.

neonatology

255. CONGENITAL SYNDROMES

1. D – Turner's syndrome

Turner's has distinctive scan features which (though not always present) are highly suggestive. Coarctation of the aorta even if present may not become apparent until the duct shuts. The size may be normal at birth. Turner's has an XO karyotype and is associated with infertility as the ovaries are vestigial. Intelligence is normal/near normal. The main long-term problem is a short stature, and Turner's is an indication for growth hormone treatment. Turner-specific growth charts are more appropriate than the standard ones for monitoring growth.

2. C – Prader–Willi syndrome

This is the classic presentation of Prader–Willi syndrome. Hyperphagia develops much later and in boys the small genitalia may not be obvious at birth. The genetic defect is a 15q deletion, in common with Angelman's syndrome and detected by a fluorescence in-situ hybridisation (FISH) method. Intelligence is always low. Recent support for growth hormone treatment has not met with widespread enthusiasm.

3. G – VATER syndrome

This baby has abnormalities of at least two systems: renal and (clinically) oesophageal. The picture is typical of an oesophageal atresia, and can be confirmed by failure of passage of an nasogastric tube into the stomach. Often there is an associated tracheo-oesophageal fistula. Additional features of VATER are:

- vertebral, eg bifid vertebrae
- ano-rectal, eg atresia
- cardiac
- oesophageal, eg tracheo-oesophageal fistula
- renal (eg horseshoe)

The additional cardiac association has led to some preferring to call this the VACTERL syndrome.

neonatology

256. NEONATAL THROMBOCYTOPENIA

1. A – Neonatal alloimmune thrombocytopenia

Neonatal alloimmune thrombocytopenia occurs due to sensitisation of a PlA-negative mother to paternal PlA-positive antigen with transplacental transfer of IgG in much the same way as rhesus sensitisation. But it is a much more benign problem. If not suspected before delivery, the diagnosis is often made initially by exclusion of more serious problems. It rarely needs any intervention as the count rises over the first few weeks to normal – like rhesus sensitisation, tends to worsen with each pregnancy but would rarely be an indication to advise against future pregnancies.

2. C – TORCH infection

This baby has features of intrauterine infection. The opacities and low platelets with IUGR are classic of congenital rubella but there is overlap with the other TORCH group of infections. Features of TORCH infections are:

- microcephaly
- cataract
- deafness
- congenital heart disease
- IUGR.

In congenital toxoplasmosis the following triad is classic:

- hydrocephalus
- intracranial calcification
- choroidoretinitis.

3. H – Maternal systemic lupus erythematosus

Congenital heart block suggested by a well baby with a profound bradycardia and low platelets strongly suggests maternal systemic lupus erythematosus . If the mother is not already known to have systemic lupus erythematosus, anti-dsDNA is diagnostic. Cardiac pacing may be necessary. Platelet transfusion is indicated if the platelet count drops below $20 \times 10^9/l$.

neonatology

NEPHROLOGY ANSWERS

257. Renin angiotensin system

Answer: C

Intravascular depletion causes a reduction in renal perfusion and release of renin from the juxta-glomerular apparatus. Renin results in angiotensinogen (in plasma) being converted to angiotensin I which is converted by angiotensin-converting enzyme to angiotensin II in the lungs. Angiotensin II causes arteriolar vasoconstriction and aldosterone release from the adrenal cortex. Aldosterone promotes sodium and chloride reabsorption in the distal tubules and collecting ducts with excretion of potassium and hydrogen ions.

258. Inappropriate ADH secretion

Answers: A B C

Anti-diuretic hormone is synthesised by the supra-optic and paraventricular neurones in the hypothalamus and then transported along the nerve axons to be released in the posterior pituitary. The release is stimulated by increased plasma osmolality or reduced plasma volume. It acts on the distal tubules and collecting ducts to increase water re-absorption. In inappropriate ADH secretion there is water retention with hypo-osmolality and hyponatraemia. The urine osmolality is inappropriately high. There is no volume depletion. Investigation is with paired plasma and urinary electrolytes and osmolality. Causes of inappropriate ADH secretion are:

- birth asphyxia
- hyaline membrane disease
- intra-ventricular haemorrhage
- meningitis (particularly pneumococcal)
- encephalitis
- other infections, eg pneumonia
- trauma, eg head injury
- tumours
- surgery
- iatrogenic
- drugs, eg vincristine, nicotine, barbiturates, carbamazepine.

Phenytoin inhibits ADH secretion. The management is with fluid restriction to 30–50% maintenance and treatment of the underlying cause.

259. Cranial diabetes insipidus

Answers: A D

This is a failure of anti-diuretic hormone secretion. It can be familial or sporadic (autosomal dominant and X-linked dominant families have been described). It can be idiopathic or due to:

- tumours, eg craniopharyngioma
- infiltration, eg histiocytosis X
- granulomatous disease, eg tuberculosis
- trauma, eg head injury, pituitary surgery.

The clinical features are:

- polyuria
- polydipsia
- nocturia
- differential diagnosis
- nephrogenic diabetes insipidus
- psychogenic polydipsia
- diabetes mellitus
- urinary tract infection.

Investigation shows inappropriate low urine osmolality with a raised plasma osmolality:

- Administer DDAVP.
- Water deprivation test – carry out for 6–8 hours or until 3% of body weight is lost. Urine osmolality of > 800 mosm/kg is normal.
- If not achieved, administer DDAVP and if urine osmolality goes to > 800 mosm/kg then the diagnosis is cranial diabetes insipidus.
- If no response to DDAVP the diagnosis is nephrogenic diabetes insipidus.
- If the water deprivation test is normal in a child with polydipsia and polyuria for which other causes such as diabetes mellitus have been excluded then the diagnosis is psychogenic polydipsia.
- Plasma osmolality often rises during the water deprivation test if the diagnosis is diabetes insipidus (cranial or nephrogenic).

For nephrogenic diabetes insipidus see Question 268.

260. Hyperkalaemia

Answers: B C

The following are useful in the emergency treatment of acute hyperkalaemia.

- Intravenous calcium gluconate which antagonises the effects of potassium on the heart by stabilising the myocardium. It does not lower the serum potassium. It should be used if either an arrhythmia or electrocardiogram (ECG) changes of hyperkalaemia are present. Dose is 0.1 mmol/kg iv.
- Salbutamol either intravenously or nebulised. Nebulised dose is 2.5–10 mg, iv dose 4 μg/kg. Salbutamol results in potassium entry into the cell.
- Intravenous sodium bicarbonate. Dose is 2.5 mmol/kg iv. Give if pH < 7.3. Sodium bicarbonate promotes the uptake of potassium into cells. In addition, acidosis will impair myocardial function and needs to be corrected. Need to check calcium as if patient is hypocalcaemic, bicarbonate may lower the ionised calcium, precipitating tetany, convulsions, hypotension or arrhythmias.
- Glucose insulin infusion. Dose of dextrose is 0.5 g/kg/h and insulin is 0.05 U/kg/h iv. Promotes the uptake of potassium into cells.
- Ion exchange resin – such as calcium resonium which facilitates sodium potassium exchange in the gut and can be given orally or by enema. Dose 1g/kg initially and then 1g/kg/day.
- Dialysis/haemofiltration.

Hydrocortisone is not useful.

Adenosine is used to control supra-ventricular tachycardia.

- ECG changes of hyperkalaemia:
  - prolongation of the PR interval
  - peaked T waves
  - widening of the QRS complex
  - ST depression
  - ventricular fibrillation.

261. Nocturnal enuresis

Answers: B C

Nocturnal enuresis is defined as bed wetting for three or more nights per month or one night per week. At age 5–6 years the prevalence is 8–10%, and at age 7–10 years the prevalence is 5–7%. The male to female ratio is 2:1. After age 10 the male to female ratio gradually reduces. About 20–30% are secondary (ie start after a period of full night time control for 6 months). The incidence doubles when the father or mother has had nocturnal enuresis and if both parents suffered there is a 70% chance that the offspring will be affected. Management of nocturnal enuresis is as follows:

- general:
  - explanation and reassurance
  - diary of wetting
- specific
  - under age 5 years – reassurance that all is normal; family therapy; practical help
  - 5–7 years – star chart; lifting; Desmospray/Desmotabs
  - Over 7 years – star chart; Desmospray/Desmotabs; enuresis alarm.

Drug treatment alleviates symptoms but will not accelerate resolution. Over 7 years of age about 60% using alarm will achieve dryness within 2 months. Children should be woken if lifted to go to the toilet otherwise they will 'learn' to pass urine while asleep. DDAVP (desmopressin) as either spray or tablets has a success rate of 60–70% but a high relapse rate when the treatment is stopped (30%). In children under 7 years of age DDAVP may relieve stress in the family in the short or long term. An adequate (not excessive) fluid intake must be maintained when on DDAVP and the medication should be stopped if vomiting occurs in order to prevent severe hyponatraemia. Dose of Desmospray is 20–40 µg at bed time and Desmotabs is 0.2–0.4 mg at night.

262. Berger's disease

Answers: A C E

Berger's disease is part of the differential diagnosis of recurrent haematuria. It is a histological diagnosis. The diagnosis is made when the predominant feature on renal biopsy is granular deposition of IgA and C3 in the mesangium of the glomerulus in the absence of systemic disease, eg systemic lupus erythematosus or abnormal plasma immunoglobulins or complement levels. The male to female ratio is 2:1. It usually presents with haematuria following an upper respiratory tract infection. Microscopic haematuria may persist. Macroscopic haematuria is associated with upper respiratory tract infections. Proteinuria occurs in 40–50%.

The prognosis for most children is good, although 5–10% will develop end-stage renal failure. Poor prognostic features include heavy proteinuria, hypertension and proliferative lesions on renal biopsy. Deafness is not a feature of Berger's but of Alport's syndrome. Berger's disease commonly recurs in transplanted kidneys.

263. Renal failure

Answer: B

In pre-renal failure there is a reduction in the intravascular volume which results in a reduced glomerular filtration rate. This activates the renin–angiotensin system and results in the secretion of aldosterone which promotes sodium reabsorption and potassium excretion in the distal tubule. Intravascular depletion results in a more concentrated urine being passed. This urine is characterised by a high osmolality (> 500 mosm/l) and a low sodium (< 20 mmol/l). The urine:plasma creatinine ratio is high (> 40).

The fractional excretion of sodium is calculated as follows:

$$\frac{\text{urine Na x plasma Cr}}{\text{urine Cr x plasma Na}} \times 100 \ (\%)$$

urine Na = urinary sodium
urine Cr = urinary creatinine
plasma Na = plasma sodium
plasma Cr = plasma creatinine.

The fractional excretion of sodium is less than 1% in pre-renal failure and greater than 1% in renal failure.

In neonates, sodium reabsorption is less efficient and the fractional excretion of sodium is nearer to less than 2.5% in pre-renal failure and greater than 2.5% in renal failure.

This approach is not helpful if either mannitol or diuretics have been given, which will interfere with the urinary electrolytes.

Diarrhoea can precede pre-renal (eg gastroenteritis) failure or renal (haemolytic uraemic syndrome) failure.

264. Renal osteodystrophy

Answers: A B

Renal osteodystrophy is a potentially life-threatening complication of chronic renal failure. A reduction in glomerular filtration rate causes a reduction in the excretion of inorganic phosphate. The decline in renal function reduces the production of 1,25-dihydroxy vitamin D from 25-hydroxy vitamin D, thus decreasing calcium absorption from the gut. Hyperphosphataemia and low serum calcium stimulate parathyroid hormone secretion (secondary hyperparathyroidism).

Parathyroid hormone:

- increases calcium reabsorption in the distal tubule
- decreases phosphate reabsorption in the proximal tubule
- stimulates the synthesis of 1,25-dihydroxy vitamin D in the proximal tubule
- promotes osteoclastic bone reabsorption.

Biochemical features of renal osteodystrophy include:

- normal or low serum calcium
- increased plasma phosphate
- increased plasma alkaline phosphatase
- markedly increased parathyroid hormone level
- normal or reduced 25-hydroxy vitamin D
- reduced 1,25-dihydroxy vitamin D.

The management is dietary phosphate restriction, use of a phosphate binder (such as calcium carbonate, aluminium hydroxide) and 1 α-hydroxy cholecalciferol or 1, 25-dihydroxycholecalciferol.

Vitamin D

Sources of vitamin D are the diet and ultraviolet radiation. Vitamin D is hydroxylated to 25-hydroxy vitamin D in the liver. 25-hydroxy vitamin D is further hydroxylated to 1,25-dihydroxy vitamin D in the kidney, which promotes:

- calcium resorption from bone
- calcium and phosphate reabsorption from the kidney
- calcium and phosphate absorption from the gut
- cell growth and differentiation.

	Vitamin D deficiency	Hypophosphataemic rickets	Renal osteodystophy
Calcium	reduced	normal	normal
Phosphate	reduced or normal	reduced	increased
Alkaline phosphatase	increased	increased	increased
PTH	increased	normal	markedly increased

nephrology

265. Henoch-Schönlein purpura

Answer: A

Around 20–50% of children with Henoch-Schönlein purpura have renal involvement. This is usually mild with microscopic haematuria and proteinuria although a nephrotic or a nephritic picture may occur in up to 2%. The renal manifestations are usually present within the first month but can present later and almost always present within 3 months. Careful follow-up of blood pressure, urine microscopy and plasma creatinine is required in patients with renal involvement until the manifestations of this disappear.

Renal biopsy should be considered if:

- there is significant and persistent proteinuria
- the patient develops frank nephrotic syndrome
- there is evidence of renal insufficiency.

High-dose immunosuppression is given to those with severe renal involvement. There is no diagnostic test for Henoch-Schönlein purpura. The differential diagnosis includes:

- systemic lupus erythematosus
- post-streptococcal glomerulonephritis
- haemolytic uraemic syndrome.

Systemic lupus erythematosus is suggested by the clinical picture, a low C3, C4 and anti-nuclear antibody (ANA) positivity. In children with post-streptococcal glomerulonephritis there is usually a history of preceding streptococcal infection. The laboratory features include a low C3 and a raised anti-streptolysin O (ASO) titre. The blood film in haemolytic uraemic syndrome is characteristic. The prognosis of Henoch-Schönlein nephritis depends on the extent of glomerular lesions. Poor prognostic factors include:

- clinical evidence of renal insufficiency
- clinical evidence of nephrotic syndrome
- glomerular sclerosis
- glomerular necrosis
- extensive crescent formation.

nephrology

266. Syndromes

Answer: B

Nephrogenic diabetes insipidus

This is an X-linked recessive condition characterised by resistance of the kidney to the anti-diuretic action of anti-diuretic hormone. The symptoms and signs include polyuria, polydipsia, dehydration, failure to thrive and mental retardation. The plasma biochemistry is characteristic and shows hypernatraemia, hyperchloraemia and hyperosmolality. Diagnosis is by a water deprivation test which demonstrates a failure to concentrate the urine despite exogenous anti-diuretic hormone. Treatment includes a low salt diet, hydrochlorothiazide and indometacin.

Alport's syndrome

Alport's syndrome is inherited as an X-linked dominant with occasional families showing an autosomal dominant inheritance pattern. It is characterised by haematuria, progressive impairment of renal function, deafness, ocular manifestations and a characteristic appearance on renal biopsy. The disease is usually silent in childhood and presents in adolescence with microscopic haematuria and proteinuria. Males are more severely affected than females.

Hartnup's disease

This condition has an autosomal recessive inheritance pattern. It is characterised by a tubular and intestinal defect in the reabsorption and absorption of cyclic and neutral amino acids. The clinical features of the condition are secondary to tryptophan malabsorption. These include a photosensitive rash and cerebella ataxia. The condition is diagnosed by the demonstration of a specific pattern of amino aciduria. Tryptophan malabsorption results in a nicotinamide deficiency and treatment with nicotinamide corrects the clinical features.

Vitamin D resistant rickets

This is an X-linked dominant condition which usually present between 12 and 18 months. The plasma biochemistry demonstrates a normal plasma calcium, low phosphate, raised alkaline phosphatase, normal parathyroid hormone level and vitamin D level. Treatment is with phosphate and vitamin D.

Cystinosis

This is an autosomally recessively inherited condition. It can present in the infant, adolescent or adult. The presentation in infancy is with failure to thrive, recurrent vomiting and dehydration. The biochemistry is of a metabolic acidosis with a low plasma potassium and a low plasma phosphate. The diagnosis is made by measurement of the white cell cystine. Treatment is with potassium and bicarbonate replacement as with other Fanconi-type syndromes and additionally with phosphocysteamine. It is important to differentiate cystinosis from cystinuria. Cystinuria is an inborn error of the metabolism of dibasic amino acids. Low cysteine solubility leads to renal stone formation. This is the only complication. The stones are radio-opaque.

267. Nephrotic syndrome

Answer: C

Minimal change nephrotic syndrome has a male predominance. It is rare in the first year of life. Peak incidence is in the age range 2–5 years. It can occur in adult life. Haematuria is usually absent. The presence of haematuria implies that a more serious form of glomerulonephritis should be considered as does the presence of hypertension or abnormal renal function tests. Complement levels are normal. Complications of nephrotic syndrome are:

- hypovolaemia
- hypertension
- infection
- thrombosis
- hyperlipidaemia
- acute renal failure.

Referral to a paediatric nephrologist should be considered if:

- age less than 12 months
- age greater than 10 years
- macroscopic or persistent microscopic haematuria
- impaired renal function not attributable to hypovolaemia
- hypertension.

Differential diagnosis of nephrotic syndrome in children aged 1–15 years includes:

- minimal change nephrotic syndrome
- focal segmental glomerulosclerosis
- mesangiocapillary glomerulonephritis
- membranous nephropathy
- Henoch-Schönlein nephritis
- systemic lupus erythematosus.

268. Metabolic acidosis

Answers: D E

Pyloric Stenosis results in hypochloraemic metabolic alkalosis due to chloride and hydrogen ion loss through vomiting.

Cystinuria

Defect in the intestinal absorption and renal tubular reabsorption of the dibasic amino acids cystine, lysine, arginine and ornithine. The consequence is the formation of renal calculi. Treatment is to alkalinise the urine.

Bartter's syndrome

The basic defect of Bartter's syndrome is impaired tubular chloride reabsorption. The biochemical features are of hypokalaemia, hypochloraemia, alkalosis, hyperreninaemia and hyperaldosteronism associated with a normal blood pressure and high urinary losses of potassium and chloride.

Cystinosis

This condition is discussed in Answer 268. The biochemical features are metabolic acidosis associated with a high plasma chloride and a low potassium and phosphate.

Pseudohypoaldosteronism

Pseudohypoaldosteronism is characterised by unresponsiveness of the distal tubule to aldosterone. Hyponatraemia, hyperkalaemia and dehydration occur. Metabolic acidosis can occur (type IV renal tubular acidosis).

269. Urinary tract infection

Answer: None are correct.

Though urinary tract infections do predispose to scarring the degree of damage is unpredictable and evidence has swung against intensive investigation. In the over 2-years group an uncomplicated UTI with a normal ultrasound probably needs no more investigation. In an infant with a normal DMSA, MCUG may not be necessary. Prophylaxis is probably not indicated beyond the age of 4 years. Avoidance of bubble bath is important as the oils alter mucosal immune defences. Further investigation is indicated in children over the age of 2 years if:

- ultrasound scan shows abnormal findings
- recurrent infections
- acute pyelonephritis
- family history of reflux.

A Mag III indirect cystogram can be used to look for vesico-ureteric reflux and for renal scars once continence has been achieved. A DMSA scan is a static scan which will detect renal scars. A DTPA is a dynamic scan to look for obstruction at any level of the renal tract and uses furosemide to promote a diuresis.

Prophylactic agents

- Trimethoprim 2 mg/kg at night
- Nitrofurantoin 1 mg/kg at night.

270. Haemolytic uraemic syndrome

Answers: C D

Haemolytic uraemic syndrome is on the increase. Peak age is 1–2 years. Peak incidence occurs during the summer months. 50% require dialysis in the acute phase and mortality is of the order of 5–10%. Hyponatraemia occurs in 70% and thrombocytopenia in 50%. The blood film shows a microangiopathic haemolytic anaemia. The majority of children recover without the need for dialysis with supportive measures and transfusion. There are two subgroups within the syndrome:

D+ (95%):

- prodromal diarrhoea
- associated with verotoxin producing *Escherichia coli* 0157:H7
- other associated infections include Coxsackie virus, *Shigella* dysentery, streptococcal infection
- 85% make a full recovery
- neutrophilia (>15) predicts a difficult course.

D– (5%):

- often familial
- no prodromal illness
- runs relapsing course
- 70% progress to chronic renal failure.

271. Renal tubular acidosis

Answers: A D E

Proximal renal tubular acidosis

This occurs as a result of a failure of reabsorption of bicarbonate in the proximal tubule. It is characterised by a high urinary pH, low plasma bicarbonate and metabolic acidosis. Most patients with proximal renal tubular acidosis manifest this tubular abnormality as part of Fanconi's syndrome. In patients with proximal renal tubular acidosis distal tubular acidification is intact. This means that following an acid load the urinary pH will drop below 5.5.

Fanconi's syndrome

This is a generalised transport abnormality in the proximal tubule characterised by excessive urinary losses of amino acids, glucose, bicarbonate, phosphate, calcium, magnesium and uric acid. It is characterised by metabolic acidosis, dehydration, hypokalaemia, hypophosphataemia, rickets and growth retardation. There are many causes, both hereditary and acquired.

Treatment

The treatment of proximal renal tubular acidosis is large amounts of alkali as sodium bicarbonate and sodium citrate. Fanconi's syndrome requires treatment as appropriate with phosphate, potassium and vitamin D.

Distal renal tubular acidosis

This occurs as a consequence of reduced hydrogen ion secretion in the distal tubule. It is not possible to lower the urinary pH below 5.5 regardless of the acid load. Children present with unexplained acidosis, failure to thrive, nephrocalcinosis, rickets and polyuria. Hypokalaemia and hypercalciuria are both common and can be severe. The treatment is with sodium and potassium bicarbonate. The condition can be autosomal dominant, sporadic or secondary.

272. Proteinuria

Answers: A B C

Orthostatic

Increased protein in the urine in the upright posture, absent when lying flat. Proteinuria is variable but can be large. It is a benign condition. Renal function is normal and family history negative.

Intermittent

Intermittent proteinuria is common after exercise or stress and with no obvious precipitant. It is rarely of serious significance.

273. Haematuria

Answers: A C D

There are many causes of haematuria:

- infection
- trauma
- glomerulonephritis
- hypercalciuria
- renal calculi
- hydronephrosis and other congenital abnormalities
- vascular problems
- tumours
- bleeding disorder
- drug induced, eg cyclophosphamide
- exercise induced
- factitious.

The haematuria itself can be macroscopic, intermittent or microscopic. Haematuria needs to be distinguished from other conditions like excessive beetroot ingestion, rifampicin, haemoglobinuria and myoglobulinuria which produce red urine. The co-existence of proteinuria with haematuria makes a renal parenchymal lesion more likely. Heavy proteinuria suggests glomerular disease. Ultrasound and plain abdominal radiography are essential to exclude obstruction, calculi or tumours. A family history of deafness suggests Alport's syndrome.

274. Hypertension

Answers: A B E

To measure the blood pressure manually the blood pressure cuff should cover half of the upper arm. A small cuff will result in a high reading.

Causes of hypertension in childhood are:

- acute glomerulonephritis
- chronic glomerulonephritis
- reflux nephropathy
- haemolytic uraemic syndrome
- polycystic renal disease
- coarctation of the aorta
- renal artery stenosis
- phaeochromocytoma
- congenital adrenal hyperplasia/11 beta hydroxylase deficiency
- acute hypovolaemia
- essential hypertension.

Drug treatment of hypertension is with:

- diuretics, eg furosemide
- calcium channel blockers, eg nifedipine
- angiotensin converting enzyme inhibitors, eg captopril
- vasodilators, eg prazosin, hydralazine, sodium nitroprusside
- β-blockers, eg propranolol
- α- and β-blockers, eg labetalol.

Complications of hypertension are:

- left ventricular failure
- retinopathy
- hypertensive encephalopathy.

Emergency treatment of hypertensive encephalopathy is with:

- nifedipine
- labetalol iv
- sodium nitroprusside.

275. Acute post-streptococcal glomerulonephritis

Answers: A C

This commonly follows group A β-haemolytic streptococcal infection. The ASOT (anti-streptolysin titre) is positive in 90% which is indicative of recent streptococcal infection. The ASOT may not rise after a skin infection whereas anti-DNAse B will rise irrespective of infection site. There are other implicated infectious agents which are less commonly seen. The usual age of presentation is between 2 and 10 years; it is commoner in males. The classical presentation is of preceding upper respiratory tract infection followed by the onset of macroscopic haematuria and oedema after 2 weeks indicating an acute nephritis. Oliguria is usually present for the first ten days of the nephritic illness. The C3 is low initially and returns to normal within 6–12 weeks. C4 is less frequently low and if so returns to normal much quicker. Problems include hypertension, pulmonary oedema and renal insufficiency. Treatment is with oral penicillin for 10 days to eradicate the *Streptococcus*. This does not influence the time course or severity of the nephritis. Diuretics may be required. Steroids are not indicated.

Feature of acute nephritis are:

- haematuria
- proteinuria
- oedema, ascites, pleural effusions
- hypertension
- renal insufficiency.

Differential diagnosis of acute nephritis in childhood includes:

- post-infectious glomerulonephritis
- Henoch-Schönlein nephritis
- IgA nephropathy
- Alport's syndrome
- lupus nephritis.

276. Undescended testis

Answers: A D E

The testes are undescended in 3% of babies born at term and 1% at the age of 12 months. Spontaneous descent is rare after the first birthday. True undescended testis must be distinguished from retractile testis which can be 'milked' down into the scrotum. Impalpable testes are not necessarily absent and may be intra-abdominal. The incidence of undescended testis is much higher in pre-term babies. Thirty per cent of cases are bilateral. There is an increased risk of infertility and of malignancy in children with undescended testis. In order to minimise these, orchidopexy should be carried out before the end of the second year. The incidence of testicular tumours in adults is 3 per 10 000. The risk in males with a history of undescended testis is 4–40 times greater. Sixty per cent of the tumours are seminomas, most of the remainder being teratomas. Important associations of undescended testis include:

- spinal muscular atrophy
- myotonic dystrophy
- X-linked ichthyosis
- Kallmann's syndrome
- prune belly syndrome.

277. Wilms' tumour

Answers: B C E

There is an increased risk of Wilms' tumour in the following conditions:

- isolated hemihypertrophy
- Beckwith–Wiedemann syndrome
- neurofibromatosis
- Drash syndrome
- WAGR syndrome
- ambiguous genitalia
- nephropathy
- aniridia
- genitourinary malformations
- mental retardation.

Wilms' tumour accounts for 10% of all paediatric tumours and 22% of abdominal masses in childhood. Ten per cent are bilateral. Ultrasound is the best investigation to make the diagnosis. The prognosis is good, with 80–90% 5-year survival.

278. Chloride

Answers: C D E

Chloride is the major anion of extracellular fluid. The reabsorption of tubular fluid must be isoelectric. Sodium and potassium transfer with chloride and bicarbonate. Chloride is actively transported in the ascending limb of the loop of Henlé and in the gut. Chloride and bicarbonate act such that if extracellular chloride is reduced then bicarbonate reabsorption is increased (hypochloraemic metabolic alkalosis) and if bicarbonate is reduced in the extracellular fluid chloride reabsorption is increased (hyperchloraemic metabolic acidosis).

Hypochloraemia (< 95 mmol/l)

Loss of hydrochloric acid from the stomach results in a metabolic alkalosis and volume depletion. This activates the renin-angiotensin system and promotes sodium reabsorption (with bicarbonate as chloride is depleted) in the proximal tubule and sodium exchange for potassium and hydrogen ions in the distal tubule.

Hyperchloraemia

Three settings:

- excessive intake
- increased absorption from the gastrointestinal tract
- renal tubular acidosis.

Excessive chloride in the extracellular fluid will suppress bicarbonate reabsorption and lead to the development of a metabolic acidosis. Renal tubular acidosis manifest by a bicarbonate leak will increase chloride reabsorption.

279. Hyponatraemia

Answers: C D E

Causes of hyponatraemia are:

- inappropriate iv fluids
- excessive loss in the urine, faeces, vomit or sweat
- prematurity
- inadequate intake
- inappropriate ADH secretion
- salt losing state, eg congenital adrenal hyperplasia, Addison's disease

- renal tubular acidosis
- diuretic therapy.

280. Membranous glomerulonephritis

Answers: A C E

Males predominate in this condition which represents under 1% of childhood nephrotic syndrome but 20–40% of adult nephrotic syndrome. It can present with full blown nephrotic syndrome or with mild proteinuria and haematuria. It can be idiopathic or secondary to other diseases such as systemic lupus erythematosus or hepatitis B. The C3 is initially low in membranous glomerulonephritis due to either of these conditions. Steroids are beneficial in the adult but rarely so in childhood. Progression to renal failure is rare. Causes of secondary membranous nephropathy are:

- hepatitis B
- malaria
- schistosomiasis
- leprosy
- systemic lupus erythematosus
- mercury
- gold
- sickle cell disease
- rheumatoid arthritis.

Other types of glomerulonephritis which present as nephrotic syndrome are:

- focal segmental glomerulosclerosis
- mesangiocapillary (membranoproliferative) glomerulonephritis
- mesangial proliferative glomerulonephritis.

281. Polycystic kidney disease

Answers: B C E

Autosomal recessive polycystic renal disease usually presents in the first year of life. The incidence is 1 in 40 000. The commonest presentation is with either respiratory distress or enlarged kidneys in the neonatal period. Ultrasound is the best method of diagnosis. Death often occurs rapidly although a number survive and those that do so beyond the first year generally do well. Autosomal dominant polycystic renal disease accounts for 8% of adults in end-stage renal failure. The incidence is between 1 in 200 and 1 in 1000. The gene is on chromosome 16. It usually presents in adult life but can, rarely, present in the neonatal period. The renal cysts are associated with cysts in other organs including the liver, pancreas spleen and lungs. 10% have a berry aneurysm in the circle of Willis.

282. Vesico-ureteric reflux

Answers: B C D

Of children who present to hospital with a confirmed urinary tract infection 30–40% have vesico-ureteric reflux (boys > girls). Of those, up to 30% develop renal scars. The diagnosis is by micturating cystography. Severity is graded from I to IV, with grade IV implying intra-renal reflux is present. A MAG 3 indirect cystogram can be used once continence has been achieved but this is both less sensitive and less specific although a better tolerated procedure. The object of management is to prevent urinary tract infections and in doing so prevent renal scarring (reflux nephropathy). This is best achieved using low dose prophylactic antibiotics to prevent infections and appropriate antibiotics if breakthrough infection occurs based on urine culture and sensitivity. Most reflux resolves by the age of 5 years. If not, and recurrent infections occur with progressive renal scarring, ureteric re-implantation is indicated. DMSA is the best investigation to look for renal scars.

Complications of reflux nephropathy are:

- hypertension
- left ventricular failure
- impaired renal function
- renal failure.

283. Hypercalciuria

Answers: A B D

Hypercalciuria is important as it is a risk factor for the production of renal calculi and can cause other urinary symptoms including polyuria, nocturnal enuresis and dysuria. It is also commonly associated with microscopic haematuria. The gold standard is to measure the 24-hour urinary calcium (upper limit of normal 0.1 mmol/kg/day); the measurement of the urinary calcium creatinine ratio is also useful (upper limit of normal 0.7). Causes of hypercalciuria can be either normo- or hypercalcaemic:

1. **normocalcaemic**
   - idiopathic (familial)
   - distal renal tubular acidosis
   - furosemide

2. **hypercalcaemic**
   - increased bone resorption
     - immobilisation
     - steroids
     - primary hyperparathyroidism
     - thyroid disease

- Cushing's disease
- increased intestinal absorption
  - calcium
  - vitamin D
- hypophosphataemia
- William's syndrome.

284. Congenital nephrotic syndrome

Answers: A E

The commonest congenital nephrotic syndrome is the Finnish type. Incidence is 12 per 100 000 live births. Babies are often born pre-term, small for gestational age and have a large placenta. Proteinuria often occurs in utero and the α-fetoprotein is raised. Thirty per cent develop oedema in the first week of life with abdominal distension and ascites. Renal function is normal initially but deteriorates to end-stage renal failure within the first 2 years of life. Renal biopsy is characteristic. There is no available treatment. Patients are managed with regular albumin transfusions followed by bilateral nephrectomy, dialysis, high calorie feeding and renal transplantation.

285. D: Admit for investigation and fluid balance

This presentation is typical of haemolytic uraemic syndrome, the commonest cause of acute renal failure in children under 2 years. It classically follows a bloody diarrhoeal illness (*Escherichia coli*, *Shigella*) but there may be non-bloody diarrhoea. Investigations show acute renal failure with thrombocytopenia and anaemia with red cell fragments and first-line treatment is that generic to acute renal failure, ie fluid management. Transfusion is often required and dialysis for those cases where conservative management fails.

286. B: Urgent renal ultrasound

This baby has renal failure secondary to posterior urethral valves until proved otherwise and the story is typical. These babies are hungry but catabolic due to the renal failure. Without urgent treatment the damage is irreversible though in many a lot of damage has already been incurred antenatally. Ultrasound confirms obstruction at the urethral level with ureteric and pelvicalyceal dilatation. Once established, catheterisation followed by diathermy correction is needed. It is also important to exclude urinary tract infection, start prophylactic antibiotics, check fluid balances, urea, electrolytes and creatinine as precise management of the biochemistry improves outcome. Pre-auricular tags are common and though there is an occasional association with renal abnormalities they do not, per se, warrant investigation. In this context, however, the sign should be an additional clue.

287. A: Start high-dose prednisolone

This is nephrotic syndrome. Most children have the minimal change histological variety of nephrotic syndrome (good prognosis). In 90% of children it is steroid sensitive though response in the form of diuresis may take several days. A regimen of 60mg/m^2 until remission of the proteinuria is followed by 40mg/m^2/day for a further 4 weeks before reduction to stop. Admission for the first episode is advisable but not always necessary. Most children have a relapsing remitting course over several years. Hypertension is due to secondary hyperaldosteronism due to reduced intravascular volume. Diet has little part in management. Malaria is a rare cause of nephritis.

288. E: Normal reaction to new siblings

The symptoms are typically non-organic. On the assumption that urine has been checked the family need reassurance that there is nothing serious amiss and that she will improve with time and attention. Starting nursery is often helpful in this sort of situation.

289. BLOOD PRESSURE

1. F – Haemolytic uraemic syndrome

This case is a typical picture of haemolytic uraemic syndrome, the commonest cause of renal failure in children aged under 2 years. It usually follows a diarrhoeal illness and most commonly is associated with verotoxin-producing *Escherichia coli* (VTEC) of the 0157 serotype. Other changes in the full blood count and film include red blood cell fragments and anaemia. Management is essentially supportive with strict renal failure fluid balance, treatment of hypertension, transfusion, and in some cases dialysis. Long-term follow-up is mandatory. Prognosis is worse in non-diarhoeal cases.

2. I – Vesico-ureteric reflux with scarring in infancy

The small kidneys and hypertension strongly suggest chronic pyelonephritis most commonly due to early reflux nephropathy. Many studies have shown a causal link between early vesico-ureteric reflux, scarring and renal failure. It is on this basis that the recommendation for investigations of and prophylaxis for urinary tract infection in young children are based.

3. G – Wilm's tumour

Wilm's tumours are associated with hemihypertrophy (easily confused with hemiatrophy) which can precede the malignancy by years. Also associated is aniridia. Children with hemihypertrophy should have annual renal ultrasonography life-long.

290. INVESTIGATIONS

1. C – DMSA isotope scan

The DMSA isotope scan. By far the best way of assessing parenchymal damage. This particular isotope concentrates well into renal tissue showing scarring which ultrasound is too insensitive to detect. DMSA scanning within 6 weeks of urinary tract infection is inadvisable due to false positive results. DMSA is also of value in quantifying differential renal function.

2. J – None of the above

The principal 'investigating' needed at presentation is confirmation of proteinuria. The diagnosis of nephrotic syndrome is based on the triad of proteinuria, peripheral oedema and hypoalbuninaemia and apart from bloods is clinical.

3. E – Renal tract ultrasound

Ultrasound is simple and effective and will show perinephric fluid in most cases. Some surgeons prefer an additional CT pre-operatively. Percutaneous drainage can be done under ultrasound guidance but open drainage is required for definitive treatment.

291. THE KIDNEY IN SYSTEMIC DISEASE

1. J – Amyloidosis

Secondary amyloidosis can result from a number of chronic inflammatory/infective conditions. These include:

- bronchiectasis
- tuberculosis
- lung abscess
- cystic fibrosis.

It leads to renal failure (by deposition) and also accumulates in the parotid glands. Diagnosis is by either showing deposition in the kidney or doing a rectal biopsy.

2. A – Systemic lupus

Though several of these conditions may have renal impairment after some years only lupus presents with involvement as a glomerulonephritis. Other features can be:

- arthritis
- malar rash
- general malaise.

nephrology

Diagnosis is made by autoantibody testing, the gold standard being anti-double-stranded DNA.

3. C – Diabetes

The classic 'herald' of renal impairment in diabetes is asymptomatic microalbuminuria. This takes 10 years to develop from diagnosis and is associated with impaired control of glycaemia (eg high HbA_1C). Annual urinary screening for microalbumin:creatinine ratio is recommended. Even after detection, further deterioration can be slowed by meticulous control.

NEUROLOGY ANSWERS

neurology

292. Sturge–Weber syndrome

Answer: D

Sturge–Weber syndrome is sporadic with an incidence of 1 in 50 000. The condition has two main features:

- An angiomatous malformation (capillary haemangioma) usually called a port wine stain present from birth over the skin of one of the branches of the trigeminal nerve; most commonly the 1st branch. It is usually unilateral.
- A similar malformation over the occipital area of the ipsilateral cerebral hemisphere which results in cerebral ischaemia giving rise to atrophy and calcification.

Clinical manifestations include:

- contralateral hemiparesis
- intractable seizures
- mental retardation
- progressive neurological deterioration.

Rail track calcification on the skull X-ray is characteristic and is due to linear calcification lines in the gyri with the intermittent sulci being spared. The blood supply to the skin and meninges is in common with that of the retina and face; therefore associated anomalies of the eyes such as glaucoma, buphthalmos and retinal defects occur. Treatment involves anti-convulsants, management of disabilities, on occasions occipital lobectomy and rarely hemispherectomy. Pulsed laser has been used for the port-wine stain.

293. Narcolepsy

Answers: A B C

Narcolepsy is characterised by episodes of sudden uncontrollable sleep occurring at any time of the day or night. It involves an abnormal sequence in the stages of sleep – REM sleep occurring within 10 minutes of falling asleep compared with 1–2 hours in normal individuals. It typically commences in adolescence, is familial and up to 90% suffer from cataplexy (sudden loss of tone in the legs, no loss of consciousness). Other associations include psychiatric problems, sleep paralysis and hypnogogic hallucinations (auditory hallucinations while falling asleep). Treatment involves stimulants for narcolepsy; clomipramine for cataplexy and multi-disciplinary management of associated problems.

294. Raised intra-cranial pressure

Answers: A B C

Rising intra-cranial pressure may present in a variety of ways including:

- headaches
- vomiting
- alteration in conscious level
- seizures
- in a trauma setting.

Causes of raised intra-cranial pressure are:

- head injury/trauma (most common)
- infection (meningitis/encephalitis)
- intracranial haemorrhages
- cerebral oedema – of which there are three 'main causes'
  - vasogenic – due to increased capillary permeability
  - cytotoxic – from hypoxia, necrosis
  - interstitial, eg from obstructive hydrocephalus.

After 18 months of age intra-cranial pressure has the potential to rise significantly, as the skull sutures are mostly closed. As this occurs, the raised intra-cranial pressure will 'squash' brain tissue against bone and this results in two syndromes:

- Central syndrome – The whole brain is forced towards the foramen magnum through which the cerebellar tonsils herniate (coning).
- Uncal syndrome – Volume increase occurs mainly supratentorially and the uncus herniates through the tentorial opening. This may lead to an ipsilateral dilated pupil due to IIIrd nerve compression.

neurology

Signs of raised intra-cranial pressure are:

- abnormal oculocephalic reflexes – doll's eyes movements
- dilated pupils (ipsilateral then bilateral)
- altered conscious level progressing to coma
- abnormal ventilation – rapid/slow/Cheyne–Stokes/apnoea
- posturing – decorticate progressing to decerebrate
- papilloedema
- absence of venous pulsation in retinal vessels
- Cushing's triad – often pre-terminal (bradycardia, high blood pressure, abnormal ventilation).

Treatment is complex and involves:

- adequate analgesia
- effective nursing
- raising head end of trolley
- hyperventilation
- mannitol
- neurosurgical referral.

295. Carpal tunnel syndrome

Answers: A C D

This results from compression of the median nerve in the carpal tunnel of the wrist. The syndrome progresses slowly resulting in:

- Pain, tingling and numbness in the lateral 3½ fingers (the thenar eminence is spared as the branch supplying the skin over this area leaves the median nerve before the carpal tunnel).
- Weakness and wasting of muscles supplied by the median nerve (lateral two lumbricals, abductor pollicis, flexor pollicis brevis, opponens pollicis).

Symptoms are initially worse at night, and are typically relieved by shaking vigorously or immersing in water. Aetiology includes causes of soft tissue swelling:

- obesity, pregnancy
- rheumatoid arthritis
- hypothyroidism
- gout
- amyloidosis
- acromegaly.

Treatment involves splints, diuretics, topical hydrocortisone injection and surgical decompression.

296. Gilles de la Tourette syndrome

Answers: A C D E

This is a severe disorder in which multiple groups of muscles are affected by tics – spasmodic, repetitive, stereotyped movements. The condition is life-long, and may start from as early as 2–3 years of age. Typical tics include:

- facial grimacing
- blinking
- violent, sudden movements
- progressing to vocalisations:
  - throat clearing
  - coughing
  - sniffing
  - forced utterances
  - swearing.

Associated learning difficulties and compulsive disorders are common. Symptoms are not present during sleep. The condition responds well to dopamine antagonists such as haloperidol and therefore can be induced in normal patients by dopamine receptor agonists. Other drugs causing similar tics include amphetamines, methylphenidate and carbamazepine.

297. Nystagmus

Answers: A D

Nystagmus is involuntary oscillation of the eyes, usually during attempted fixation. It must be sustained for a few seconds to be significant. The direction of the fast or rapid phase describes the direction of the nystagmus. The fast phase in fact is an attempt by the eyes to correct the drift from fixation that has occurred, and it is the slow phase which is pathological. Nystagmus fall into three categories:

Jerk nystagmus – distinct fast and slow phases, more obvious on gaze towards the rapid phase. Aetiology includes:

- Vestibular lesions – VIIIth nerve, inner ear, vestibular pathway. Horizontal or rotatory. Fast phase away from the side of the lesion. Usually transient.
- Central lesions – brain stem, cerebellum. Horizontal, rotatory or vertical. Fast phase towards the side of the lesion. Usually last weeks or longer.
- Positional nystagmus – benign positional vertigo. Occurs in one direction only. Induced by rapid head movements but delayed. Fatigues after short time.

neurology

NB: vertical nystagmus originates only from central lesions.

Pendular nystagmus – No fast and slow phases. Aetiology includes:

- Congenital lesions – X-linked or autosomal dominant
- Secondary to poor visual fixation, such as severe visual impairment/blindness, albinism, cataracts, optic atrophy.

Ataxic nystagmus – as in internuclear ophthalmoplegia. A gaze palsy exists – on looking to one side there is nystagmus in the abducting (contralateral to lesion) eye, but no movement in the 'adducting' (ipsilateral to lesion) eye. It is usually due to damage to the medial longitudinal fasciculus (multiple sclerosis).

Other causes of nystagmus include drugs – alcohol, barbiturates, phenytoin.

298. Head injuries

Answers: A C D

Head injuries are the commonest cause of death in children, usually as a result of a road traffic accident. Damage to the brain in head injuries occurs as result of:

- primary damage from the injury itself
- secondary damage from the cerebral injury or as result of associated physiological changes.

After 18 months of age, when a child's skull sutures have closed, there exists very limited space in which the brain can expand. Hence any space-occupying lesion, such as blood, has the potential to cause the intra-cranial pressure to increase significantly following the failure of early compensatory mechanisms. These include decreased cerebrospinal fluid (CSF) and venous blood volume within the cranium. Before the sutures have closed there is considerable 'give' to allow intra-cranial pressure to remain relatively normal. Following initial resuscitation and cervical spine immobilisation, various neurological parameters should be assessed such as conscious level, pupils, fundi and peripheral nervous system examination. For children of 4 years and over the traditional Glasgow Coma Scale is used, but for those younger than 4 years the modified Children's Coma Scale is essential for accurate scoring. You should be roughly familiar with both of these. A score of 8 or less should prompt intubation and ventilation. Appropriate radiological investigations include skull X-rays, cervical spine X-rays and a computed tomography (CT)/magnetic resonance imaging (MRI) scan if indicated. Referral to a neuro-surgical centre may be necessary. Adequate pain control should be administered particularly as there are often other injuries. Poor pain control can lead to a further increase in intra-cranial pressure which will result in a drop in the cerebral perfusion pressure. Intravenous morphine may be appropriate.

neurology

299. Guillain-Barré syndrome

Answers: A B C

The pathology of Guillain-Barré syndrome is inflammation with segmental demyelination in peripheral nerves. It is commonly preceded by an upper respiratory tract infection (10–14 days) and can follow gastroenteritis. The implicated infectious agents are:

- Epstein–Barr virus
- Coxsackie virus
- influenza virus
- ECHO virus
- cytomegalovirus
- *Mycoplasma pneumoniae*
- *Campylobacter.*

The initial symptoms are of numbness and paraesthesia followed by progressive weakness. This generally starts in the lower limbs and 'ascends' over days or weeks. Weakness is usually symmetrical (90%). Power and tone are reduced with absent or reduced reflexes. About 50% have bulbar involvement. Myalgia may occur early in the disease. Autonomic involvement can occur with flushing and hypotension. Bladder dysfunction may occur early in the disease in about 20%. Fifty per cent have cranial nerve involvement. Cerebrospinal fluid protein rises with a normal CSF white cell count and glucose. Close monitoring of the vital capacity is essential. Type II respiratory failure can occur secondary to muscle weakness. Recovery is usually complete and treatment largely supportive. Relapses can occur in up to 5% of children. Plasmapheresis, intravenous immunoglobulin, steroids and immunosuppressive drugs are used in patients with rapidly progressive ascending paralysis.

300. Spinal muscular atrophy (SMA)

Answers: A B

There are three types of anterior horn cell disease:

- acute infantile spinal muscular atrophy, SMA type I, Werdnig–Hoffmann disease.
- intermediate spinal muscular atrophy (late infantile), SMA type II, chronic Werdnig–Hoffmann disease.
- juvenile spinal muscular atrophy – which is Kugelberg–Welander disease.

All three are usually inherited in an autosomal recessive manner. The gene locus for all three types is on chromosome 5 and they are all variants of the same disease. The age of presentation varies with each disorder. SMA type I presents

neurology

between 0 and 6 months, SMA type II between 3 and 15 years and Kugelberg–Welander between 5 and 15 years. Survival of children with SMA type I is rare beyond 3 years. Clinical features are:

- hypotonia
- weakness
- absent reflexes
- fasciculation of the relaxed tongue
- normal intelligence.

Diagnosis is by:

- DNA studies
- creatine phosphokinase raised but can be normal
- Electromyography (EMG) – fibrillation potentials
- Muscle biopsy – characteristic

Differential diagnosis of Kugelberg–Welander disease includes:

- Duchenne's muscular dystrophy
- fascioscapulohumeral muscular dystrophy
- limb girdle dystrophy
- inflammatory myopathies.

301. Epilepsy

Answers: A C

Simple and complex differentiates between seizures in which consciousness is retained (simple) and those in which consciousness is impaired or lost (complex).

Partial seizures begin focally. They can become generalised (secondary generalisation). Symptomatic epilepsy is when the cause is known. Cryptogenic is when there is a likely but unidentified cause and idiopathic is when no cause is known. Most childhood epilepsy is idiopathic. An aura is not necessary for the diagnosis of childhood epilepsy.

302. Tuberous sclerosis

Answers: A B C D

This shows an autosomal dominant inheritance with a 50% recurrence risk in offspring; 70% are new mutations. The prevalence in children is 1 in 10 000–15 000. The gene is on chromosomes 9 and 11. Seizures are common, often presenting as infantile spasms. All seizure types except petit mal have been described in tuberous sclerosis. Tuberous sclerosis is a cause of symptomatic epilepsy. The age of seizure onset and the severity of mental handicap are directly

neurology

related, with most children in whom seizures develop under the age of 2 years suffering mental handicap. Seizures respond well to anti-convulsants but rarely with complete seizure control. Vigabatrin is indicated particularly in seizures associated with hypsarrhythmia on the EEG. Prevalence of mental handicap is 30–50%. Clinical features include:

- skin
  - hypopigmented macules
  - adenoma sebaceum present in 85% over the age of 5 years
  - periungual fibromas
  - shagreen patches
  - café-au-lait spots
- teeth – enamel hypoplasia
- eyes – choroidal hamartomas
- central nervous system – cerebral astrocytoma, malignant glioma, hydrocephalus
- kidney – renal angiomas and polycystic kidneys
- cardiac – rhabdomyomas
- gastrointestinal – rectal polyp.

Investigations required are:

- Echocardiography
- skull X-ray
- EEG
- CT
- MRI.

Early death may occur due to seizures or tumours affecting the central nervous system, heart or kidney.

Causes of calcification on skull X-ray:

- arteriovenous malformation
- tuberous sclerosis
- Sturge–Weber syndrome
- toxoplasmosis
- cytomegalovirus infection
- glioma
- astrocytoma
- craniopharyngioma.

303. Cerebral palsy

Answers: A B C

Cerebral palsy is the commonest cause of severe neurological disability in childhood. It is a disorder of posture and movement that results from a static injury to the developing brain. Although the injury is static the manifestations will change as the child develops and diagnosis is not always clear until late infancy. About 20% have mental retardation. Prevalence is 2–4 per 1000 live births. Male to female ratio is 1.5:1. It is idiopathic in 75% of cases. Known aetiologies are divided into pre-, peri- or post-natal onset. These include hypoxia, infection, trauma, genetic and cerebral malformation. There is a strong association with low birth weight (51 per 1000 live births under 1500 g will have cerebral palsy), but these only account for a small amount of the total number of children with cerebral palsy. Perinatal asphyxia accounts for no more than 8%.

There are several different classifications of cerebral palsy. The Swedish classification is generally used:

- diplegic
- quadriplegic
- hemiplegic
- dyskinetic (athetoid)
- ataxic.

304. Petit mal epilepsy

Answers: D E

This accounts for 5% of childhood epilepsy. The peak age is 3–12 years. It is commoner in females. It shows an abnormal ictal EEG with three per second spike and generalised wave discharges. The inter-ictal EEG is normal. Hyperventilation will provoke seizures. There is no known aetiology. Clinically, it is characterised by sudden cessation of speech and motor activity with a blank facial expression and flickering of the eyelids. There is no aura or post-ictal state. Tone is not lost but the head may fall forwards. The drugs of choice are sodium valproate and ethosuximide. The long-term prognosis is good with most patients becoming seizure free by adolescence although a number do develop generalised seizures.

305. Cerebral palsy

Answers: D E

Prenatal causes are:

- genetic forms – autosomal recessive and autosomal dominant
- cerebral malformation
- alcohol
- substance abuse
- infection (TORCH)
- intra-uterine growth retardation.

Peri-natal causes are:

- hypoxic ischaemic encephalopathy
- ventricular haemorrhage (pre-term babies)
- postnatal causes
- meningitis
- encephalitis
- head injury.

Pre-term delivery is a risk factor for, but not a cause of, cerebral palsy.

306. Infantile spasms

Answers: A C D E

These represent 1–5% of childhood epilepsy. The incidence is 1–3 per 10 000 live births. It is commoner in boys. Onset is usually between 4 and 9 months. The spasms are brief and transient but often occur in clusters. A spasm is due to a sudden muscular contraction which is usually generalised and a mixture of flexion and extension. Clusters of as many as 100 spasms can occur. The EEG is characteristic and shows hypsarrhythmia (high voltage with multifocal spikes, spike and wave discharges, chaotic slowing and asynchrony). This is an inter-ictal appearance and may be suppressed during seizure activity. The EEG can be normal, and it is not of prognostic value in individual children. Aetiology of infantile spasms may be:

- symptomatic – 70–80%
  - hypoxic-ischaemic encephalopathy
  - dysgenesis, eg tuberous sclerosis, Sturge–Weber syndrome
  - infection pre-, peri- or post-natal
  - haemorrhage intraventricular haemorrhage
  - metabolic, eg neonatal hypoglycaemia
- idiopathic – 20–30%.

Traditional treatment is with high-dose prednisolone or adrenocorticotropic hormone (ACTH) to which 70% have a good response. More recently vigabatrin has been used at doses of up to 200 mg/kg/day with good effect and a better safety profile. In many centres vigabatrin has now become the drug of first choice. Its effect is particularly good in seizures secondary to tuberous sclerosis. Other drugs often used are:

- nitrazepam
- sodium valproate
- lamotrigine.

The prognosis is worse in the symptomatic group. Early recognition and early treatment of seizures is of benefit.

- 70% have severe developmental delay.
- 50–60% develop chronic epilepsy which will be part of a chronic epilepsy syndrome.
- 25–30% go on to develop the Lennox–Gastaut syndrome.

307. Hypotonia

Answers: B D E

Hypotonia in the infant can be as a result of neurological abnormality or systemic disease, and the differential diagnosis is wide. Infants implies less than 12 months and the age of presentation needs to be considered when the correct answers are selected. Becker's muscular dystrophy presents in late childhood (6–16 years) as does subacute sclerosing panencephalitis. The latter is more likely to manifest with hypertonia. Neurological causes of hypotonia are:

- cerebral
  - encephalopathy, eg birth asphyxia presenting as hypotonic cerebral palsy
  - Abnormal brain structure – trisomy 21, Prader–Willi syndrome, hydrocephalus, agenesis of corpus callosum
  - degenerative disease, eg metachromatic leukodystrophy
  - neurometabolic disease, eg Zellweger's syndrome
- spinal cord
  - transection, eg following complicated breech delivery
  - spina bifida
- anterior horn cell disease
  - spinal muscular atrophy (Werdnig–Hoffmann's disease)
  - type ii glycogen storage disease
  - poliomyelitis
- peripheral nerve disease
  - Guillain-Barré syndrome
- disease of the myoneural junction
  - myasthenia gravis
- diseases of the muscle
  - congenital muscular dystrophy
  - congenital myotonic dystrophy.

Systemic causes of hypotonia – most acute and chronic childhood illnesses will cause hypotonia; particular examples include:

- hypercalcaemia
- renal tubular acidosis
- rickets
- hypothyroidism
- coeliac disease

neurology

- cystic fibrosis
- failure to thrive.

308. Cerebral lesions

Answers: A D E

Features of a frontal lobe lesion are:

- disinhibition
- presence of the grasp reflex
- impaired memory
- abnormal micturition behaviour.

The pre-frontal lobe is concerned with aspects of psychological reactions, the ability to make intelligent anticipation of the future and the emotional consequence of thought. Features of a pre-central gyrus lesion are:

- pyramidal tract lesion (upper motor neurone lesion)
- contralateral hemiparesis
- features of a parietal lobe lesion
- spatial disorientation
- apraxia (loss of the ability to perform a pattern of movements although the purpose is known)
- agnosia (loss of the ability to recognise a previously familiar object)
- sensory inattention
- receptive dysphasia
- contralateral homonymous hemianopia (lower quadrant or both).

Features of an occipital lobe lesion are:

- flashing lights
- contralateral homonymous hemianopia
- features of a temporal lobe lesion
- visual sensations
- auditory/gustatory/olfactory hallucinations
- receptive dysphasia
- contralateral homonymous hemianopia (upper quadrant).

309. Benign rolandic epilepsy

Answers: C D

This is commoner in boys with a peak incidence at age 2–14 years. It represents 15–20% of childhood epilepsy. It is often called benign partial epilepsy with centro-temporal spikes. The fits are often preceded by an aura. The seizures themselves are short lived (1–2 minutes) and include paraesthesia and unilateral

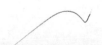

tonic-clonic convulsions involving the face, lips, tongue, pharyngeal and laryngeal muscles. Consciousness is usually preserved and seizures usually occur on wakening. Generalised (nocturnal) seizures often occur especially in children under the age of five years. There are a proportion of children with this syndrome who only have nocturnal seizures. Inter-ictal EEGs often show centro-temporal spikes. Carbamazepine is the drug of choice and fits are well controlled on it. In some children treatment is not required. Seizures generally disappear around puberty.

310. Cranial nerves

Answers: A B D

Features of a IIIrd (oculomotor) nerve lesion are:

- complete ptosis
- diplopia
- downward and lateral gaze (unopposed lateral rectus and superior oblique muscles)
- pupil dilatation
- failure of the pupil to react to light or to accommodation.

Features of a IVth (trochlear) nerve lesion are:

- diplopia
- failure of infero-lateral gaze (failure of the superior oblique muscle).

Features of a VIth (abducent) nerve lesion:

- diplopia
- failure of lateral gaze
- features of Horner's syndrome
- partial ptosis
- pupil constriction
- anhydrosis
- entophthalmia
- heterochromia iridis
- normal direct and consensual reflex.

Causes of ptosis:

- congenital
- Horner's syndrome
- oculomotor nerve palsy
- myasthenia gravis.

311. Ataxia

Answers: A E

Clinical features of ataxia are:

- inco-ordination of voluntary movement
- abnormal speech – dysarthria
- ocular inco-ordination – nystagmus
- hypotonia
- intention tremor.

Aetiology of congenital ataxia includes:

- cerebellar malformation
- dysgenesis of the cerebellar vermis, eg Joubert's syndrome
- cystic malformation of the posterior fossa, eg Dandy–Walker syndrome
- peri-natally acquired, eg hypoxic ischaemic encephalopathy.

Aetiology of acquired ataxia includes:

- acute
  - infectious and post-infectious, eg mycoplasma, chickenpox, measles
  - structural lesions, eg tumours, hydrocephalus
  - toxic, eg lead, phenytoin
  - metabolic disorders
  - vascular – basilar artery thrombosis
- intermittent
  - migraine
  - epilepsy
  - inherited recurrent ataxia (eg Hartnup disease)
- progressive
  - structural, eg tumours
  - DNA repair abnormalities, eg ataxia telangiectasia, xeroderma pigmentosa
  - metabolic, eg Wilson's disease, leucodystrophies, abetalipoproteinaemia
  - spinocerebellar degeneration, Friedreich's ataxia.

Friedreich's ataxia is a progressive ataxia with pyramidal tract dysfunction. Inheritance is usually autosomal recessive. The gene locus is known and is on chromosome 9. It usually presents before the fifteenth birthday with loss of position and vibration sense. Other features include absent tendon reflexes, extensor plantars, nystagmus, pes cavus, kyphoscoliosis, cardiac abnormalities (hypertrophic cardiomyopathy) and an increased risk of diabetes mellitus. Treatment is largely supportive. Death is usually secondary to cardiac complications.

neurology

Ataxia telangiectasia is an autosomal recessively inherited condition. The gene locus is known and is on chromosome 11. The ataxia usually presents in early childhood with characteristic telangiectasia. A third of these children develop malignancy. There is an increased risk of recurrent infection with a low IgA and IgG. The α-fetoprotein is usually raised. There is a 50–100-fold greater chance of developing lymphoreticular malignancy as well as brain tumours.

312. Patterns of inheritance

Answers: A E

This is an important question. Patterns of inheritance are often asked in Multiple Choice Questions and should be learnt. The inheritance of the conditions listed are as follows:

- tuberous sclerosis – autosomal dominant
- ataxia telangiectasia – autosomal recessive
- colour blindness – X-linked recessive
- haemophilia A – X-linked recessive
- myotonic dystrophy – autosomal dominant.

Genetic anticipation

Genetic anticipation refers to the situation by which successive generations are more severely affected by a particular disease process and at a younger age. Examples of this include:

- fragile X syndrome
- myotonic dystrophy
- Huntingdon's chorea.

313. Duchenne's muscular dystrophy

Answers: B E

The incidence of Duchenne's muscular dystrophy is 1 in 3000 live born males. The inheritance is X-linked recessive. The gene locus known and is at Xp21. A third of cases represent a new mutation. Females may be symptomatic as a consequence of the random inactivation of one of the X chromosomes. Cases usually present between the ages of 3 and 5 years with weakness and calf muscle hypertrophy. The reflexes disappear early in the disease apart from the ankle jerk which disappears late. Creatinine phosphokinase is usually raised at birth and high at diagnosis. Diagnosis is made by electromyography and muscle biopsy both of which show typical features. In addition, DNA studies can be done looking for the dystrophin gene. Complications arise from cardiac, respiratory and skeletal muscle involvement.

neurology

Becker's muscular dystrophy

This presents later than Duchenne's muscular dystrophy, but the gene defect is known and is at the same locus as Duchenne's muscular dystrophy. Cardiac and respiratory muscle involvement is rare. The creatinine phosphokinase is high at diagnosis. EMG and muscle biopsy are helpful in establishing a diagnosis.

McLeod's syndrome

This a benign non-progressive late onset myopathy in which the creatinine phosphokinase is usually mildly raised. It is X-linked. Symptoms are usually mild. Splenomegaly is often seen.

314. Febrile convulsions

Answers: C E

Febrile convulsions occur in 3–4% of children. The age range is variably quoted but usually between 6 months and 5 years. Simple (75%) febrile convulsions last less than 15 minutes and are associated with a good prognosis. Complicated (25%) are either focal in origin or prolonged. These have a worse prognosis. Risk factors for recurrent febrile seizures include previous febrile seizures and a positive family history of febrile seizures. The risk factor for siblings of an index case is 10% and the risk if either parent had febrile convulsions is 15%. There is no sex difference. There is no increased risk if there is a family history of epilepsy. A third of children who have a first fit will have a second and a third of these will have a third. Risk factors for the development of epilepsy are:

- positive family history of epilepsy
- prolonged or atypical seizure
- pre-existing neurological problem
- abnormal neurological examination.

Prophylactic anti-convulsants are not helpful in children with recurrent simple febrile seizures. The use of oral diazepam at the time of fever is controversial. An inter-ictal EEG is usually normal and the investigation is unhelpful, except in children presenting with atypical febrile seizures.

315. Complex partial seizures

Answers: A D

Complex partial seizures originate as focal (partial) seizures usually in the fronto-temporal region. They can become generalised and consciousness is impaired.

The symptomatology is complex. Possibilities include:

- transient blankness, staring or confusion

- abrupt alteration of mental state in the form of time relationships and memory
- déjà vu
- semi-purposeful automatisms, eg lip smacking, chewing, swallowing.

The EEG changes are characteristic with focal discharges from the fronto-temporal region. The drugs of choice are carbamazepine, vigabatrin and sodium valproate. There is often a past history of febrile convulsions. Surgery may be helpful in a number of children with resistant seizures.

316. Myoclonus

Answers: A B D

Myoclonus is a simple jerk-like movement that is not co-ordinated or suppressible. The jerks are usually flexor and occur at an extremity. If the legs are involved a child may be thrown to the ground. In childhood epilepsy myoclonic jerks can either present as the main seizure type (benign myoclonic epilepsy of infancy) or be one of several seizure types seen in an epilepsy syndrome.

West's syndrome

- infantile spasms
- mental handicap
- hypsarrhythmia on the EEG.

Lennox–Gastaut syndrome

- extension of West's syndrome occurring between the ages of 1 and 5 years
- atypical absences, myoclonic, tonic and atonic seizures
- EEG shows slow spike and wave discharges
- 90% show moderate to severe mental handicap.

Landau–Kleffner syndrome

This is rare and is characterised by the near complete or complete loss of previously acquired language before the onset of seizures which develop in 70–80%. The EEG is usually abnormal and the outlook poor. Myoclonic jerks are not usually seen.

Janz syndrome

This is juvenile myoclonic epilepsy and is characterised by myoclonic episodes with preserved consciousness. The episodes often occur on wakening or following sleep deprivation. EEG abnormalities are usually seen and the response to sodium valproate is good. Prolonged treatment is required.

neurology

317. Peripheral nerve injuries

Answers: C E

Peripheral nerve injuries need to be revised as they are often the subject of questions. The small muscles of the hand are supplied by the median and ulnar nerves. The radial nerve (C5 to C8) supplies two muscle groups:

- those that supinate the forearm
- the extensors of the fingers, wrist and elbow.

The radial nerve also supplies sensation to the back of the hand. Injuries to the radial nerve occur either at the axilla or the elbow. Injury at the axilla will result in an inability to extend the elbow and wrist drop. Involvement at the elbow will result only in wrist drop. Klumpke's paralysis results from an injury to the lower part of the brachial plexus (C8–T1). Clinically this manifests as a claw hand with failure of forearm flexion.

318. Primitive reflexes

Answers: B C

The Moro reflex

This is initiated by sudden movement of the neck and consists of a rapid abduction and extension of the arms with opening of the hands. Eliciting it helps to assess muscle tone. It usually disappears by 3 months. A decrease in it on one side may be an early sign of a hemiparesis.

The startle reflex

This is similar to the Moro reflex, but is elicited by a loud noise. There is no opening of the hands.

The grasp reflex

Stimulation of the palm causes it to close. This reflex usually disappears by 3 months.

The asymmetric tonic neck reflex

When a baby lies with its head to one side, the arm and leg are extended to the same side, and the arm and leg on the contralateral side are flexed. This appears by 2–3 weeks and disappears by 3 months. Its persistence is suggestive of cerebral palsy.

The parachute reflex

This appears between 6 and 9 months and persists. It is elicited by holding the infant in ventral suspension and suddenly lowering them. The arms extend as a defence reaction. Asymmetry may be a sign of hemiparesis.

The Babinski (extensor plantar) response is normal up until about 1 year of age.

319. Hydrocephalus

Answers: B C D

Macrocephaly is defined as a head circumference larger then two standard deviations from the normal age corrected mean. Normal/familial large head is the commonest cause of macrocephaly. Other causes are hydrocephalus, megalencephaly (large brain) and a thickened skull. Hydrocephalus occurs due to an excess volume of cerebrospinal fluid in the skull vault. This can result from either increased production or impaired reabsorption and circulation. CSF is formed in the choroid plexus principally within the lateral ventricle. It flows from the lateral ventricles through the foramen of Munro into the third ventricle and from there via the aqueduct of Sylvius into the fourth ventricle. It exits the fourth ventricle via the foramina of Luschka and Magendie for reabsorption principally through the arachnoid villi. Hydrocephalus can be either communicating or non-communicating. Non-communicating occurs as a consequence of obstruction at some point in the ventricular system. Megalencephaly is enlargement of the brain substance. Hydrencephaly refers to the replacement of the brain substance by CSF.

Causes of communicating hydrocephalus are:

- meningitis
- post-haemorrhagic
- choroid plexus papilloma
- meningeal malignancy.

Causes of non-communicating hydrocephalus are:

- aqueduct stenosis
- Arnold–Chiari malformation
- Dandy–Walker syndrome
- Klippel–Feil syndrome
- mass lesion
- Warburg's syndrome.

Causes of megalencephaly are:

- genetic
- Sotos' syndrome
- achondroplasia
- incontinentia pigmenti

neurology

- neurofibromatosis
- tuberous sclerosis
- Alexander disease
- Canavan disease
- galactosaemia
- mucopolysaccharidosis.

Causes of macrocephaly due to a thickened skull are:

- anaemia
- rickets
- renal dwarfism
- hyperphosphataemia
- osteogenesis imperfecta.

320. Microcephaly

Answers: A B C D

Microcephaly refers to a small head due to a small brain, the head circumference being less than two standard deviations below the mean when corrected for age and sex. There are other causes of a small head including craniosynostoses (premature suture fusion). Microcephaly can be primary or secondary. Primary microcephaly refers to the situation whereby there is a genetic or chromosomal abnormality that causes the brain to be small. Secondary microcephaly refers to the situation whereby the brain was initially normal but because of a disease process subsequent growth has been impaired.

Causes of primary microcephaly are:

- familial – autosomal dominant or autosomal recessive
- chromosomal/syndromes
  - trisomy 13,18 and 21
  - cri-du-chat syndrome
  - Cornelia de Lange syndrome
- holoprosencephaly.

Causes of secondary microcephaly are:

- intrauterine infection
- drugs
- placental insufficiency/alcohol/drugs
- hypoxic ischaemic encephalopathy
- meningitis/encephalitis.

321. Brain tumours

Answers: A B

Primary brain tumours are the second commonest malignancy in childhood after leukaemia. Metastatic tumours are rare in childhood. Between the ages of 2 and 12 years infratentorial (posterior fossa) tumours are the commonest. Under the age of 2 years and in adolescence supra- and infra-tentorial tumours occur with the same frequency. Tumours within the posterior fossa produce symptoms and signs of raised intracranial pressure. Supra-tentorial tumours produce focal signs dependent on the tumour site. Personality changes can occur as a consequence of either. Infra-tentorial (posterior fossa) tumours include:

- medulloblastoma – commonest brain tumour in children under the age of 7 years
- brain stem glioma
- ependymoma
- astrocytoma.

Supra-tentorial tumours include:

- craniopharyngioma – common, present with bitemporal visual field defect, treatment is surgical and radiotherapy, residual hypothalamopituitary problems are common
- optic glioma
- pineal tumour
- oligodendroglioma.

322. Neurofibromatosis

Answer C

Eight types of neurofibromatosis have been described at the time of writing. Types 1 and 2 are the commonest.

Type 1:
- 1 in 4000
- 90% of all cases of neurofibromatosis
- autosomal dominant inheritance
- 50% new mutations
- gene locus on chromosome 17.

Diagnosis of type 1 – if two of the following features are present:

- axillary or inguinal freckling
- optic gliomas (15%)
- distinctive osseous lesion, eg kyphoscoliosis, tibial bowing
- two or more neurofibromas or one plexiform neurofibroma

neurology

- two or more Lisch (iris) nodules (90%, do not occur in type 2)
- pre-pubertal child – five or more café-au-lait spots greater than 5 mm diameter
- post-pubertal child – six or more café-au-lait spots greater than 15 mm diameter
- a first-degree relative with neurofibromatosis.

Café-au-lait spots are usually present at birth. Less than 10% of patients are mentally retarded. There are many other clinical manifestations and these should be reviewed. Maternal folate deficiency is a risk factor for spina bifida. There is an increased incidence of the following in type 1 neurofibromatosis:

- phaeochromocytoma
- rhabdomyosarcoma
- leukaemia
- Will's tumour
- seizures
- neurofibrosarcoma
- Schwannoma.

Conditions associated with café-au-lait spots include:

- neurofibromatosis
- tuberous sclerosis
- ataxia telangiectasia
- Fanconi's anaemia
- McCune–Albright syndrome
- Russell–Silver dwarfism
- Bloom's syndrome
- Gaucher's disease
- Chédiak-Higashi syndrome
- normal variant.

Type 2:

- represents 10% of all cases of neurofibromatosis
- autosomal dominant inheritance
- mostly new mutations
- gene locus on chromosome 22.

Diagnosis of type 2:

- bilateral acoustic neuromas

or

- unilateral acoustic neuroma and first-degree relative with neurofibromatosis type 2 or

- two of the following – neurofibroma, meningioma, glioma, schwannoma, juvenile posterior subcapsular lenticular opacities.

323. Bell's palsy

Answers: A B D E

This is an acute unilateral facial palsy (lower motor neurone lesion). It usually occurs two weeks after a viral infection. Causes include:

- Epstein–Barr virus
- herpes virus
- mumps
- hypertension.

Prognosis is excellent with full recovery in more than 85% and permanent weakness in around 5%. Steroids have not been proved to be helpful although they are often prescribed.

Other causes of facial nerve palsy:

- tumour invasion
- trauma
- birth injury.

Other causes of facial weakness are:

- myotonic dystrophy
- fascioscapulohumeral muscular dystrophy
- myasthenia gravis.

324. Microcephaly

Answer: E

Uncontrolled phenylketonuria in the mother can be neurotoxic ante-natally. There are various mechanisms which include disruption of normal metabolism by phenylalanine metabolites, phenylethylamine and phenylpyruvic acid. There may also be associated congential heart disease and good control (maintaining phenylalanine levels < 10 mg/dl) is of great importance. Chickenpox late in pregnancy can cause disseminated disease in the baby if delivery happens < 1 week after maternal illness, ie before adequate maternal antibody is passed to the fetus. It does not, however, cause microcephaly at this stage. Dandy–Walker is fourth ventricular hydrocephalus and associated with a normal or large head. Neither myotonia nor neurofibromatosis is linked to microcephaly.

325. A first afebrile tonic-clonic seizure

Answers: B D

Blood glucose, full blood count and chemistry are arguably the only essential tests after a first afebrile seizure. Unless the fit is focal or associated with developmental delay or regression a CT is not indicated. EEG is usually carried out after a second fit though management tends to be clinically based even with a normal EEG, with the latter guiding treatment rather than leading it. Blood and CSF culture is needed if infection/meningitis suspected.

326. A: Posterior plagiocephaly

Craniosynostosis is the premature fusion of one or more cranial sutures. Sutures are normally kept open by ongoing brain growth, with skull growth occurring perpendicular to suture lines. Craniosynostosis may be classified as primary (when it is due to an ossification defect – <10% of cases) or secondary (due to failure of brain growth – >90% of cases). If only 1 suture is affected it is termed simple craniosynotosis, while compound or complex craniosynostosis affects multiple sutures. It is seen as part of a variety of syndromes including Crouzon's and Apert's.

In simple primary synostosis, the cosmetic defect is the primary morbidity while in secondary synostosis, the major morbidity is due to the underlying disorder causing failure of brain growth, typically neurodevelopmental delay. Raised intracranial pressure can result if multiple sutures fuse while brain is still increasing in size, but is rare if only 1 or 2 sutures are affected. Scaphocephaly is the commonest form of craniosynostosis and is caused by premature fusion of the sagittal suture (as seen in preterm infants).

Posterior plagiocephaly is most commonly caused by positional moulding but may also be due to synostosis of the lambdoid suture. The former can be differentiated from the latter by the more anterior position of the ear on the side of the flattening and frontal bossing seen ipsilateral to the flattening in the positional form.

Individuals with craniosynostosis should be followed up for developmental assessment, monitoring of growth of head circumference and for signs and symptoms of raised intracranial pressure (ICP). Surgery is indicated in the presence of elevated ICP and for cosmetic purposes in the more severaly affected individual. Best results are obtained in children with syndromic craniosynostosis if surgery is performed early (before 6 months of age). A multidisciplinary approach is required.

327. D: Abnormal posturing

Lumbar puncture has diagnostic (meningitis, encephalitis, demyelination, malignancy, benign intracranial hypertension) and therapeutic (intra-thecal antibiotics and chemotherapy, and CSF drainage) uses. Complications include headache, bleeding, infection, damage to cord/nerves, cardio-respiratory compromise and cerebral/cerebellar herniation. Should not be performed in the presence of the following without further evaluation:

- signs of raised intracranial pressure or herniation
- recent (within 30 min) convulsive seizures
- prolonged (> 30 min) convulsive seizures
- focal or tonic seizures
- focal neurological signs
- Glasgow Coma Scale score < 13 or deteriorating conscious level
- cardiovascular or respiratory compromise
- coagulopathy/thrombocytopenia
- local superficial infection
- strong suspicion of meningococcal infection (ie typical purpuric rash).

Even with normal appearances of the brain on imaging, the presence of signs of herniation means it is not safe to perform a lumbar puncture. Cellular and biochemical changes persist in CSF for 48–72 hours after treatment, although cultures may be rendered negative by administration of appropriate antibiotics within 2 hours (meningococcus), 6 hours (pneumococcus), 8 hours (group B Strep) and 48 hours (coliforms). In cases of suspected meningitis/encephalitis where any of the above contraindications or relative contraindications to lumbar puncture are present, administration of antibiotics or antiviral agents should not be postponed pending further evaluation of the patient.

328. E: Propranolol and sodium valproate can be used as prophylaxis

Migraine may or may not be associated with aura in childhood – indeed in some cases, headache may not even feature. Variant migraine types include hemiplegic migraine (where neurological deficit can persist for hours or even days and may precede the onset of the headache), abdominal migraine and basilar migraine. The child normally looks pale and ill during an attack – which is typically relieved by sleep. Boys more commonly affected than girls until the age of 7 years. Incidence continues to increase throughout adolescence, but more so in girls. It affects 5–10% of school-age children, but can also affect pre-schoolers. Diagnosis usually made through history and detailed physical examination – both general and neurological. Neuroimaging and EEG not required routinely. Treatment involves education regarding potential triggers (eg caffeine, citrus fruits and chocolate), plan for treatment during an acute attack and prophylaxis for frequent episodes. None of the prophylactic medications are fully effective in preventing all attacks – drugs that can be tried include pizotifen, amitriptyline, propranolol and sodium valproate, but all have potential side-effects.

329. A: Myoclonic jerks, generalised tonic-clonic seizures and absence seizures

An idiopathic generalised epilepsy syndrome accounting for up to 10% of all cases of epilepsy. It is characterised by myoclonic jerks, generalised tonic-clonic seizures and sometimes absence seizures. Jerky movements are typically experienced in the morning — perhaps interfering with breakfast or brushing teeth. It is associated with normal intelligence, onset around adolescence and seizures occurring shortly after wakening. About a third of patients with JME have a positive family history of epilepsy. Precipitating factors for seizures include sleep deprivation, psychological stress, alcohol use, photic stimulation and menses. Neuroimaging studies are typically normal. Sleep-deprived EEG is investigation of choice with typical interictal EEG findings of generalised 4–6 Hz spike and slow-wave discharges lasting up to 20 seconds. These changes are not, however, pathognomonic of JME. A normal study is also possible. Monotherapy is usually adequate to control seizures, 80% of patients becoming seizure free with sodium valproate. Lamotrigine and topiramate can also be used. Carbamazepine may increase number of myoclonic jerks and also precipitate absences, but can be useful in combination therapy with other agents in difficult to control cases. Withdrawal of anticonvulsants, even after a prolonged seizure free period, leads to seizure recurrence in >80% of cases. Hence life-long treatment is usually required.

330. B: Screening for sickle cell disease

Peri-natal stroke defined as cerebrovascular event occurring from 28 weeks' gestation to 28 days' post-natal age. Risk factors are the presence of cardiac disorders, infection and coagulation disorders. Recurrence risk of neonatal stroke is much less than that occurring in childhood (3–5%). Risk factors for childhood stroke are as above plus sickle cell disease (up to 400x greater risk of stroke), moya-moya (accounts for 10–20% of arterial infarcts) and arterial dissection (most commonly secondary to trauma). Cardiac disorders account for up to 50% of cases. In more than a third of cases, no cause is found. Ischaemic events (due to thromboembolism or angiopathy) are commoner than haemorrhagic events, which may be secondary to vascular malformations (most commonly arterio-venous malformations), malignancy, trauma, haemophilia or thrombocytopenia. Recurrence risk is up to 1 in 3 but depends on cause — the presence of multiple risk factors indicating a worse long-term outcome.

Evaluation of a child with a stroke should include neuroimaging (CT, MRI and MR angiography) as well as investigations to rule out non-vascular causes (haematological and metabolic studies). Cranial ultrasound is inadequate to identify ischaemic stroke, especially cortical or posterior infarcts. Surgical intervention may be required in some cases , eg embolisation of an arterio-venous malformation. Aspirin at a dose of 5mg/kg/day can be used for cases of non-haemorrhagic stroke, but not in children with sickle cell disease. No adequate trials have been performed into the use of thrombolytic agents in children although case reports do exist. Mortality rates are up to 10%, with more than half of survivors developing some degree of neurological or cognitive deficit. Seizures at presentation are associated with a poor outcome.

331. Hypotonia

1. F – Plasma very long chain fatty acids

This child has features of Zellweger's syndrome (hypotonia, large anterior fontanelle, hepatomegaly and seizures), which is one of the peroxisomal disorders which include adrenoleukodystrophy, Refsum's disease and rhizomelic chondrodysplasia punctata. Functions of peroxisomes include β-oxidation of fatty acids longer than C22 (ie very long chain fatty acids), the abnormal accumulation of which are the disease hallmark. Other features of Zellweger's syndrome include:

- high forehead
- large anterior fontanelle
- hypoplastic supraorbital ridges
- epicanthal folds
- psychomotor retardation
- hypotonia
- seizures
- retinal degeneration
- impaired hearing
- hepatomegaly
- death within first year of life.

2. I – Cri-du-chat syndrome

The presence of a distinctive high-pitched cat-like cry is suggestive of cri-du-chat syndrome. Other features of this syndrome include growth failure, microcephaly, facial abnormalities and learning difficulties. The child may also have associated cardiac anomalies and cleft lip and palate. The syndrome is caused by deletion of chromosome 5p. The distinctive high-pitched cry in infancy is typically lost by age 2 years. It is commoner in females. Swallowing difficulties and poor suck cause failure to thrive in infancy and may require placement of a gastrostomy. Affected individuals have severe cognitive, speech and motor delays. Behavioural problems include hyperactivity, aggression and tantrums with hypersensitivity to sound. Females are fertile and therefore have a 50% risk of passing on the condition to their offspring. Males have small testes but spermatogenesis is thought to be normal. Other medical problems encountered include recurrent upper respiratory tract infections, otitis media and severe constipation. Affected children usually attain developmental and social skills consistent with those of a 5–6-year-old.

3. A – Muscle biopsy for congenital myopathy

Congenital myopathies

Reduced muscle bulk in association with generalised hypotonia and hyporeflexia are the typical characterisitics of congenital myopathies. These are a group of conditions including nemaline rod myopathy and central core disease. Affected individuals suffer generalised weakness, often affecting proximal more than distal muscle groups. Typical characteristics include onset in early life with hypotonia, hyporeflexia, reduced muscle bulk and generalised weakness, often affecting proximal more than distal muscle groups. Dysmorphic features may be present secondary to the weakness. They are often relatively non-progressive and hereditary (may be autosomal dominant, recessive or X-linked). Both sexes equally affected. May be a history of reduced fetal movements or breech presentation. Other features may include poor suck/swallow and respiratory failure. Arthrogryposis may also be a feature. Creatine kinase levels either in reference range or mildly elevated. EMG and nerve conduction studies can also be normal. Therefore muscle biopsy required for diagnosis.

Treatment is supportive in all cases. Prognosis depends on type. Can be fatal in the neonatal period or associated with a normal life span. Cardiopulmonary insufficiency is the usual cause of death. Duchenne's and Becker's muscular dystrophies are characterised by elevated creatine kinase levels but do not present in the neonatal period. Features of congenital hypothyroidism are generally not present at birth but develop within the first few weeks of life.

332. MENINGITIS

1. E *Haemophilus influenzae* type B

The CSF picture is consistent with a bacterial meningitis. In a baby of this age the presence of Gram-negative rods is most likely to represent infection with *Haemophilus influenzae* (see below).

2. C Pneumococcus

The CSF picture is consistent with partially treated bacterial meningitis (see below). Given the presence of the preceding upper respiratory tract infection and that the child has sickle cell disease, the most likely infecting organism is pneumococcus.

3. B *Listeria monocytogenes*

This CSF picture in a neonate is consistent with a bacterial or viral meningitis. However, the presence of Gram-positive rods on Gram staining makes *Listeria* the most likely infective agent. (See also Answer 198.)

Meningitis

Neonates

Commonest infecting organisms are Group B Streptococcus, *Escherichia coli*, *Listeria*, and herpes simplex and varicella zoster viruses. Pre-term babies are at greatest risk. Symptoms are often non-specific and require a high index of suspicion. Interpretation of CSF findings complicated by higher levels of glucose and protein normally seen in neonates. Bacterial meningitis typically causes a white cell count > 1000/mm^3. In cases secondary to *Listeria*, this is typically a lymphocytosis. Viral meningitis causes a less dramatic pleocytosis. Results should be interpreted in conjunction with any results available from the mother. Poor prognostic indicators include low birth weight, significant leucopenia or neutropenia, high CSF protein, coma and seizures lasting more than 72 hours. Appropriate empirical treatments for neonatal bacterial meningitis include combinations of either ampicillin and an aminoglycoside, or ampicillin and a third-generation cephalosporin. Treatment should be reviewed in the light of culture results and response to treatment and continued for 10–21 days.

Infants and children

Seventy per cent of cases of bacterial meningitis occur in those under 2 years of age. Commonest infecting agents are pneumococcus, meningococcus and *Haemophilus influenzae* type b, although since the introduction of the vaccination programme against the latter organism, its incidence has fallen significantly. In 1 in 2 cases of pneumococcal meningitis there is a parameningeal focus or pneumonia is also present. Individuals with sickle cell disease, other haemoglobinopathies or functional or anatomical asplenia are at increased risk. Incidence of penicillin resistance varies from < 10% to 60% worldwide. Meningococcus causes peaks of incidence in the 6–12 month and adolescent age groups. *H. influenzae* type b primarily affects the unimmunised, with 80–90% of cases occurring between the ages of 1 month and 3 years.

CSF should be obtained in all cases of suspected meningitis, unless performing a lumbar puncture is contraindicated. Opening pressure should be recorded. CSF glucose and protein estimation, total and differential cell counts, Gram stain and culture should always be requested. Also consider agglutination tests or polymerase chain reaction (PCR) evaluation. Patients with early or fulminant disease and those with poor immune response may not show 'normal' CSF changes. Partially treated meningitis may cause culture results for pneumococcus and meningococcus in particular to be unreliable, but protein, glucose and cell count abnormalities can persist even after treatment with antibiotics. Lymphocytosis may be seen in partially treated patients.

neurology

Cefotaxime or ceftriaxone provides coverage against the three commonest causes of meningitis – vancomycin should be added in areas where penicillin resistant pneumococcus is prevalent. Duration of treatment varies but is usually continued for a minimum of 7–10 days. Dexamethasone has been shown to be of benefit if given prior to antibiotics in cases of Hib meningitis, but not in any other form of meningitis.

neurology

RESPIRATORY
ANSWERS

333. Oxygen dissociation curve

Answers: B C D

Oxygen is transported in blood in two ways:

- by reversibly combining with the haem portion of haemoglobin in red cells (oxyhaemoglobin)
- a very small amount is dissolved (approximately 3 ml/l arterial blood).

The oxyhaemoglobin dissociation curve is sigmoid in shape, with oxygen saturation of haemoglobin on the y axis and partial pressure of oxygen on the x axis. It demonstrates a progressive increase in the amount of haemoglobin that is bound with oxygen as the Po_2 increases. Above a Po_2 of 7 kPa the curve flattens off. Arterial blood leaving the lungs has a Po_2 of ˜13 kPa, equivalent to an oxygen saturation of Hb of 97%; 100 ml of arterial blood carries approximately 20 ml of oxygen. Venous blood has a Po_2 of ˜5kPa, equivalent to an oxygen saturation of haemoglobin of 70%; 100 ml of venous blood carries approximately 15 ml of oxygen. Therefore each 100 ml of blood liberates approximately 5 ml of oxygen during one cycle to the tissues. During heavy exercise venous blood oxygen saturation can fall to 20% – releasing over 10 ml more oxygen per 100ml blood to active tissues.

The oxyhaemoglobin dissociation curve represents an important oxygen buffer function of haemoglobin. In order for the resting state amount of oxygen to be given up to the tissues (5 ml/100 ml blood), the capillary Po_2 must not exceed 5 kPa. In heavy exercise massive amounts of oxygen are required and this can be achieved with very small drops in capillary Po_2 – because of the steep slope of the curve. Also, at the other extreme when the alveolar Po_2 drops (eg to 8 kPa, which occurs at an altitude of 3218–4828 m), arterial haemoglobin is still ˜89% saturated. This enables the tissues to easily extract their required amount of oxygen from haemoglobin by dropping the Po_2 of venous blood minimally. Even if the alveolar Po_2 rises to levels way in excess of 13 kPa, the amount of oxygen binding to haemoglobin barely rises (as demonstrated by the flat part of the curve). So haemoglobin acts by maintaining tissue Po_2 levels in a narrow range for cellular homoeostasis.

respiratory

As blood passes through the tissues, the physiological oxyhaemoglobin dissociation curve develops. As blood gains carbon dioxide from active tissues, P_{CO_2} rises. This causes haemoglobin to liberate its oxygen more readily – supplying necessary oxygen to active tissues. This causes the curve to shift to the right (Bohr's effect). Factors causing the curve to shift to the right are present when tissue activity is increased and therefore more oxygen is required. These include:

- increased temperature
- increased acidity
- increased concentration of 2,3 DPG (occurs at increased altitude and with tissue hypoxia).

The curve is shifted to the left by:

- changes opposite to the above
- carboxyhaemoglobin (haemoglobin has stronger affinity for carbon monoxide)
- fetal haemoglobin (binds oxygen with strong affinity).

334. Lymphocytic interstitial pneumonitis

Answers: A E

Lymphocytic interstitial pneumonitis is defined as reticulonodular pulmonary infiltrates that persist for 2 months or more, with or without associated lymphadenopathy, that do not respond to antimicrobials in an human immunodeficiency virus (HIV)-infected patient. It is an acquired immune deficiency syndrome (AIDS)-defining diagnosis. It occurs in 15% of children with vertically acquired HIV infection. The aetiology is not known but co-existent infection with Epstein–Barr virus may have a role. The onset is usually insidious but can be acute and rarely presents before the age of 2 years. The disease can be asymptomatic. Early symptoms are of dry cough and exertional dyspnoea. Long-standing disease is accompanied by finger clubbing and chronic bronchiectasis. Acute deterioration of chronic disease occurs with superimposed bacterial or viral infections. In this instance, hypoxia and respiratory decompensation can occur. The chest X-ray appearance is of hilar lymphadenopathy with diffuse bilateral interstitial infiltrates more prominent in the lower lobes. Other causes of interstitial infiltrates include tuberculosis, cytomegalovirus infection and *Pneumocystis* infection. A lung biopsy is occasionally required for the diagnosis. Treatment with azathioprine is not of proved benefit. For severe disease, treatment should be with high-dose oral steroids for 6–12 weeks followed by a maintenance dose with oxygen therapy if required.

335. Theophylline

Answers: C D

Increased clearance	Decreased clearance
Cigarette smoking	Prematurity
Phenytoin	Obesity
Phenobarbital	Cirrhosis
Alcohol	Congestive cardiac failure
Rifampicin	Fever
Carbamazepine	Acute viral illness
	Pneumonia
	Cimetidine
	Erythromycin
	Ciprofloxacin
	Allopurinol
	Verapamil
	Propranolol

[handwritten: PC BRAS] *[handwritten: ODENCES]*

336. *Pneumocystis carinii* pneumonia

Answers: D E

Pneumocystis carinii has attributes of fungi and protozoa. *Pneumocystis carinii* pneumonia occurs in 40% of children with acquired immune deficiency syndrome (AIDS). It is commonest in the first year of life when it is associated with a poor outcome. Overall the mortality from childhood infection is high. Signs and symptoms are often non-specific and diagnosis is often delayed. The chest X-ray may be normal or show a diffuse interstitial infiltrate. Diagnosis is by isolation of the organism from respiratory secretions or lung biopsy. Treatment is with co-trimoxazole and steroids. Prophylaxis is given to HIV–infected infants routinely. Extrapulmonary infection is rare (retina, spleen, bone marrow). Eighty per cent of children with HIV infection develop pulmonary disease. The most important respiratory pathologies are *Pneumocystis carinii* pneumonia, lymphocytic interstitial pneumonitis and tuberculosis. The incidence of normal childhood respiratory illness is also increased. The CD4 count is a good marker of immune dysfunction and the risk of opportunistic infection rises as it falls. *Mycobacterium tuberculosis* infection is common in HIV–infected children. The tuberculin skin test is often negative but the response to therapy good.

respiratory

337. Asthma

Answers: A B C D

Pulsus paradoxus is the difference between systolic blood pressure in inspiration and expiration. Patients with a difference greater than 20 mmHg have severe asthma or cardiac tamponade. Pulse oximetry is a good indicator of the severity of an acute attack of asthma. It is also a good predictor of the duration of the attack if done on admission to hospital with an episode of acute asthma. Features of severe asthma are:

- inability to talk in sentences
- intercostal recession
- peak flow less than 50% expected
- reduced level of consciousness
- oxygen saturation less than 85% in air
- silent chest
- cyanosis.

338. Pulmonary hypoplasia

Answers: A B D E

Pulmonary hypoplasia occurs in 1 in 1000 births. It can be unilateral or bilateral. Causes can be primary (rare) or secondary.

Reduced volume of the affected hemithorax

- Congenital diaphragmatic hernia
- Pleural effusion
- Thoracic dystrophy
- Congenital cyst

Oligohydramnios

- Prolonged rupture of membranes .
- Potter's syndrome
- Renal tract anomalies

Reduced pulmonary vascular perfusion

- Hypoplastic left heart
- Pulmonary artery agenesis
- Tracheo-oesophageal fistula.

Outcome is variable. Babies who are ventilated have a high risk of pulmonary interstitial emphysema. Unilateral hypoplasia usually presents late and can be asymptomatic.

respiratory

Potter's syndrome

This is a sporadic condition and consists of oligohydramnios with consequent pulmonary hypoplasia. In its most severe form the oligohydramnios is due to renal agenesis. The baby has a classic appearance with a squashed face, hypertelorism, prominent epicanthic folds, micrognathia, lowset ears and large floppy hands and feet. All of these babies die although some survive for up to 48 hours.

Other developmental anomalies of the lung

- Congenital lung cysts
- Cystic adenomatoid malformation
- Congenital lobar emphysema
- Lobar sequestration

339. Acute stridor in childhood

Answers: A B E

Causes of acute stridor in childhood are:

- acute laryngotracheobronchitis
- acute epiglottitis
- foreign body
- bacterial tracheitis
- retropharyngeal abscess
- tonsillitis (quinsy)
- angioneurotic oedema
- diphtheria
- thermal, mechanical (eg post extubation) or chemical trauma

Steroids and croup

Recent evidence suggests that it is beneficial to give nebulised steroid (as budesonide) or oral steroid (as dexamethasone) on admission to children with croup (acute laryngotracheobronchitis) and that this both shortens the illness and reduces disease severity. In severe croup intravenous steroids:

- reduce the need for intubation
- reduce the duration of intubation and ventilation if required
- reduce the incidence of subglottic stenosis in ventilated babies.

Adrenaline and croup

Nebulised adrenaline 1 ml of 1 in 1000 solution will provide temporary relief in croup lasting 20–30 minutes. Other therapies, such as steam, although widely used are not of proved benefit.

respiratory

340. Bronchiolitis

Answers: A D E

Respiratory syncytial virus infection is responsible for 50–70% of cases. Other aetiological agents include adenovirus, parainfluenza virus, rhinovirus, mumps, influenza virus and *Mycoplasma pneumoniae*. It is commonest during the first 6 months of life. Peak incidence in the winter months. Risk factors include maternal smoking, poor social circumstances, not being breast fed and male sex. Inappropriate antidiuretic hormone secretion can occur during the acute phase of the illness. Treatment is mainly supportive. Nebulised ipratropium bromide or nebulised salbutamol may be but are not always beneficial. Antibiotics are only indicated for secondary bacterial infection. Steroids are unhelpful. Ribavirin is occasionally of benefit in selected cases including children with pre-existing cardiac or respiratory disease such as bronchopulmonary dysplasia or congenital heart disease. Palivizumab is licensed for the prevention of respiratory syncytial virus infection in a highly selected group of at risk patients. The neutrophil count is usually normal. Chest X-ray shows hyperinflation with scattered areas of atelectasis in 30%. Respiratory syncytial virus can be demonstrated in nasopharyngeal secretions. Complications during the acute phase include:

- difficulty feeding
- apnoea
- bacterial infection
- respiratory failure.

Recurrent wheeze after bronchiolitis occurs in 40–50%. Duration of attack, family history of asthma and cigarette smoking are risk factors.

341. Respiratory failure

Answers: B D E

Type I

Reflects ventilation perfusion mismatch and presents with hypoxia and normo- or hypocapnia. Aetiologies include:

- pulmonary oedema
- pneumonia
- pulmonary embolus
- acute asthma
- adult respiratory distress syndrome

respiratory

Type II

Reflects hypoventilation and presents with hypoxia and hypercapnia. Aetiologies include:

- Head injury/encephalitis/meningitis
- Muscle disease
- Drugs
- Kyphoscoliosis
- Severe asthma
- Respiratory obstruction
- Pneumothorax

Patients with type I respiratory failure can progress to type II when respiratory muscle fatigue occurs or with CNS depression from hypoxia.

342. Laryngomalacia (Congenital Laryngeal Stridor)

Answer: A

In infancy 60–70% of persistent stridor is due to laryngomalacia. This usually presents at birth, but can present at any stage up to 4 weeks. Most children with laryngomalacia thrive and feed normally. The condition usually resolves by 18 months of age. Specific indications for investigation include stridor at rest, late presentation (>4 months) and failure to thrive. In addition any stridor that is persistent, severe and biphasic should be further investigated. Investigations that should be considered include chest X-ray, lateral neck X-ray, barium swallow and direct laryngoscopy. The aetiology is unknown, with histologically normal cartilage.

Differential diagnosis of laryngomalacia:

- Neonatal tetany
- Subglottic stenosis
- Subglottic haemangioma
- Laryngeal nerve palsy
- Laryngeal web
- Vascular ring
- Goitre

respiratory

343. Asthma

Answers: A B D E

Salmeterol is a long-acting β stimulant. It is useful for prominent night cough, exercise-induced symptoms and as an add on treatment in refractory chronic asthma when control is poor despite other therapies. The duration of action following administration is 12 hours. Fluticasone propionate is a corticosteroid which exhibits almost complete first-pass metabolism in the liver and therefore has minimal systemic absorption. It is available in inhaler and dischaler form. Sodium cromoglycate inhaled shortly before exercise can prevent exercise-induced asthma.

344. Bronchoscopy

Answers: A E

Bronchoscopy can be carried out with either a flexible or a rigid endoscope. A rigid endoscope is an open tube and therefore a child can be ventilated through it. It can be left in situ and is therefore appropriate for the removal of foreign bodies, clots and mucous plugs and in massive haemoptysis. A flexible endoscope is solid and requires ventilation to occur around it. There is a suction and biopsy channel – larger objects cannot be removed through it. Bronchoscopy can be either diagnostic or therapeutic.

Indications for bronchoscopy are:

- diagnostic
    - congenital stridor
    - foreign body
    - persistent atelectasis
    - unexplained interstitial disease
    - undiagnosed infection particularly in an immunocompromised host
    - haemoptysis
- therapeutic
    - bronchopulmonary lavage
    - removal of clot, mucous plug, foreign body

Investigation of suspected foreign body

- clinical history of inhalation.
- inspiratory/expiratory films or screening to look for unilateral hyperinflation.
- ventilation perfusion scan
- bronchoscopy
- fluoroscopy.

respiratory

Commonest site of impaction is the right main stem bronchus.

Complications of bronchoscopy include:

- hypoxia
- cardiac arrhythmias
- bronchospasm
- laryngospasm
- infection
- haemorrhage
- pneumothorax.

345. Sweat test

Answers: B C

The sweat test is the most appropriate diagnostic test for cystic fibrosis. Diagnostic values are of a sweat sodium greater than 70 mmol/l or a sweat chloride of greater than 70 mmol/l on a sample weighing more than 100 mg. A number of books quote a sweat chloride of greater than 60 mmol/l as being diagnostic. In normal individuals the sodium is greater than the chloride and the sum of the two is less than 140 mmol/l. In patients with cystic fibrosis the chloride is usually greater than the sodium and the sum greater than 140 mmol/l. In the general population over the age of 16, 10% have a sweat sodium greater than 60 mmol/l. In these patients a fludrocortisone test can be performed in order to confirm the diagnosis. Plasma immunoreactive trypsin (IRT) is useful until the age of 3 months. Pancreatic function tests are sometimes required and typically show normal enzyme values with a low bicarbonate concentration. A number of children with cystic fibrosis get a pseudo-Bartter's syndrome with hyponatraemia and hypokalaemia due to excessive salt losses in the sweat. Causes of a raised sweat sodium are:

- cystic fibrosis
- adrenal insufficiency
- pseudohypoaldosteronism
- hypothyroidism
- nephrogenic diabetes insipidus
- glycogen storage disease type one
- mucopolysaccharides
- glucose 6-phosphate dehydrogenase deficiency
- ectodermal dysplasia
- nephrotic syndrome
- severe malnutrition
- HIV infection
- anorexia nervosa.

respiratory

Causes of a false-negative sweat test are:

- oedema
- hypoproteinaemia.

346. Cleft lip and palate

Answers: A D E

This is a defect of mesodermal development. The lips usually fuse between the fifth and seventh weeks of gestation and the palate between the ninth and twelfth. Antenatal ultrasound is helpful. Cleft lip can be detected by skilled operators by 17 weeks. Cleft palate is more difficult to see. The incidence is 1 in 700 births. Cleft lip 1 in 600, cleft palate 1 in 1000. The recurrence risk if there is an affected sibling is 1 in 25. If one parent is affected the risk is 1 in 20. Cleft lip and palate is an isolated abnormality in 75%. A third of patients have cleft lip only and a quarter have cleft palate only. Associations are commoner in children with cleft palate alone (20–50%) than children with cleft lip only (7–13%) or cleft lip and palate (2–11%). Submucous cleft palate (3% of all clefts) is suggested by a bifid uvula and central translucent zone in the palate. Problems associated with cleft lip and palate are:

- feeding difficulties with poor weight gain
- difficulty with bonding
- respiratory disease
- speech delay
- hypernasal speech
- glue ear with impaired hearing
- dental caries
- problems with secondary dentition
- cosmetic appearance

micrognathia occurs as part of the pierre robin syndrome.

Aetiology of cleft lip and palate

- idiopathic
- polygenic
- maternal drugs, eg steroids, phenytoin
- environmental
- chromosomal, eg Patau's syndrome
- Pierre Robin syndrome.

It is current practice to do early lip closure between 0 and 3 months and often in the neonatal period. The palate is closed subsequently between 6 and 12 months. Grommets are usually required. The advice of a speech therapist is essential early on to help with feeding and later with the development of speech.

Pierre Robin syndrome

This occurs in 1 in 30 000 live births. Features are:

- micrognathia due to mandibular dysplasia
- midline cleft palate or high arched palate
- glossoptosis (causing pseudomacroglossia).

The most serious and potentially life-threatening problem in children with Pierre Robin syndrome is apnoea due to upper airway obstruction.

The mandibular profile improves with age.

347. Epiglottitis and croup

Answers: A D E

Factors that suggest epiglottitis rather than croup

- short history
- high pyrexia with toxaemia
- absence of cough
- drooling
- neck extension.

Factors that suggest croup rather then epiglottitis include:

- several days' history
- low-grade pyrexia without toxaemia
- barking cough
- absence of drooling.

Acute epiglottitis

This life-threatening condition is caused by *Haemophilus influenzae* type b. Peak age is 6 months to 6 years. Hib immunisation has dramatically reduced the incidence. Treatment involves protection of the airway combined with high-dose antibiotic therapy.

Croup

Croup (acute laryngotracheobronchitis) is caused by a number of viruses including para-influenza, influenza, respiratory syncytial virus and rhinovirus. The peak age is 6 months to 4 years. A number of patients have recurrent attacks.

respiratory

Bacterial tracheitis

Bacterial tracheitis (pseudomembraneous croup) runs a more prolonged course. It usually occurs in children under 3 years of age. The presenting features are of a barking cough associated with severe toxaemia and the absence of drooling. Causative organisms include *Staphylococcus aureus* and *Streptococcus pneumoniae*. High-dose antibiotics are required and up to 80% of patients need intubation and ventilation.

348. Management of asthma

Answers: A B

It is essential to have a good knowledge of asthma management for the exam and to be clear about what devices should be used in children of different ages. The aim of asthma management is to reduce the number of acute attacks and to prevent chronic symptoms. This is achieved by general measures (patients education, allergen avoidance and exercise prophylaxis) and drug therapy. Drug therapy is preventative and to control acute symptoms. Acute attacks are principally treated with inhaled or nebulised bronchodilators and oral steroids. Other therapies used in severe attacks include ipratropium bromide, intravenous aminophylline and intravenous salbutamol. Prophylactic agents include sodium cromoglycate, leukotriene receptor antagonists and inhaled steroids. It is principally the latter which are used in children. The device used to administer the drug is important. There are many different devices and it is appropriate for the candidate to be familiar with them all. In general a spacer device with a face mask or a nebuliser is used under the age of two and a spacer device without a face mask in older children. The oral route is not recommended. Dry powder devices like the turbo haler and accuhaler along with older devices such as the dischaler, autohaler and Rotahaler are best used in the over fives. It is essential to ensure that a child is able to use a particular type of device before prescribing it. The reader must be familiar with the most recent asthma guidelines (see answer to Question 365).

349. Primary ciliary dyskinesia

Answers: A B C E

This is an autosomal recessive group of disorders, the commonest being Kartagener's syndrome. The incidence of primary ciliary dyskinesia is 1 in 16 000 live births. Clinical features are:

- chronic bronchiectasis
- nasal polyposis
- recurrent sinusitis
- recurrent otitis media
- infertility, subfertility.

Diagnosis is by:

- saccharin test which assesses mucociliary clearance.
- light or phase contrast microscopy of scraping from the nasal mucosa.
- electron microscopic examination of cilia obtained from the nasal turbinates or tracheobronchial tree.

Treatment is with:

- normal saline nebulisers
- bronchodilators
- mucolytics such as acetylcysteine
- physiotherapy
- regular antibiotics
- immunisation
- avoidance of cigarette smoke.

Complications include:

- pneumothorax
- haemoptysis
- failure to thrive
- male infertility
- respiratory failure.

A normal lifespan is possible if appropriately treated. Symptoms tend to improve after adolescence. The classic Kartagener's syndrome is present in 50% of children with primary ciliary dyskinesia. Features of Kartagener's syndrome include:

- chronic sinusitis
- bronchiectasis
- visceral situs inversus.

350. Cystic fibrosis

Answers: A B D

351. Cystic fibrosis

Answers: A B C

Inheritance of cystic fibrosis is autosomal recessive. In the UK, the incidence of the carrier state is 1 in 20 and incidence of the disease 1 in 2500. The gene locus is on chromosome 7. The gene codes for the cystic fibrosis transmembrane regulator (CFTR) that facilitates the transport of chloride across cell membranes. Mutations in the CFTR gene leads to reduced epithelial chloride ion permeability. More than 450 mutations have been identified. The commonest is ΔF 508 (70%) which is invariably associated with pancreatic insufficiency – this is due to a deletion of phenylalanine at position 508.

- 10–15% present with meconium ileus. Meconium ileus can occur in children without cystic fibrosis.
- 85% have clinically obvious pancreatic insufficiency in infancy.
- 99% of males are infertile.
- 50% of children with cystic fibrosis have recurrent wheeze.
- 20% have atopic asthma.
- 10% have rectal prolapse.

Distal intestinal obstruction syndrome is common in older children. Diabetes mellitus occurs in 24% of 20-year-olds and 75% of 30-year-olds. *Staphylococcus aureus* is the commonest pathogen in infancy, followed by non-capsular *Haemophilus*. In older children *Pseudomonas aeruginosa* becomes a significant pathogen. A thorough knowledge of the clinical features, genetic aspects and management of cystic fibrosis will be required for the exam.

Causes of clubbing include:

- congenital
- cyanotic congenital heart disease
- cystic fibrosis
- primary ciliary dyskinesia
- bronchiectasis
- inflammatory bowel disease
- cirrhosis
- chronic active hepatitis.

352. Bronchiectasis

Answers: B C D E

This is defined as persistent dilation of the bronchi, resulting from inflammatory destruction of its walls, associated with chronic cough with sputum production. It is characterised by periods of relapse and remission and poor weight gain is

respiratory

often a feature. Clubbing is a common finding. The commonest cause is cystic fibrosis. High resolution computed tomography (CT) scanning is useful for diagnosis. Other causes of bronchiectasis are:

- immunodeficiency
- α_1-anti-trypsin deficiency
- primary ciliary dyskinesia
- foreign body
- lobar sequestration
- previous infection – measles, pertussis, pneumonia
- asthma.

The management is with antibiotics and physiotherapy. Surgery is occasionally required if a defined lobe is affected and the patient unresponsive to medical treatment.

353. Obstructive sleep apnoea

Answers: A B C E

Hypoventilation occurs resulting in hypoxia and hypercarbia (type II respiratory failure). This occurs until the central arousal mechanism operates and stimulates breathing by hypoxia. A definition of obstructive sleep apnoea has been offered which is 30 apnoeic episodes of 10 seconds or longer in a 7-hour period which occur secondary to airway obstruction. The peak age is 2–6 years, with equal incidence in boys and girls. About 1% of snoring children have obstructive sleep apnoea. About 10% of children snore. The symptoms and signs that occur as a consequence of nocturnal hypoxia and hypercapnia include:

- apnoea
- failure to thrive
- excessive day time sleepiness
- behavioural problems
- polycythaemia
- right ventricular hypertrophy
- pulmonary hypertension.

The diagnosis is made by clinical assessment and by overnight monitoring of respiratory rate, heart rate and oxygen saturations. Adenotonsillectomy and not just adenoidectomy may be curative in some cases. Tracheostomy is occasionally required. Obstructive sleep apnoea is associated with active sleep. Nocturnal enuresis is common. There is an increased risk of obstructive sleep apnoea in children with:

- Down's syndrome
- hypotonia from any cause
- developmental delay

respiratory

- craniofacial anomalies
- sickle cell disease
- obesity.

354. *Mycoplasma pneumoniae*

Answers: A B C

Mycoplasma pneumoniae is a bacterium without a cell wall. It is spread by droplets and humans are the only host. Incubation period is 3 weeks. The commonest clinical manifestation of infection is an atypical pneumonia presenting with cough. Infection is usually preceded by headache and sore throat. Wheeze is common. The chest X-ray appearance is usually worse than the symptoms and signs suggest. Peak incidence is in school age children. Diagnosis is by serology with a positive *Mycoplasma* IgM in the acute illness and a convalescent rise in the *Mycoplasma* IgG titre. Culture is difficult. Cold agglutinins will be positive in 50%. White cell count is often normal. Treatment is with erythromycin, bronchodilators and physiotherapy. Azithromycin and clarithromycin are other appropriate antibiotics. Tetracyclines can be given in adolescence. Associations and complications of *Mycoplasma* infection are:

- skin – erythema multiforme; Stevens–Johnson syndrome
- central nervous system – meningoencephalitis; aseptic meningitis; cerebellar ataxia; Guillain-Barré syndrome
- joints – monoarticular arthritis
- cardiac – myocarditis; pericarditis
- blood – haemolysis; thrombocytopenia
- gut – hepatitis; pancreatitis; protein-losing enteropathy.

355. **Acute tonsillitis**

Answers: C E

Acute tonsillitis is rare in infancy. The peak incidence is around the age of 5 years. There is a second peak in adolescence. Viral infections are much commoner than bacterial. The commonest viral agent is the adenovirus. Others include influenza, parainfluenza, respiratory syncytial virus. The commonest bacterium is Group A β-haemolytic *Streptococcus*. Other agents include pneumococcus, *Haemophilus* and *Mycoplasma*. Tonsillar hypertrophy with exudate does not help to distinguish between a bacterial or a viral aetiology. The differential diagnosis of tonsillitis includes diphtheria, agranulocytosis and infectious mononucleosis. The indications for tonsillectomy are controversial but are often asked.:

- recurrent tonsillitis associated with failure to thrive and frequent school absence

- quinsy
- sleep apnoea
- to exclude a tonsillar tumour.

Complications of tonsillectomy include haemorrhage. This can be either primary (within a few hours) or secondary (within a few days). Secondary haemorrhage is usually due to infection of the tonsillar bed and resolves once the infection is treated.

356. Anaphylaxis

Answers: B C D

Anaphylaxis is a type 1 immediate hypersensitivity reaction. It is IgE mediated. Features include itching, facial swelling, urticaria, abdominal pain, diarrhoea, wheeze and stridor which may precede shock. It is potentially life-threatening, with airway impairment due to laryngeal oedema and shock due to acute vasodilatation and capillary fluid leak. Management is as follows:

- remove allergen
- assess airway, breathing then circulation and intervene as appropriate
- adrenaline 10 μg/kg im, hydrocortisone 4 mg/kg iv
- repeat adrenaline every 15 minutes until sustained response seen – an infusion may need to be given
- consider aminophylline 5 mg/kg then 15 μg/kg/min
- consider colloid 20 ml/kg
- if stridor severe give adrenaline 5 ml 1:1000 nebulised
- if bronchospasm is severe then salbutamol 5 mg nebulised can be given every 15 minutes – an infusion can be given.

357. Pulmonary tuberculosis

Answers: B C

Mycobacterium tuberculosis is a Gram-positive acid-fast bacillus which turns red when stained with the Ziehl–Nielson stain and is difficult to culture. The reservoir for infection is the mammalian host (unlike atypical mycobacteria). Children are not normally infectious. Infectivity is highest in adults with cavitating open lung lesions. The clinical features of infection are very variable and depend on the balance between bacterial multiplication and host response. Symptoms can either be from a primary complex or as a consequence of reactivation. The primary complex is a peripheral lung lesion (Ghon focus) with associated hilar lymphadenopathy. The diagnosis of tuberculosis in childhood is difficult. Sputum is difficult to obtain and is rarely positive to acid-fast bacilli. Early morning gastric aspirates can be used instead of sputum. Pointers include the clinical picture,

respiratory

history of contact, suggestive radiology and a positive tuberculin test. A positive mycobacterial culture may not be available and usually takes 6 weeks although it is diagnostic. Bronchoscopy with lung biopsy is sometimes required. Recent work has been done using the polymerase chain reaction to identify mycobacterial DNA. Tuberculin testing is best done using Mantoux's test. This is often difficult to interpret. It can be negative in fulminating disease in its early stages and in children with HIV infection. In addition a cohort of children will have been given bacille Calmette Guérin (BCG). A strongly positive Mantoux's (>15 mm induration in response to 0.1 ml of 1 in 1000 preparation) is suggestive of infection even if BCG has previously been given. Treatment is with isoniazid, rifampicin (6 months) and pyrazinamide (2 months). Side-effects of antituberculous therapy are:

- isoniazid – peripheral neuropathy (preventable with pyridoxine), skin rashes, abnormal liver function tests
- rifampicin – skin rashes, abnormal liver function tests (LFTs)
- pyrazinamide – skin rashes, abnormal LFTs, photosensitivity
- ethambutol – ocular toxicity
- streptomycin – ototoxicity, nephrotoxicity.

358. Lung development

Answers: C D

Lung development is divided into four stages according to microscopic appearance:

- Embryonic – 0–7 weeks. Lung foundation is laid down. Lung bud develops as a ventral diverticulum of the foregut (endodermal). Surrounding mesenchyme also derived from the foregut. All segmental bronchi are developed by the end of the embryonic phase.
- Pseudoglandular – 7–17 weeks. Conducting airways are developed with continuous branching of bronchial buds. Adult number of airways proximal to the acini are present by the 16th week of gestation. Epithelial lining differentiates. Goblet and serous cells are identifiable by 16 weeks. All pre-acinar vessels are present by 17 weeks.
- Canalicular – 17–26 weeks. This phase sees the maturing of the conducting airways and the development of the terminal respiratory units. There is an increase in size of the proximal airways with an increase in cartilage, muscle and glandular tissue. By 22 weeks type I and type II pneumocytes are seen.

respiratory

- Alveolar – 27 weeks to term. This period sees the further development of gas exchange units such that by term a third to a half of the adult number of alveoli are present. Pre acinar airways increase in size and there is a continued increase in the number of goblet cells. The acinus is a functional unit comprising alveoli, alveolar ducts and respiratory bronchioles.
- Alveoli increase in number up until 4–8 years of age.

359. Peak expiratory flow rate

Answers: D E

The peak expiratory flow rate is the maximum expiratory flow rate following a full inspiration. It is dependent upon the diameter of the airways at the narrowest point and the intrathoracic pressure generated. It is effort dependent. Few children under the age of 5 years can do a peak flow. Forced expiratory volume (FEV_1) is the volume of air that can be forcibly expired in 1 second. It is less effort dependent and more reproducible than the peak expiratory flow rate. In asthma the residual volume will increase reducing the forced vital capacity.

360. C: Po_2 – 11 kPa

The gas shows an uncompensated metabolic acidosis. Key features are the low pH, low HCO_3, negative base excess and lack of respiratory compensation which would include a low CO_2 and longer term a rise in HCO_3. Likeliest cause in a child of this age would be sepsis and shock for other reasons eg severe gastroenteritis. Other causes include congenital heart disease, inborn metabolic errors and ingestions and (in an older child) diabetic keto-acidosis.

361. B: Tachypnoea and signs of respiratory distress in the neonatal period

Congenital lobar emphysema is a rare congenital lung abnormality caused by overexpansion of a pulmonary lobe with resulting compression of the remaining ipsilateral and sometimes contralateral lung. Intrinsic cartilaginous deficiencies or extrinsic compressive lesions may be the cause (eg large pulmonary artery). The left upper lobe is most likely to be affected. Approximately 10% have associated abnormalities, the commonest being cardiac. Congenital lobar emphysema usually presents in the neonatal period with increasing respiratory difficulty although may be an incidental finding in an older child. The chest X-ray findings are typically that of over inflation and/or hyperlucency of the affected segment. The differential diagnosis includes:

respiratory

- pneumothorax
- bronchial mucus plug with associated hyperinflation
- agenesis/hypoplasia of the contralateral lung
- congenital cystic adenomatoid malformation.

The diagnosis should be confirmed with further imaging such as computed tomography (CT) or magnetic resonance imaging (MRI) scanning. Those with significant symptoms should be considered for surgery (lobectomy), but conservative management is appropriate for those who have only mild symptoms.

362. A: Infants with bronchopulmonary dysplasia

While ribavirin is the only agent licensed in the UK for the treatment of respiratory syncytial virus infection, palivizumab is the only agent currently licensed in the UK for the prevention of respiratory syncytial virus lower respiratory tract infection requiring hospitalisation. It is a humanised monoclonal IgG antibody that prevents the uptake of respiratory syncytial virus into host cells.

It is licensed for use in:

- children born at less than 35 weeks gestation who are less than or equal to 6 months old at the start of the respiratory syncytial virus season
- children less than 2 years old who have received treatment for BPD within the last 6 months
- children less than 2 years with haemodynamically significant congenital heart disease.

Monthly intramuscular injections are required during the respiratory syncytial virus season at a dose of 15mg/kg. Side effects include injection site reactions and fever (similar to placebo). Cost is prohibitive with a course of 5 injections costing upward of £2500 per patient depending on weight.

363. C: Initial catarrhal phase

Bordetella pertussis (a Gram negative bacillus) is the cause of > 90% of cases of whooping cough. There are three stages to the illness – catarrhal, paroxysmal and recovery phases. The child is most infectious during the catarrhal phase when symptoms are indistinguishable from those caused by viruses such as RSV, para-influenzae and adenovirus. Erythromycin may attenuate the disease if given early enough and may shorten the period of infectivity. Immunisation has greatly reduced the incidence of whooping cough but outbreaks still occur. Bronchopneumonia (sometimes due to secondary infection) may occur as a complication, but lower respiratory tract signs are not always present.

respiratory

364. D: Treatment with oral amoxicillin

The British Thoracic Society (BTS) published guidelines for the management of community acquired pneumonia (CAP) in childhood in 2002. The commonest bacterial cause of pneumonia is *Streptococcus pneumoniae,* although in younger children, viruses are more commonly found and a significant proportion of cases of CAP (up to 40%) represent mixed infection. According to the BTS guidelines referred to above, unless a child (who is otherwise fit and well with no underlying chest, cardiac or immunodeficiency syndrome) is hypoxaemic, tachypnoiec, having difficulty in breathing, dehydrated or unable to tolerate oral medication, or has insufficient family support, admission to hospital is **not** required. Amoxicillin is recommended as first line treatment for those children in whom pneumococcus is considered the most likely pathogen and who meet the above criteria for management at home (with advice to the carers regarding identifying signs of deterioration). Macrolide antibiotics can be used as first line treatment in children aged greater than 5 years of age due to the increased incidence of mycoplasma in this age group. Repeat chest X-rays are recommended only in those children with lobar collapse or apparent round pneumonia on initial chest X-ray and in those whose symptoms fail to resolve. It is therefore important that children are reviewed (either by their GP or in a hospital follow up appointment) to ensure the child does not have continuing symptoms. Randomised controlled trials have demonstrated that physiotherapy is not beneficial in reducing the length of hospital stay or improving chest X-ray findings.

365. B: Add montelukast

The BTS/Scottish Intercollegiate Guidelines Network (SIGN) guidelines describe five steps in the management of asthma. The treatment this child is receiving would be equivalent to step 3. His control is suboptimal and therefore needs to be reviewed. At 250 µg/day of fluticasone, which is equivalent to 500 µg/day of beclomethasone or budesonide, he is already on more than the recommended dose of inhaled steroids for a child (400 µg/day of beclomethasone equivalent). A further increase in inhaled steroid dose would therefore not be the change of choice. He is also on a maximal long-acting β-agonist dose. At the age of 5 years, a child's ability to use a dry powder device must be carefully assessed as it is possible that he is still too young to take this form of medication reliably. At all ages, the use of a large volume spacer maximises the amount of drug deposited in the airways and should be recommended. The most appropriate addition to this child's therapy would be the introduction of montelukast, a leukotriene receptor antagonist (LTRA). It is licensed for use from the age of 6 months. Only about a third of people appear to benefit from the use of these agents and it would therefore be important to reassess the child's asthma control having commenced this treatment and discontinue it should no benefit be gained. LTRAs are administered orally rather than in inhaled form. Side effects include headache,

respiratory

sleep disorders and gastrointestinal disturbance. In all children whose symptoms do not improve on appropriate anti-asthma treatment, review the diagnosis, inhaler technique and treatment compliance.

366. RESPIRATORY DISEASES

1. E – Pulmonary haemosiderosis

This is a rare disorder that typically has its onset prior to 10 years of age. It is characterised by a triad of iron deficiency anaemia, haemoptysis (rarely overt in childhood) and diffuse parenchymal infiltrates on chest X-ray. The majority of cases in childhood are idiopathic, but some are due to cow's milk protein hypersensitivity or secondary to systemic disease (cardiac, pneumonia, autoimmune disease). Bronchoalveolar lavage yields haemosiderin laden macrophages secondary to diffuse alveolar haemorrhage. The swallowing of this sputum results in positive faecal occult blood testing. Peripheral eosinophilia and failure to thrive are seen usually secondary to intolerance to cow's milk protein and symptoms improve on an elimination diet. In idiopathic cases, the prognosis is more variable. Treatment with iron replacement, steroids and sometimes other immunosuppressive agents is required. If left untreated, pulmonary fibrosis will develop and the condition can prove fatal. NB α_1-anti-trypsin deficiency rarely presents with chest symptoms in infancy. Hepatomegaly and jaundice may be presenting features in infancy but portal hypertension is rare in early childhood. Gastrointestinal bleeding is not a feature of α_1-anti-trypsin deficiency.

2. A – Bronchiolitis obliterans

In childhood cases of bronchiolitis obliterans, there is usually a preceding history of infection with adenovirus, measles, pertussis, influenza or mycoplasma. It can also be related to connective tissue disease, malignancy, drugs and as part of graft-versus-host disease after bone marrow transplantation. Progressive symptoms of dyspnoea, cough, general malaise and weight loss are characteristic. Examination usually reveals the presence of inspiratory crepitations. Clubbing is unusual. Chest X-ray changes are variable and can range from normal appearances through to air space consolidation with air bronchograms to findings consistent with miliary tuberculosis. High resolution CT scanning provides a more sensitive assessment of disease pattern and severity. Pulmonary function tests are likely to reveal severe obstruction although a restrictive picture is sometimes seen. Treatment with antibiotics is of no benefit. Some forms of bronchiolitis obliterans in adults respond well to corticosteroids, but this is seen less commonly in children. A trial of treatment with inhaled steroids is reasonable to rule out a diagnosis of asthma although sufficient dose must be given to ensure that lack of response is not due to inadequate dosage.

3. G – Lobar sequestration

Lobar sequestration refers to a mass of non-functioning pulmonary tissue that is supplied by the systemic rather than pulmonary circulation and has no identifiable bronchial communication. They are classified as either extralobar (ELS) or intralobar (ILS) sequestrations. ILS accounts for 75% of sequestrations. ELS usually present in infancy with respiratory distress and cough, and 90% are left sided. They are four times commoner in males. They can be associated with other congenital abnormalities in 40–60% of patients, including diaphragmatic hernias, vertebral anomalies and congenital heart defects. ILS more commonly presents in older childhood with infection or haemoptysis. They are usually found in a lower lobe, 60% being left sided.

Patients need to be investigated to confirm the diagnosis and provide further anatomical information facilitating treatment. In addition to cross-sectional imaging of the chest, angiography (conventional, CT and MR) is used to identify the blood supply to the lesion. In certain cases, embolisation of the feeding vessel can be performed as a curative procedure. In other cases, surgical resection is required. The normal sweat chloride in the presence of an adequate amount of sweat collected is sufficient to rule out cystic fibrosis. (See also Question 347).

367. Management of acute respiratory illness

1. B – Nebulised adrenaline

This child is unwell with evidence of upper airway obstruction. You are unable to obtain a clear history and given that the child has only recently arrived in the UK it is important to remember that she probably hasn't been immunised against *Haemophilus influenzae* type b. She is therefore at increased risk of epiglottitis. The immediate management must centre on maintaining patent airway which is obviously compromised. Therefore, nebulised adrenaline with oxygen should be given. Intravenous cefotaxime would also be required but you must not cause the child more distress by inserting a cannula until you are certain her airway is secure.

2. E – Supportive treatment only

This baby has a history and examination findings consistent with bronchiolitis, typically seen in the winter months and in 70% of cases secondary to respiratory syncytial virus. Although auscultation reveals wheeze, bronchodilators have not been proven to reduce admission rates or produce a clinically important improvement in oxygen saturations. Antibiotics are only required if secondary bacterial infection is suspected. Supportive treatment with oxygen and nasogastric feeding would be appropriate.

respiratory

3. C – Oral erythromycin

This child has signs and symptoms suggestive of infection with *Mycoplasma pneumoniae*, the second commonest cause of CAP in the UK in children above the age of 5 years. Typically, in addition to the chest signs, you may elicit a history of headache, wheeze, myringitis and abdominal pain. The treatment of choice is with a macrolide antibiotic such as erythromycin or azithromycin. His presentation is not of sufficient severity to require admission for intravenous antibiotics (see BTS guidelines for the management of CAP, Answer 366). If there is sufficient wheeze to require treatment with bronchodilators, an inhaler and large volume spacer would be the appropriate method of drug delivery. It would be important to ensure the child is instructed and tested on how to use the device prior to discharge.

respiratory

INDEX

Note to reader: Entries are indexed by question number, not page number.

t test 68
tuberculosis 221
tuberous sclerosis 302
tumour necrosis factor 187
Turner's syndrome 11, 81, 105, 255

ulcerative colitis 139
undescended testis 276
urinary frequency 126, 290
urinary tract infection 269

vaccines, live 218
VATER syndrome 255
venous hum 26
ventricular fibrillation 27
ventricular septal defects 14
vesico-ureteric reflux 282, 289
viruses, DNA-containing 195
vitamin A 115, 142
vitamin B_{12} 156
vitamin C deficiency 163

vitamin D 264
vitamin D resistant rickets 266
vitamin K 117
von Willebrand's disease 167

warfarin, as teratogen 20
Werdnig-Hoffman disease 253, 300
West's syndrome 316
whooping cough 363
William's syndrome 2, 105
Wilm's tumour 277, 289
Wilson's disease 128
Wiskott-Aldrich syndrome 155
Wolff-Parkinson-White syndrome 28
Wolf-Hirschhorn syndrome 70

X-linked agammaglobulinaemia 170
xylose tolerance test 118

Zellweger's syndrome 331
zoster immunoglobulin 222